Neonatal Cardiology

Neonatal Cardiology

Second Edition

Michael Artman, MD
Joyce C. Hall Distinguished Professor of Pediatrics
Chairman, Department of Pediatrics
Pediatrician-in-Chief, Children's Mercy Hospitals and Clinics
Children's Mercy Hospital and Clinics
Department of Pediatrics
Kansas City, Missouri

Lynn Mahony, MD
Professor, Pediatrics
University of Texas Southwestern Medical Center
Dallas, Texas

David F. Teitel, MD
Professor, Department of Pediatrics and the Cardiovascular Research Institute
Chief, Division of Pediatric Cardiology
Medical Director, Pediatric Heart Center
University of California, San Francisco
San Francisco, California

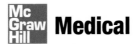

New York   Chicago   San Francisco   Lisbon   London   Madrid   Mexico City
Milan   New Delhi   San Juan   Seoul   Singapore   Sydney   Toronto

Neonatal Cardiology, Second Edition

Copyright © 2011, 2002 by The McGraw-Hill Companies, Inc. All rights reserved. Printed in the United States of America. Except as permitted under the United States Copyright Act of 1976, no part of this publication may be reproduced or distributed in any form or by any means, or stored in a data base or retrieval system, without the prior written permission of the publisher.

1 2 3 4 5 6 7 8 9 0   CTP/CTP   14 13 12 11 10

ISBN 978-0-07-163579-0
MHID 0-07-163579-3

This book was set in Minion by Glyph International.
The editors were Alyssa Fried and Christine Diedrich.
The production supervisor was Catherine Saggese.
The illustration manager was Armen Ovsepyan.
Project management was provided by Arushi Chawla, Glyph International.
The designer was Mary McKeon; the cover designer was Thomas DePierro.
China Translation & Printing Services Ltd. was printer and binder.

This book is printed on acid-free paper.

Library of Congress Cataloging-in-Publication Data

Artman, Michael, 1952-
    Neonatal cardiology / Michael Artman, Lynn Mahony, David F. Teitel.—2nd ed.
        p. ; cm.
    Includes bibliographical references and index.
    Summary: "A full-color guide to understanding, evaluating, and treating heart disease in fetuses and newborns, Neonatal Cardiology is the trusted go-to guide for pediatricians and neonatologists needing concise, practical guidance on the evaluation and management of newborns with heart disease and other cardiac functional abnormalities. Focusing on physiology, mechanics, and presentation of congenital heart disease, this full-color resource provides a succinct, yet complete overview of neonatal cardiology. Neonatal Cardiology opens with discussions of basic aspects of embryology of the heart and a review of normal and abnormal muscle function. From there, you are led through the clinical assessment of patients with an array of cardiac abnormalities. Management and treatment follow, beginning with a basic chapter on the principles of medical management, followed by drug therapy and postoperative care. The book concludes with a chapter on Epidemiology, Etiology, and Genetics of Congenital Heart Disease. Features: Full-color presentation with new radiographic images and explanatory illustrations of normal and abnormal anatomy, blood flow patterns, and the effects of various treatment options. Suggested readings appear at the end of each chapter for more in-depth study. Includes coverage of: Excessive pulmonary blood flow, cyanosis, inadequate systemic perfusion, cardiomyopathies, and arrhythmias, Cardiovascular drug therapy, Neurology of congenital heart disease, and Perinatal Cardiovascular Physiology"—Provided by publisher.
    ISBN-13: 978-0-07-163579-0 (alk. paper)
    ISBN-10: 0-07-163579-3 (alk. paper)
    1. Congenital heart disease in children.   2. Pediatric cardiology.   3. Newborn infants—Diseases.
    4. Fetal heart—Diseases.   I. Mahony, Lynn.   II. Teitel, David F.   III. Title.
    [DNLM: 1. Cardiovascular Diseases.   2. Infant, Newborn.   WS 290]
    RJ269.N46 2010
    618.92′12043—dc22
                                                                                    2010033468

McGraw-Hill books are available at special quantity discounts to use as premiums and sales promotions, or for use in corporate training programs. To contact a representative please e-mail us at bulksales@mcgraw-hill.com.

This book is dedicated to our families for their unwavering support, understanding, and sacrifices. It is from them that we gain our balance.

We are grateful to the many teachers from whom we were fortunate to learn more than mere facts. Each of us continues to benefit from the wisdom of our mentors, who prepared us so well for our lives, careers, and academic endeavors.

Contents

Contributors

Patrick McQuillen, MD
Associate Professor, Departments of Pediatrics and
  Neurology
University of California, San Francisco
San Francisco, California

Kathleen Ruppel, MD
Assistant Adjunct Professor, Department of Pediatrics and
  the Cardiovascular Research Institute
University of California, San Francisco
San Francisco, California

Foreword to the First Edition

The incidence of congenital heart disease is generally stated to be about 8 per 1000 births. However, most reports worldwide have not included individuals whose lesions were not recognized by clinical examination alone. In recent years it has become evident, based on ultrasound studies, that the incidence is considerably higher than that usually quoted. Thus bicuspid aortic valve is thought to occur in 1% or more of the population. Prenatal ultrasound examination has documented not only congenital heart lesions, but also cardiac arrhythmias and myocardial dysfunction as important causes of fetal morbidity and mortality. In fact, cardiac anomalies and arrhythmias are the dominant cause of non-immune hydrops fetalis. Although there is such a high prevalence of heart disease, it was recognized, prior to the modern era of early evaluation and treatment, that the major mortality occurred during infancy. Thus, of all deaths related to congenital heart disease, 50% occurred by 6 months, and 80% by 1 year of age. It is thus appropriate that attention should be focused on heart disease in the neonate.

Previous books devoted to neonatal heart disease were published 10 years ago or more. During the intervening period, major advances in diagnostic and therapeutic approaches and in the developmental biology of the heart and circulation have occurred. This volume presents an update on these aspects of perinatal cardiology. Michael Artman, Lynn Mahony, and David Teitel are eminently qualified to review current knowledge of neonatal cardiology. They have all been engaged in research on various aspects of perinatal changes in myocardial performance and adjustments of the circulation after birth. In addition, they have extensive experience in clinical assessment and management of infants with heart disease.

This book comprises four major sections. The first section reviews basic aspects of embryology of the heart, developmental changes in myocardial contraction and relaxation, and mechanisms involved in the circulatory changes after birth. The contribution by Deepak Srivastava provides a unique approach to embryology of the heart with an emphasis on current knowledge of the various genes involved in different aspects of cardiac morphogenesis. The second section is concerned with clinical assessment. The first chapter discusses the use of ultrasound techniques in evaluation and management of the fetus suspected to have heart disease. The next four chapters present a symptom-complex approach to the evaluation of the neonate with heart disease. Unlike most publications, in which disease entities are presented, this approach is particularly useful because it considers neonatal heart disease from the perspective of the diverse clinical presentations. The initial chapter reviews general aspects of the evaluation and management of neonates with cardiovascular symptoms; subsequent chapters consider approaches to the neonate with cyanosis, the infant with high pulmonary blood flow, and the infant with poor peripheral perfusion. The section is completed by discussions of cardiomyopathy and arrhythmias in the neonate. The third section reviews general principles of treatment, pharmacological aspects of therapy, and management of neonates following surgery for cardiac anomalies. The final section includes a presentation of nursing aspects of the neonate with heart disease by anomalies.

This book, presenting current knowledge of basic biology related to cardiac development and of the evaluation and management of the neonate with heart disease, will be invaluable to neonatologists, pediatric cardiologists, and obstetricians. The illustrations are excellent and extremely helpful in defining myocardial physiology and in appreciating the abnormal hemodynamics of various congenital heart lesions. The symptom-complex approach to clinical presentation will have particular appeal to medical and nursing students, as well as to residents and nurses caring for the infant with heart disease.

Abraham M. Rudolph, MD

Foreword to the Second Edition

During the 8 years since the publication of the first edition of *Neonatal Cardiology* in 2002, many remarkable advances in our understanding of normal cardiovascular development and of mechanisms, resulting in congenital cardiovascular malformations, have been achieved.

The concept that these malformations had little impact on normal fetal development was widely accepted; the influence of congenital cardiovascular malformations on fetal blood flow patterns and oxygenation, as well as their effect on fetal cardiac and vascular development, is increasingly being recognized. Furthermore, the potential effects of these defects on other organ systems, particularly the brain, has engendered great interest and study.

In this second edition, Drs. Michael Artman, Lynn Mahony, and David Teitel have continued the general philosophy of the first edition; they have presented clinical and hemodynamic manifestations of congenital and acquired cardiovascular disturbances, based on biological information regarding development and function. All chapters have been significantly modified to address the increased understanding of basic biology and factors affecting normal development and performance. As in the first edition, the graphic material largely presents diagrams that help to explain basic physiological concepts and pathophysiology. The quality of the diagrams has been greatly improved, making the information presented more readily assimilable.

The first chapter, on cardiac embryology, contributed by Dr. Kathleen Ruppel, reviews the advances in the understanding of genetic pathways involved in cardiac morphogenesis. Also, the revolutionary changes in our appreciation of the embryology of the heart and great vessels are presented. It was widely accepted that all structures developed from the primitive heart tube; it is now recognized that other primitive cells from the anterior or secondary heart field, as well as neural crest cells, are major contributors to cardiac and great vessel formation. Their importance in development of congenital cardiovascular malformations is now being explored.

The association of neurological abnormalities with congenital cardiovascular malformations has been recognized for many years; in many genetic syndromes, both developmental delay and cardiac defects are encountered. In recent years, concern has been raised regarding intellectual and behavioral impairment in children with several congenital cardiac anomalies. The possibility that this was related to surgical procedures during infancy was considered, but recent evidence suggests interference with brain development occurs during fetal life. In a most interesting new chapter, authored by Dr. Patrick McQuillen, neurological development and mechanisms by which congenital cardiovascular malformations could affect it are presented. This topic is of great importance, because it is suggested that in some infants with these cardiac lesions, correction during the neonatal period may not improve the neurological deficit. This would support the concept of intervention to correct the circulatory disturbance during fetal life.

The use of nonsurgical approaches to cardiac lesions has become standard practice over the past decade. Many of these procedures are not yet applicable to neonates, but as discussed in this edition, interventions to relieve aortic and pulmonary stenoses by balloon valvuloplasty have now become standard practice, thus avoiding the high risks of surgery in critically ill infants.

This edition of *Neonatal Cardiology* continues to provide pediatric cardiologists, neonatologists, and obstetricians with an invaluable resource for the differential diagnosis of cardiovascular disturbances and their management in newborn infants. The symptom-complex approach is particularly helpful to students and residents in understanding the mechanisms responsible for clinical manifestations.

Abraham M. Rudolph, MD

Acknowledgments

We are grateful to Alyssa Fried at McGraw-Hill for stimulating us to revise this book. She was the primary force in launching the project and we appreciate her encouragement in helping us bring the effort to completion. It was a pleasure to work with Alyssa and her team of professionals.

We are indebted to Dr. Ian Law at the University of Iowa Children's Hospital for his helpful comments in revising Chapter 10.

Molecular and Morphogenetic Cardiac Embryology: Implications for Congenital Heart Disease

■ INTRODUCTION

Cardiogenesis involves a precisely orchestrated series of molecular and morphogenetic events that combines cell types from multiple lineages. Subtle perturbations of this process can result in life-threatening illnesses in the form of congenital heart defects. As the organ most essential for life, the heart is the first organ to form and functions to support the rapidly growing embryo before it becomes a four-chambered organ. The combination of the complex

morphogenetic events necessary for cardiogenesis and the superimposed hemodynamic influences may contribute to the exquisite sensitivity of the heart to perturbations. This phenomenon is reflected in the estimated 10% incidence of severe cardiac malformations observed in early miscarriages. The fraction of congenital heart malformations that are capable of supporting the intrauterine circulation comprises the spectrum of congenital heart disease observed clinically.

Although congenital heart disease was classified in the 18th and 19th centuries based on embryologic considerations, the advent of palliative procedures and clinical management led to a descriptive nomenclature founded on anatomic and physiologic features that directed surgery and medical therapy. However, seemingly unrelated defects may share common embryologic origins from a mechanistic standpoint, and thus the etiology of various defects may be better understood from a developmental standpoint. Recent advances in genetics and molecular biology have stimulated a renaissance in studies designed to define an embryologic framework for understanding congenital heart disease. The ability to go beyond descriptions of the anatomical defects to developing an understanding of the genes responsible for distinct steps of cardiac morphogenesis is necessary for more directed therapeutic and preventive measures.

Although human genetic approaches are important in understanding congenital heart disease, detailed molecular analysis of cardiac development in humans has been difficult. The recognition that cardiac genetic pathways are highly conserved across vastly diverse species from flies to man has resulted in an explosion of information from studies in more tractable and accessible biological models. Chemical mutagenesis studies of the fruit fly (*Drosophila*) and of the simple vertebrate, zebra fish, have resulted in the identification of many genes that are required for normal cardiac development. Although genetic approaches are not feasible in chick embryos, they have four-chambered hearts and the embryos are easily accessible within the egg for surgical and molecular manipulation during cardiogenesis. Such approaches have been useful for defining the role of populations of cells during development. Finally, the laboratory mouse, a mammal with a cardiovascular system nearly identical to that in humans, has been an invaluable model system for understanding the mechanisms underlying human disease. Advances in technology have made it possible to mutate or to delete specific genes in the mouse genome, either globally or in a tissue-specific manner, and to study the effects of such mutations in mice heterozygous or homozygous for the disrupted gene of interest. Thus, each biological system offers unique opportunities to enhance understanding of cardiogenesis.

Mapping and identification of human congenital heart disease genes is equally important. Correlation of particular amino acid mutations with the associated cardiac malformations has provided insights into the structure-function relationships of the encoded proteins in vivo.

Many disease-causing genes associated with human congenital heart disease encode either transcription factors or signaling molecules. Transcription factors are proteins that contain DNA-binding domains that allow them to regulate the expression of one or more genes. Signaling molecules are proteins that enable cells to respond to their environment and are thereby involved in regulation of many important biological functions, including cell-cell interactions. The pathogenic mechanisms by which identified mutations in specific transcription factors and signaling molecule cause defects can then be analyzed in model systems. Together, human molecular genetic studies and model systems provide complementary approaches to investigating the etiology of congenital heart disease.

In this chapter, anatomic, molecular, and clinical aspects of cardiac embryology will be interwoven to develop a framework in which to consider the etiology of human congenital cardiac defects. In this framework, defects in particular regions of the heart may arise from unique genetic and environmental effects during specific developmental windows of time. To simplify the complex events of cardiogenesis, unique regions of the developing heart will be considered individually in the context described earlier.

■ EARLY CARDIOGENESIS: FROM MESODERM TO HEART TUBE

Specification and Determination of Cardiogenic Mesoderm

The first step in cardiac development is the specification of the cells that will ultimately give rise to the functioning heart. Cardiac progenitors derive from a small population of mesodermal cells that arises in the anterior portion of the primitive streak at gastrulation. As the progenitor cells migrate into the anterior lateral plate mesoderm, they become specified to a cardiac fate as a result of complex interactions with the surrounding tissues. A variety of signaling molecules emanating from the adjacent endoderm promote cardiac specification, while inhibitory signals from the neural plate and axial mesoderm delineate the medial and lateral borders of the cardiogenic region. By day 15 in the human embryo, this region, termed the cardiogenic mesoderm, adopts a bilaterally symmetric crescent shape in the lateral plate mesoderm (Figure 1-1).

Cells within the cardiogenic mesoderm become committed to a myocardial fate through the interactions of a network of transcription factors that regulate expression of

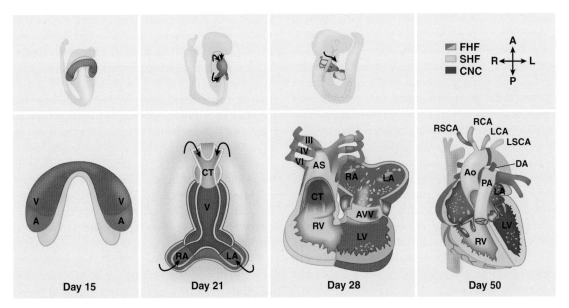

FIGURE 1-1. Schematic of cardiac morphogenesis. Oblique views of whole embryo and frontal views of cardiac precursors during human cardiac development are shown. **Day 15:** First heart field cells form a crescent shape in the anterior embryo with second heart field cells medial to the first heart field. **Day 21:** Second heart field cells lie dorsal to the straight heart tube and begin to migrate (arrows) into the anterior and posterior ends of the tube to form the right ventricle, conotruncus, and part of the atria. **Day 28:** After rightward looping of the heart tube, each cardiac chamber balloons out from the outer curvature of the looped heart tube. Cardiac neural crest cells also migrate (arrow) into the outflow tract from the neural folds to septate the outflow tract and pattern the bilaterally symmetric aortic arch arteries (III, IV, and VI) of the aortic sac. **Day 50:** Remodeling, alignment, and septation of the ventricles, atria, and atrioventricular valves, and alignment and rotation of the conotruncus, result in the four-chambered heart. Mesenchymal cells form the cardiac valves from the conotruncal and atrioventricular valve segments. Remodeling of the aortic arch arteries results in the mature aortic arch and ductus arteriosus. Corresponding days of human embryonic development are indicated. Abbreviations: A, atria; Ao, aortic arch; AS, aortic sac; AVV, atrioventricular valve; CNC, cardiac neural crest; CT, conotruncus; DA, ductus arteriosus; FHF, first heart field; LA, left atrium; LCA, left carotid artery; LSCA, left subclavian artery; LV, left ventricle; PA, pulmonary artery; RA, right atrium; RCA, right carotid artery; RSCA, right subclavian artery; RV, right ventricle; SHF, second heart field; V, ventricle. *Reproduced with permission from Srivastava D. Cell. 2006;126(6):1037-1048.*

cardiomyocyte specific genes. Nkx2.5, a transcription factor expressed in the earliest cardiac progenitors, plays an evolutionarily conserved central role in myocardial determination. First identified in fruit flies, the Nkx homologue *tinman* was found to be essential for commitment to the myocardial lineage and formation of the primitive heart-like structure in flies known as the dorsal vessel. Gene deletion studies in mice revealed a central role for Nkx2.5 in vertebrate heart development, as mice lacking Nkx2.5 died early in embryogenesis secondary to failure of the heart tube to undergo looping. Cardiomyocytes from Nkx2.5-deficient embryos showed reduced expression of genes encoding several myocardial structural proteins and other cardiac transcription factors, confirming the importance of Nkx2.5-mediated transcriptional regulation of multiple sets of cardiac specific genes.

The transcriptional activity of Nkx2.5 is modulated through its interaction with other transcription factors, including members of the GATA and T-box (Tbx) families of transcriptional regulators. Like Nkx2.5, GATA4 and Tbx5 are among the earliest markers of committed myocardial precursors, and loss of function of either protein during mouse embryogenesis results in the arrest of heart development prior to the looping stage. Nkx2.5, GATA4, and Tbx5 physically associate to synergistically stimulate transcription of myocardial specific genes. The complex interactions among these and other transcription factors during myocardial fate determination have yet to be fully elucidated but are the subject of investigation in a number of laboratories. In particular, the role of transcriptional regulation in myocardial fate determination is currently a subject of intense inquiry, as it has implications for both cardiac development and potential cardiomyocyte regenerative therapies. Transcription factors, identified in model systems as being important for cardiac determination, have become candidate genes for the discovery of genetic defects underlying congenital heart disease in humans. Mutations in *NKX2.5*, *GATA4*, and *TBX5* have been found in patients with a spectrum of structural and conduction defects, as discussed in the following paragraphs.

Cardiomyocyte Precursor Populations and Heart Field Patterning

Cells of the cardiogenic mesoderm begin to express Nkx2.5 and other markers of committed cardiomyocyte precursors at the cardiac crescent stage. During the third week of gestation, crescent cells begin to differentiate and coalesce in the ventral midline to form a primitive heart tube. Classic cell-labeling studies in chick embryos led to the theory that these cardiac progenitor cells were prepatterned along the anterior-posterior axis of the cardiac crescent (and thus heart tube) to give rise to specific regions of the mature heart. In this segmental model of cardiogenesis, it was assumed that all of the building blocks of the mature heart were present in the heart tube in a linear array (outflow tract, right ventricle, left ventricle, atria, systemic veins) of precursor components. In the last several years, a more complete understanding of the patterning of cardiac progenitor cells has emerged that fundamentally alters this model. Recent experimental advances that allow the tracking of specific groups of cells and their progeny during development have revealed the existence of two distinct but related regions of cardiogenic mesoderm that contribute progenitor cells to the developing heart in a spatially and temporally specific fashion. The first region, termed the first heart field (FHF), is comprised of the cells of the classically studied cardiac crescent that differentiate to form the initial heart tube (Figure 1-1). The more recently discovered

second heart field consists of a population of cardiogenic mesodermal cells that lie medial to and contiguous with the first heart field-derived cardiac crescent (Figure 1-1). As the cardiac crescent fuses in the ventral midline, the second heart field cells migrate within the pharyngeal mesoderm to a position dorsal to the developing heart tube. At the onset of rightward looping of the heart tube, second heart field cells are added to both the arterial and venous poles and proliferate to populate a large portion of the developing heart previously thought to be derived from the primitive heart tube, or first heart field. Myocardial precursors from this region give rise to the left ventricle and part of the atria, while the rest of the atria, the right ventricle, and the outflow tract are derived from the second heart field.

FHF cells at the cardiac crescent stage quickly begin to differentiate into functioning cardiomyocytes and form the primitive heart tube. In contrast, cells of the second heart field remain in a committed but undifferentiated cardiac progenitor state until they are incorporated into the growing heart tube. The second heart field lies medial to the first heart field at the crescent stage and thus closer to signals emanating from the midline of the embryo that may inhibit cardiac differentiation of the second heart field. *Nkx2.5* is expressed in both first and second heart field cells at the crescent stage and marks both populations as committed cardiomyocyte precursors. In contrast, the transcription factor Islet1 (Isl1), while also initially expressed in all cardiac progenitors, is quickly downregulated in the first heart field as those cells begin to express markers of differentiation. Expression of *Isl1* is maintained in the second heart field and is required for the expansion and migration of this progenitor population prior to addition to the heart tube. Gene deletion of *Isl1* in mice results in embryonic hearts lacking a right ventricle, outflow tract, and much of the atria, consistent with a central role for Isl1 in the regulation of second heart field cells that populate these structures. Isl1 expression in the second heart field is lost as the progenitor cells begin to differentiate upon addition to the heart tube.

The identification of two distinct heart fields is likely to have an important effect on the classification and interpretation of human congenital heart disease. Until now, these malformations have been considered mainly in the context of the segmental model of heart development. The knowledge that different populations of myocardial precursors contribute to the left (first heart field-derived) and right (second heart field-derived) ventricular chambers may be important for understanding the molecular basis of diseases that differentially affect the ventricles. Furthermore, malformations of the outflow region, which are observed in 0.3% of live births, can now be examined by a candidate-gene approach based on what is known about the genes that regulate the second heart field, as the outflow tract is derived almost exclusively from these precursors.

■ CARDIAC MORPHOGENESIS: FROM HEART TUBE TO MATURE HEART

Heart Tube Formation and Cardiac Looping Morphogenesis

Once the cells of the first heart field–derived cardiac crescent differentiate into cardiomyocytes, they migrate ventrally and converge in the midline to create a beating linear heart tube consisting of an outer layer of myocardial cells and an inner layer of endothelial cells separated by an extracellular matrix known as cardiac jelly (Figure 1-1). It is the first functioning organ of the embryo.

The linear heart tube then undergoes a series of morphogenetic changes that result in rightward looping of the heart tube and movement of its caudal end to a more cranial and dorsal position. As the tube bends along the anterior-posterior axis, it rotates to the right such that the ventral surface of the linear heart tube becomes the outer curvature of the looped heart, and the dorsal surface becomes the inner curvature. In the "ballooning model" of chamber formation, the outer curvature is the site of active chamber growth, while the inner curvature remodels to appropriately align the developing inflow tract, atrioventricular canal (AVC), and the outflow tract with the nascent chambers (Figure 1-2). As cells from the second heart field are added to both ends of the tube during looping, the ventricular chambers begin to develop along the cranial aspect of the outer curvature, followed slightly later by formation of the atria more caudally. With further bending along the anterior-posterior axis, the forming atria assume a more cranial and dorsal position, and active tissue remodeling of the inner curvature begins to bring the inflow and outflow portions of the heart into proper alignment.

The cellular and biomechanical mechanisms that underlie cardiac looping morphogenesis are not well understood. The process is intrinsic to the heart, as the heart is capable of looping when removed from the embryo and grown in culture. Looping is prevented by inhibition of contractile protein synthesis and by cytochalasin-mediated disruption of myofibril and actin cytoskeleton assembly. Proposed mechanisms include differential rates of proliferation within the heart tube, as well as localized changes in cell adhesion, cell migration, cell shape, and cytoskeletal contraction.

Abnormalities in the process of cardiac looping may underlie a number of defects. Folding of the heart tube positions the inflow cushions adjacent to the outflow cushions and involves extensive remodeling of the inner curvature of the looped heart tube. In the primitive looped heart, the segments of the heart are still in a linear pattern and must be repositioned considerably for alignment of the atrial chambers with the appropriate ventricles, and the ventricles with the aorta and pulmonary arteries. The atrioventricular septum (AVS) begins to divide the AVC into right and left components that subsequently shift to the right to position the AVS over the ventricular septum (Figure 1-2A-C). This allows the right AVC and the left AVC to be aligned with the right and left ventricles, respectively. Simultaneously, the conotruncal region is septated into the aorta and pulmonary trunks as the conotruncus moves toward the left side of the heart such that the conotruncal septum is positioned over the AVS. The rightward shift of the AVS and leftward shift of the conotruncus converts the single-inlet, single-outlet heart into a four-chambered heart that has separate atrial inlets and ventricular outlets.

Arrest or incomplete movement of the AVS or conotruncus might result in malalignment of the inflow and outflow tracts (Figure 1-2). If the AVS fails to shift to the right, both of the right and left AVCs would communicate with the left ventricle, a condition known as double-inlet left ventricle. Incomplete shifting may be the basis for "unbalanced" AVC defects where the right AVC only partly communicates with the right ventricle. Similarly, if the conotruncal septum fails to shift to the left, both the aorta and pulmonary artery would arise from the right ventricle resulting in a double-outlet right ventricle. From this embryologic perspective, it is not surprising that double-outlet left ventricles and double-inlet right ventricles are rarely seen clinically. In contrast, any abnormality in cardiac looping can be associated with double-inlet left ventricle or double-outlet right ventricle, along with other manifestations of improper alignment of specific regions of the heart. If the conotruncus shifts appropriately to lie over the AVS but fails to twist, transposition of the great arteries may result (Figure 1-2G). In this defect, the pulmonary artery communicates with the left ventricle and

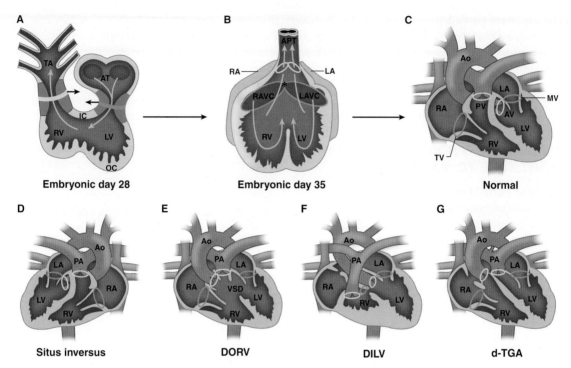

FIGURE 1-2. Normal and abnormal cardiac morphogenesis associated with left-right signaling. A. As the linear heart tube loops rightward with inner curvature (IC) remodeling and outer curvature (OC) proliferation, the endocardial cushions (dark blue) of the inflow (green) and outflow (light blue) tracts become adjacent to one another. Subsequently, the atrioventricular septum shifts to the right, while the aortopulmonary trunk shifts to the left. **B.** The inflow tract is divided into the right (RAVC) and left atrioventricular canal (LAVC) by the atrioventricular septum (∗). The outflow tract, known as the truncus arteriosus, becomes the aortopulmonary trunk (apt) upon septation. **C.** Ultimately, the left and right atria are aligned with the left ventricle and right ventricle, respectively. The left ventricle and right ventricle become aligned with the aorta and pulmonary artery, respectively, after 180° rotation of the great vessels. **D.** If the determinants of the left-right axis are coordinately reversed, then a condition known as situs inversus results. **E.** If the aortopulmonary trunk fails to shift to the left, then double-outlet right ventricle (DORV) results, in which the right ventricle is aligned with both the aorta and pulmonary artery. **F.** Likewise, if the atrioventricular septum fails to shift to the right, both atria communicate with the left ventricle causing double-inlet left ventricle (DILV). **G.** Transposition of the great arteries (TGA) results if the aortopulmonary trunk fails to twist resulting in communication of the right ventricle with the aorta and left ventricle with the pulmonary artery. Abbreviations: Ao, aorta; LA, left atrium; LV, left ventricle; PA, pulmonary artery; PV, pulmonary valve; RA, right atrium; RV, right ventricle; TA, truncus arteriosus. *Reproduced with permission from Kathiriya IS, Srivastava D. Am J Med Genet. 2001;97:271-279.*

the aorta communicates with the right ventricle, resulting in two separate circuits in which blood in the systemic circulation is not oxygenated.

Control of Left-Right Asymmetry in the Heart

Cardiac looping represents the first overt break in the bilateral symmetry of the embryo; however, the left/right axis patterning events that underlie the asymmetry of the heart, lungs, liver, spleen, and gut occur during gastrulation before these organs are ever formed. The usual arrangement of these asymmetric organs is referred to as "situs solitus," whereas "situs inversus" implies the complete reversal, or mirror image. Any other arrangement is considered "situs ambiguous" or heterotaxy (from the

Greek "heteros" meaning "other" and "taxy" meaning "order" or "arrangement"). Defects in establishment of left/right asymmetry in humans (heterotaxy syndromes) are associated with a wide range of cardiac alignment defects, suggesting that the pathways regulating left/right asymmetry dramatically affect cardiac development.

Left/right pattern formation requires propagation and amplification of an initial break in bilateral symmetry to the surrounding tissue, followed by translation of left/right axis information from the developing tissue into anatomical asymmetries during organogenesis. In vertebrate embryos, asymmetric expression of the transforming growth factor-β (TGF-β) family member nodal in the node is amplified by a cascade of positive and negative regulatory loops to generate robust *nodal* expression exclusively in left-sided tissues. Left-sided expression of *nodal* is required for normal laterality in all species thus far examined. Bilateral, absent, or randomized *nodal* expression patterns are observed in *iv/iv* mice. These animals exhibit randomization of the left/right orientation of the heart and viscera typically seen in human heterotaxy syndromes and are homozygous for a mutation in the gene encoding a ciliary motor protein. Left-sided nodal-dependent pathways induce expression of the transcription factor, Pitx2c, in the left lateral plate mesoderm. Pitx2c expression persists in committed cardiogenic mesoderm, and Pitx2c-expressing precursors are found in the left limb of the cardiac crescent and subsequently the left side of the primitive heart tube. Pitx2c is required for normal cardiac development, and mice lacking Pitx2c and its related isoforms (Pitx2a, Pitx2b) exhibit gut malrotation, right pulmonary isomerism, and a spectrum of cardiac defects usually associate with heterotaxy, including common atrioventricular canal, double-outlet right ventricle, and anomalous systemic and pulmonary venous return. The outflow tract defects in these mutant mice reflect the fact that Pitx2c is also expressed in the second heart field, where it again affects laterality. Thus, Pitx2c is clearly an important link between nodal-mediated left/right axis determination and asymmetric development of both inflow and outflow regions of the heart.

More detailed knowledge of the effects of left/right patterning on heart development has advanced our understanding of defects linked to human laterality defects. Kartagener syndrome is a genetically heterogeneous disorder resulting from loss of function of various proteins within the primary ciliary apparatus, and is associated with a 50% incidence of *situs inversus*. In those patients with *situs inversus*, there is a well-ordered reversal of left/right asymmetry and a relatively low incidence of congenital heart disease (3%-9%). In contrast, the majority of patients with left/right asymmetry defects have visceroatrial heterotaxy with randomization of cardiac, pulmonary, and gastrointestinal situs, similar to the *iv/iv* mouse, in which coordinated signaling is absent. Virtually any aspect of heart development can be affected, and complex CHD is commonly present. Often either the right- or left-sided signals appear to predominate with patients having either bilateral expression of right-sided (asplenia syndrome) or left-sided (polysplenia syndrome) structures. Analysis of kindreds with an X-linked form of heterotaxy led to the discovery that mutations in the transcription factor gene *ZIC3*, which has been shown to affect formation of midline structures in model organisms, can cause both familial and sporadic cases of the syndrome. Using a candidate approach that involves searching for alterations in genes implicated in left-right axis determination in model organisms, a small number of heterotaxy patients harboring mutations in nodal pathway genes (*CFC1, LEFTY A, NODAL, ACVR2B*) have been identified. Whether these mutations account for a significant portion of heterotaxy syndrome awaits further study.

Cardiac Chamber Development

In the "ballooning model" of cardiac chamber formation, the outer curvature of the looping heart tube is the site of active chamber growth, while the inner curvature remodels to appropriately align the developing inflow tract, AVC, and outflow tract with the nascent chambers. Chamber formation is initiated when myocytes in distinct regions along the outer curvature of the looping heart tube begin to increase in size and proliferate. Expression of genes encoding gap junctions and myofibrillar proteins allow this chamber myocardium (also referred to as "working" myocardium) to increase contractile function by building organized sarcomeric structures, as well as to increase conduction velocity by forming gap junctions. Chamber myocardial gene expression is induced by a transcriptional network that includes Nkx2.5, GATA4, and Tbx5. This program is repressed in the inner chamber myocardium by other T-box family members.

Superimposed upon the pathways controlling differentiation of chamber myocardium are the regulatory networks that coordinate formation of the specific chambers. Atrial and ventricular cardiac myocytes express distinct subsets of cardiac muscle genes that confer specific contractile, electrophysiological, and pharmacologic properties unique to each chamber. More strikingly, separable regulatory networks of genes are responsible for gene expression in specific chambers of the heart.

Ventricular Development

Certain transcription networks are common to both the left and right ventricles and direct expression of ventricle-specific genes such as that encoding ventricular myosin heavy chain. However, as the left ventricle is derived almost exclusively from the first heart field and the right ventricle from the second heart field, significant differences in transcriptional control of their development exist. Left ventricular development is regulated by transcription factors expressed in the primitive heart tube during chamber formation, including Nkx2.5, Hand1, and Tbx5 (Figure 1-3). Loss of any of these factors in mouse models affects development of the left ventricle.

In contrast, many of the transcription factors implicated in regulation of the second heart field are required for normal right ventricle formation (Figure 1-3). Loss of the central second heart field transcription factor Isl1 results in failure of second heart field cells to proliferate and incorporate into the primitive heart tube. In *Isl1*-deficient embryos, a two-chambered heart expressing atrial and left ventricular markers is seen—neither the right ventricle nor the outflow tract form. Loss of factors downstream of Isl1, including transcription factors Mef2c and Hand2, results in failure of the right ventricle to form in embryonic mouse hearts.

Clinically, hypoplasia of either the right or left ventricle is a severe congenital defect that primarily affects one chamber of the heart; remarkably, the remaining three chambers are typically well formed and are physiologically and electrically intact. Because growth of each chamber is likely dependent upon hemodynamic influences, primary

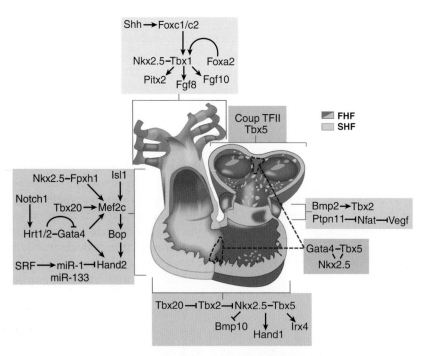

FIGURE 1-3. Pathways regulating region-specific cardiac morphogenesis. A partial list of transcription factors, signaling proteins, and miRNAs that can be placed in pathways that influence the formation of the regions of the heart. Positive influences are indicated by arrowheads, and negative effects by bars. Physical interactions are indicated by direct contact of factors. In some cases relationships of proteins are unknown. See text for details. Abbreviations: FHF, first heart field; SHF, second heart field. *Reproduced with permission from Srivastava D. Cell. 2006;126(6):1037-1048.*

defects that affect blood flow into either ventricle may result in secondary hypoplasia. For example, in chick embryos, ligation of the mitral valve results in a phenotype similar to hypoplastic left heart syndrome. However, there is also strong evidence for a genetic etiology—almost 20% of first-degree relatives of infants with hypoplastic left heart syndrome have a congenital heart defect, and 10% of infants born with a terminal 11q chromosomal deletion have a hypoplastic left heart. Interestingly, mutations in the NKX2.5 gene have been found in a small number of patients with hypoplastic left heart syndrome. In addition, there are case reports in the literature of patients with hypoplastic left heart syndrome who also have Holt-Oram syndrome (Chapter 15). Although these patients were not genotyped, Holt-Oram syndrome is associated almost exclusively with mutations in TBX5. Tbx5 and Nkx2.5 are both expressed in the developing left ventricle and are required for its development in animal models. Whether some cases of hypoplastic right ventricle formation in humans are secondary to mutations in genes important for regulating second heart field development remains to be determined.

Atrial Development

Considerably less is known about the genetics of atrial development. In contrast to the ventricle-specific transcription factors, the orphan nuclear receptor, Coup-TFII, is expressed specifically in the atrial precursors and is required for atrial but not for ventricular growth. Tbx5 is expressed most strongly in the caudal portion of the heart tube, and Tbx5-null mice have severely hypoplastic atria. Second heart field-derived cells give rise to part of the atria, and mice lacking certain transcription factors important in second heart field development also exhibit defective atrial formation.

Myocardial Growth

Growth of chamber myocardium is a complex process that requires coordination of signaling networks from the epicardial, myocardial, and endocardial layers of the developing heart. At the heart tube stage, the myocardial layer is one or two cells thick. Primitive trabecular ridges are evident in the chamber outgrowths along the outer curvature of the looped heart by the end of the fourth week of gestation. As chamber formation proceeds, the ridges become a "spongy" meshwork of fenestrated trabecular sheets that grow into the chamber in a centripetal fashion. Early trabeculations effectively increase surface area for myocardial

oxygenation, enabling the myocardial mass to increase in the absence of a coronary circulation. The outer compact layer, still only 3 to 4 cells thick, has a higher proliferative index than the trabecular myocardium and serves as a source of new cells for the trabecular layer. Retinoic acid signaling in the epicardium results in secretion of soluble mitogens such as Fgfs that are required for proliferation of the compact layer. Cardiac trabeculation is dependent on endocardial-myocardial interactions involving both secreted and membrane-bound signaling proteins. For example, neuregulin growth factors are expressed in the endocardium and signal to their receptors, erbB2 and erbB4, which are expressed on ventricular myocytes. In mice lacking neuregulin, erbB2, or erbB4, the trabecular layer fails to form. Recent mouse studies have suggested a central upstream role for the Notch signaling pathway in regulating trabecular myocardial formation.

As the coronary vasculature develops and invades the compact layer from the epicardium, the compact layer thickness increases significantly, because of compaction of the trabeculae and cell proliferation. Failure of the trabecular layer to compact results in isolated ventricular noncompaction, a cardiomyopathy characterized by persistence of "spongy" myocardium (Chapter 9). Although the clinical presentation varies, at its most severe, ventricular noncompaction can cause hydrops fetalis in utero and congestive heart failure in neonates. A strong familial inheritance pattern for this disease suggested a genetic etiology, and subsequent mapping studies have shown it to be genetically heterogenous. Interestingly, it has recently been discovered that mutations in genes encoding β-myosin heavy chain (MYH7) and cardiac actin (ACTC1), genes that are also mutated in hypertrophic cardiomyopathy, account for a significant percentage of patients with ventricular noncompaction. The "spongy" myocardium phenotype is also seen in a wide variety of knockout mice. The diversity of genes affecting myocardial growth suggests that this aspect of cardiac development is particularly sensitive to perturbations.

Conotruncal and Aortic Arch Development and the Cardiac Neural Crest

Congenital defects involving the cardiac outflow tract, aortic arch, ductus arteriosus and proximal pulmonary arteries account for 20% to 30% of all congenital heart disease. This region of the heart undergoes extensive and complex morphogenetic changes that require precise interactions between the second heart field, migrating neural crest cells, and surrounding pharyngeal tissue.

Conotruncal Formation

The cardiac outflow tract consists of the muscularized conus and the adjacent truncus arteriosus, collectively termed the conotruncus, as it arises from the primitive right ventricle. The conotruncus normally shifts to the left to override the forming ventricular septum (Figure 1-2). Mesenchymal cells then septate the truncus arteriosus into the aorta and pulmonary artery; the muscular ridge that forms between the two vessels is known as the conotruncal septum. However, at this stage, the aorta communicates with the right ventricle and the pulmonary artery with the left ventricle. Subsequent rotation of the two vessels in a spiral fashion places the aorta more dorsal and leftward and the pulmonary artery more ventral and rightward. This spiraling event results in the normal alignment of the aorta and pulmonary artery with the left and right ventricles, respectively.

Abnormalities in septation or incomplete spiraling of the conotruncus result in several different defects (Figure 1-4). For example, failure of septation of the truncus arteriosus results in persistent truncus arteriosus. If the truncus septates, but fails to rotate, transposition of the great arteries occurs. Partial but incomplete rotation might result in an aorta and pulmonary artery that arise from the right ventricle (double-outlet right ventricle) or tetralogy of Fallot if the aorta lies above the ventricular septum. The conotruncal septum between the aorta and pulmonary artery forms in tetralogy of Fallot, but because of malalignment of the great vessels, the conotruncal septum fails to connect to the muscular ventricular septum, resulting in a ventricular septal defect. Similarly, malalignment of the conotruncus results in an obligatory ventricular septal defect that, unlike muscular ventricular septal defects, does not have the potential to close spontaneously after birth.

The outflow tract is derived from the last of the second heart field progenitors to be added to the heart tube, and these progenitors give rise to all of the outflow tract myocardium, as well as to smooth muscle of the truncus arteriosus. Not surprisingly, gene and tissue ablation studies of the second heart field in model organisms result either in outflow tract defects or complete failure of outflow tract formation. Ablation of a subset of second heart field cells in chick embryos results in tetralogy of Fallot and pulmonary atresia. Many of the second heart field regulatory genes implicated in right ventricle formation (see earlier) also play important roles in conotruncal development (Figure 1-3). Loss of the central second heart field transcription factor *Isl1* completely inhibits outflow tract formation,

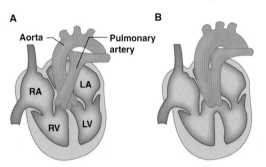
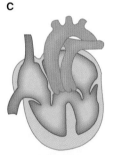
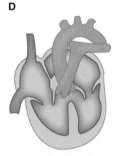

FIGURE 1-4. Cardiac defects involving conotruncal development. Many congenital heart diseases resemble a normal developmental stage of the cardiac outflow tract and great vessels during embryogenesis. **A.** Normal mature heart with the aorta arising from the left ventricle and the pulmonary artery arising from the right ventricle. **B.** Persistent truncus arteriosus represents an arrest around day 35 of human gestation due to a lack of truncal septation into a pulmonary artery and aorta. **C.** Transposition of the great arteries may result from lack of rotation of the great vessels after septation, as seen around day 45 in human embryos. **D.** Tetralogy of Fallot may represent incomplete rotation of the great arteries, which occurs around human embryonic day 45, resulting in malalignment of the vessels with rightward deviation and a narrowed right ventricular outflow tract. Regions populated by neural crest cells are shown in blue. Abbreviations: LA, left atrium; LV, left ventricle; RA, right atrium; RV, right ventricle. *Adapted by permission from Macmillan Publishers Ltd. copyright 1996; Nature Medicine. 10(2):1069-1071.*

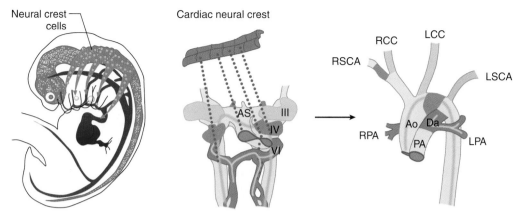

FIGURE 1-5. Migration and contribution of the cardiac neural crest. Neural crest cells arise from the crest of the neural folds between the otic placode and the third somite. Subsequent migration of the neural crest into the aortic arch arteries and cardiac outflow tract is required for arch and conotruncal development. Abbreviations: Ao, aorta; DA, ductus arteriosus; LCC, left common carotid; LPA, left pulmonary artery; LSCA, left subclavian artery; PA, pulmonary artery; RCC, right common carotid; RPA, right pulmonary artery; RSCA, right subclavian artery. *Reproduced with permission from Srivastava D, Baldwin HS. Molecular determinants of cardiac development. In: Allen HD, Gutsgell HP, Clark EB, Driscoll DJ, eds.* Heart Disease in Infants, Children, and Adolescents, *6th ed. Baltimore, MD: Williams and Wilkins; 2000:3-23.*

as the second heart field progenitor pool fails to proliferate and incorporate into the heart tube. Loss of other transcription factors expressed in the second heart field results either in formation of a truncated outflow tract (Mef2c, Foxh1), or in outflow tract defects such as persistent truncus arteriosus or double-outlet right ventricle (Tbx20).

Cardiac Neural Crest and Conotruncal Development
Other second heart field regulatory genes that more specifically affect outflow tract development may do so in part by perturbing the interactions between the second heart field–derived myocytes and the cardiac neural crest cells that migrate into the developing outflow tract. Neural crest cells are a unique population of pluripotent cells derived from the crest of the neural folds that migrate away from the neural folds and differentiate into multiple cell types. They contribute to diverse embryonic structures, including the cranial ganglia, peripheral nervous system, adrenal glands, and melanocytes. The cardiac neural crest is comprised of those cells originating from the level of the otic placode to the third somite that migrate through the developing pharyngeal arches and populate the mesenchyme of each of the pharyngeal and aortic arch arteries, the conotruncus, and conotruncal

septum (Figure 1-5). Tissue ablation studies of premigratory cardiac neural crest in chick embryos revealed a critical role for neural crest cells in outflow tract septation, great vessel formation, and aortic arch patterning. Embryos deficient in cardiac neural crest cells have a variety of cardiac outflow tract defects including tetralogy of Fallot, persistent truncus arteriosus, double-outlet right ventricle, and conotruncal ventricular septal defects; aortic arch patterning defects are seen as well (discussed in following text). These defects closely mirror the spectrum of defects seen in patients with microdeletions of chromosome 22q11.

The deletion 22q11 syndrome is the most common chromosomal microdeletion syndrome and is thought to represent a disorder of neural crest migration. Variable phenotypic features include thymic, parathyroid, craniofacial, renal, and cardiovascular anomalies. A variety of mouse studies have shown that loss of the gene encoding the T-box transcription factor Tbx1, which is expressed in the second heart field but not the neural crest, results in cardiac outflow tract and pharyngeal arch artery anomalies reminiscent of those observed in the 22q11 deletion syndrome in a gene dosage-dependent manner. Furthermore, mutations within the *Tbx1* gene were found in several patients with features of the 22q11 deletion syndrome who lacked the deletion by fluorescence in situ hybridization (FISH). Animal studies show that Tbx1 plays a central regulatory role in outflow tract development (Figure 1-3). *Tbx1* expression in the second heart field is important for second heart field cell proliferation and formation of outflow tract myocardium. Tbx1 also regulates the expression of a family of fibroblast growth factor (Fgf) signaling molecules that influence the cardiac neural crest cells that migrate into the second heart field. Thus, Tbx1 likely regulates outflow tract development via direct effects on the second heart field and indirect effects on the neural crest cells. Conversely, defects of cardiac neural crest development have been shown to indirectly influence the second heart field. Ablation studies in chick showed that a subset of second heart field cells failed to migrate into the developing outflow tract of cardiac neural crest ablated embryos. In the absence of the neural crest cells, excess Fgf signaling in the pharynx caused the second heart field cells to proliferate rather than migrate and differentiate into outflow tract myocardium. Thus, the outflow tract defects seen in these embryos reflect both a direct loss of cardiac neural crest cells and an indirect loss of second heart field cells. These studies highlight the intricate interactions that must take place between these two populations of cells for normal conotruncal development to occur.

Mouse models have also provided insight into genes that affect the proliferation, migration, differentiation, and patterning of the neural crest cells that populate the outflow tract and aortic arches. For example, the naturally occurring mutant *Splotch*, which harbors a mutation in the homeobox gene *pax3*, has persistent truncus arteriosus and aortic arch defects. Neural crest cells in *Splotch* mice migrate properly but too few cells reach the outflow tract and arch, suggesting a proliferation or survival defect. Semaphorins are secreted ligands important for axon guidance. *Semaphorin 3C*-null mice have persistent truncus arteriosus and interrupted aortic arch, suggesting that these molecules may also play a role in guiding migration of neural crest cells to the outflow tract. Sema3C is expressed in outflow tract myocardium and its receptors, PlexinA2 and Neuropilin1, are expressed in neural crest cells. Deletion of the gene encoding either receptor also results in persistent truncus arteriosus and interrupted aortic arch. Neural crest cells do not migrate as individual cells, but rather as organized streams or sheets of cells that are functionally coupled via gap junctions. Mice lacking the gap junction protein Connexin43 have abnormal

outflow tract formation, and the cardiac neural crest cells in these mice exhibit decreased directionality and speed of migration. Neural crest cell-specific inhibition of the signaling protein Notch in mice is sufficient to recapitulate many of the cardiac outflow tract defects seen in patients with Alagille syndrome, an autosomal dominant disorder caused predominantly by mutations in the gene encoding the Notch ligand Jag1 (Chapter 15). Studies of the mouse model revealed that loss of Notch function caused a post-migratory defect in the ability of neural crest cells to differentiate into vascular smooth muscle, which is important for great vessel and aortic arch development. These studies illustrate the fact that conotruncal malformations may result from perturbations of many different aspects of cardiac neural crest cell biology.

Aortic Arch Patterning

The aortic sac lies distal to the conotruncus and gives rise to six bilaterally symmetric vessels known as aortic arch arteries. The aortic arch arteries arise sequentially along the anterior-posterior axis, each traversing a pharyngeal arch before joining the paired dorsal aortae. The first and second arch arteries involute and the fifth arch artery never fully forms. The third, fourth, and sixth arch arteries undergo extensive asymmetric remodeling to ultimately form distinct regions of the mature aortic arch and proximal pulmonary arteries (Figure 1-5). The majority of the right-sided dorsal aorta and aortic arch arteries undergo programmed cell death resulting in a left-sided aortic arch. The third aortic arch artery contributes to the proximal carotid arteries. The left fourth aortic arch artery forms the transverse aortic arch between the left common carotid and left subclavian arteries, whereas the right fourth aortic arch artery provides the proximal part of the right subclavian artery. Finally, the proximal sixth arch arteries contribute to the proximal pulmonary arteries and the distal left sixth aortic arch artery contributes to the ductus arteriosus. Extrapolating from their embryologic origins, subtle arch anomalies are likely the result of third aortic arch defects, interrupted aortic arch and aberrant right subclavian arteries arise from fourth arch defects, and patent ductus arteriosus and proximal pulmonary artery hypoplasia/discontinuity result from defects in sixth arch artery development.

Development of the aortic arch artery system involves stabilization of the initial endothelial network by acquisition of neural crest-derived smooth muscle cell layer, followed by a remodeling process in which discrete segments expand or involute. Complex interactions between neural crest cells, pharyngeal ectoderm, mesoderm, and pouch endoderm have been implicated in these processes. In chick embryos that undergo premigratory neural crest ablation, a broad spectrum of aortic arch anomalies are observed, including interruption of the aortic arch, aberrant origins of the right subclavian artery and persistence of the right aortic arch rather than the left aortic arch. As might be expected, many of the regulatory genes and signaling pathways that affect neural crest contributions to the outflow tract (discussed earlier in the text) also affect aortic arch vessel development.

As is the case for chamber development, the development of specific segments of the mature aortic arch can be affected by distinct regulatory genes or networks. Disruption of the transcription factor Hoxa3, which is expressed in the third pharyngeal arch endoderm and in the neural crest cells that invade the third arch, results in anomalies specifically of the carotid arteries. Deletion of a variety of mouse genes specifically affects the fourth aortic arch artery and results in absence of the transverse aortic arch, resembling the type B interruption of the aortic arch seen clinically. A recent paper proposes a model for TGF-β signaling within this segment that involves alterations in angiogenic signals that lead to decreased flow. Lower flow causes down-regulation of sheer stress responsive genes resulting in accelerated apoptosis of that segment. The relative role of blood flow, apoptosis, and angiogenesis in arch remodeling is an area of active investigation.

Finally, the fact that failure of the ductus arteriosus to close after birth is the third most common congenital heart defect is suggestive that the sixth aortic arch artery is independently regulated. Ductus arteriosus closure requires migration, proliferation, and contraction of distal left sixth arch smooth muscle cells at birth. Interestingly, recent analysis of two kindreds with thoracic aortic aneurysm and PDA revealed causative mutations in the smooth muscle myosin heavy chain gene *MYH11*. Heterozygous mutations of the gene encoding the transcription factor, TFAP2β, can result in familial patent ductus arteriosus (Char syndrome, Chapter 15). TFAP2β is expressed in developing neural crest, and the mutated protein may alter the function of the neural crest-derived medial layer, preventing the postnatal constriction that leads to ductal closure.

Cardiac Valve Formation

Appropriate placement and function of cardiac valves is essential for chamber septation and for unidirectional flow of blood through the heart. The first evidence of valvulogenesis during embryonic development is the formation of the endocardial cushions in the atrioventricular canal and outflow tract of the looped heart tube. The endocardial cushions are regional swellings of extracellular matrix that provide valve-like function in the primitive heart. They form the anlage of the semilunar and atrioventricular valves and ultimately contribute to formation of the definitive valve leaflets. In the AVC, the superior and inferior cushions fuse to form the atrioventricular septum and divide the single tube into the right (tricuspid) and left (mitral) inlets. Mesenchyme from the endocardial cushions extends anteriorly and inferiorly to form the inlet portion of the ventricular septum and posteriorly and superiorly in the plane of the primary atrial septum to complete atrial septation. The endocardial cushions in the outflow region form the aortopulmonary septum, contribute to semilunar valve development, and contribute to formation of the conal and perimembranous septums, in conjunction with cardiac neural crest-derived cells.

The molecular pathways that regulate valvulogenesis are becoming increasingly well understood. Both the atrioventricular canal and the outflow tract cushions are derived from the primary myocardium of the inner curvature of the looped heart tube. The same regulatory networks that repress chamber myocardial gene expression along the inner curvature also act to stimulate synthesis of extracellular matrix components such as hyaluronan and versican in the regions of incipient valve formation. This increase in cardiac jelly formation causes a localized protrusion into the lumen of the heart tube, resulting in endocardial cushion formation. Reciprocal signaling between the myocardium and the endocardium overlying the cushion results in a subset of endocardial cushion cells undergoing an endothelial-to-mesenchymal transformation migrating into the cushion extracellular matrix. These cells will differentiate into the fibrous tissue of the valves. Mouse studies have revealed crucial roles for the bone morphogenetic protein (Bmp) and Notch signaling pathways in endothelial-to-mesenchymal transformation. Mutations in the genes encoding Notch and its receptor Jag in humans are associated with abnormal semilunar valve development (see following discussion and Chapter 15). Once endothelial-to-mesenchymal transformation has occurred, the newly formed mesenchymal cells proliferate within the extracellular matrix in response to a variety of signals. Proper balance of positive and negative regulatory signals is essential for normal valve development, as loss of inhibitory signals results in formation of hyperplastic, thickened, gelatinous valves in mice. The Ras-mitogen activated protein kinase (MAPK) pathway has been implicated in mesenchymal cell proliferation, and activating mutations in a number of pathway genes in humans cause Noonan syndrome, an autosomal dominant disease in which the cardiac manifestations include pulmonic stenosis secondary to thickened, dysplastic pulmonary valves (Chapter 15).

The valve primordia undergo elongation into thin valve leaflets over a period of many weeks. Differential gene expression is observed within distinct regions of the developing valve tissue. Elastin expression is localized to the side of the valves exposed to unidirectional blood flow, whereas collagen fibrils predominate on the fibrous layer away from blood flow. The intervening spongiosa layer is rich in proteoglycans, while increased tenascin-X expression is observed in the chordae tendineae and other supporting structures. Expression of these and other proteins during valve maturation allows different regions of the valve apparatus to develop biomechanical properties suitable to their functional roles. Hemodynamic flow is thought to play a role in valve maturation; however, the role of hemodynamic influences on these changes in gene expression is presently unclear. One attractive hypothesis is that shear stress on the flow side of the valve initiates valve polarity and differential gene expression.

Defective development of cardiac valves occurs in 20% to 30% of patients with congenital heart disease. In addition to the previously mentioned mutations in Notch and Ras-MAPK signaling pathways, altered expression and function of a variety of structural proteins are associated with developmental valvular disease in humans. Haploinsufficiency for the elastin gene (*ELN*), either isolated or as part of a larger chromosomal deletion (Williams-Beuren syndrome, Chapter 15), is associated with valvar aortic stenosis as well as the more prevalent supravalvar arteriopathies. Mutations in the fibrillin gene (*FBN1*) cause Marfan syndrome and are associated with mitral valve prolapse, in addition to aortic dilatation. Mitral valve prolapse is also seen in certain patients with Ehlers-Danlos syndrome and Stickler syndrome. These connective tissue disorders are caused by mutations in the genes encoding tenascin-X or one of several different collagen isoforms that are involved in valve maturation and homeostasis. The role of other extracellular matrix proteins in developmental valvular disorders is being studied both in animal models and through candidate gene approaches in human genetic analysis.

Finally, trisomy 21 (Down syndrome) in humans is commonly associated with incomplete septation of the atrioventricular valves. Studies of rare individuals with congenital heart defects and partial duplications of chromosome 21 have identified a Down syndrome–critical region associated with the presence of cardiac defects. However, the specific genes responsible for the cardiac anomalies have yet to be defined. A recent study suggests that gene dosage changes in two genes within the Down syndrome–critical region may affect NFATc1 function and disrupt key gene regulatory circuits, resulting in the pleiotropic effects of trisomy 21. Data from various mouse models, including the evidence of endocardial cushion maturation abnormalities in *NFATc1*-null mice, are consistent with this hypothesis, but further studies are needed. Although 70% of patients with complete atrioventricular septal defect have Down syndrome, analysis of kindreds with autosomal dominant atrioventricular septal defect has excluded linkage to chromosome 21, suggesting that distinct genetic etiologies account for this cardiac defect in Down syndrome as compared to nonsyndromic patients.

Cardiac Conduction System Development

The myocardium of the embryonic tubular heart initially beats irregularly in an uncoordinated fashion. Homogenous contraction is subsequently achieved, but at a slow rate reflecting the low density of gap junctions in the myocardial cells of the primitive heart tube. After cardiac looping, some of the primary myocardium of the inflow tract and atrioventricular canal retains aspects of the primary myocardial phenotype, namely high automaticity and slow conduction. Myocytes from these regions will eventually form the sinoatrial and atrioventricular nodes of the conduction system. In the ventricular conduction system, the atrioventricular (His) bundle forms from the crest of the interventricular septum, while the bundle branches and subendocardial peripheral Purkinje network forms from the early ventricular chamber myocardium. The heart tube is initially polarized along the craniocaudal axis with the dominant pacemaking activity found at the inflow, or caudal pole. This pacemaker activity, the first element to function in the cardiac conduction system, gives rise to the dominant sinoatrial node. After cardiac looping, this caudal to cranial depolarization sequence translates to base-to-apex activation. The activation sequence is reversed to the apex-to-base pattern of the mature heart before completion of ventricular septation in the mouse.

Formation of the conduction system requires repression of chamber myocardial gene expression in the myocytes destined to become conduction tissue. The transcriptional repressor Tbx3 is expressed in SA node precursors, where it functions to induce and maintain SA node cells as pacemaker cells, while repressing expression of genes that confer the atrial myocyte phenotype. Ectopic expression of Tbx3 within the atria is sufficient to induce ectopic pacemaker sites characterized by suppression of normal atrial gene expression and induction of the pacemaker channel Hcn4. Similarly, formation of the ventricular conduction system requires a network of transcription factors, including Nkx2.5, Tbx5, and Id2, that act to inhibit sarcomere differentiation and promote conduction tissue differentiation. Mutations in some of these transcription factors underlie certain human arrhythmias. Patients with mutations in *NKX2.5* can manifest progressive AV conduction disorders, with or without associated structural defects (see subsequent discussion). Mutations in *TBX5* cause the structural and atrioventricular nodal disease seen in patients with Holt-Oram syndrome (Chapter 15).

Epicardial and Coronary Vascular Development

The epicardium derives from a specialized group of mesothelial cells associated with the sinus venosus called the proepicardial organ. In addition to the epicardium, the proepicardial cells ultimately give rise to the coronary vasculature and interstitial fibroblasts of the heart. Lineage studies show that the proepicardial organ consists of a mixed population of fibroblast, vascular smooth muscle, and endocardial progenitor cells that migrate to the looped heart. Upon reaching the heart, the vascular smooth muscle and fibroblast progenitors envelop it to form the epicardium. Removal of the epicardium in avian species leads to the arrest of both cardiomyocyte proliferation and coronary artery development. Mice deleted for genes important for proepicardial organ formation, epicardial progenitor cell survival, or epicardial cell migration and attachment show similar phenotypes. Organ culture and animal studies show that retinoic acid signaling in the epicardium promotes cardiomyocyte proliferation by inducing secretion of mitogens such as Fgfs into the subepicardial space to promote proliferation of the compact layer of the myocardium.

Coronary vascular development involves formation of a vascular plexus followed by angiogenic remodeling that gives rise to the mature vascular tree. The proepicardial organ and the epicardium that is derived from it play several essential roles in this process, including contributing the cellular components of the coronary vasculature, and providing essential paracrine signals. Coronary vasculogenesis begins when endocardial progenitor cells from the proepicardial organ begin to coalesce into tubes within the extracellular matrix-rich area between the epicardium and myocardium called the subepicardial space. Endocardial cells also invade the myocardium from the subepicardial space and begin to form tubular networks that extend from the epicardial to the endocardial surface of the myocardium. The subepicardial and myocardial networks connect to form a vascular plexus. Experiments using mouse models and organ culture have shown that this endothelial network forms in response to a cascade of Fgf and hedgehog signaling between the epicardium and myocardium that results in the expression of pro-angiogenic signals in the myocardium. As the endothelial networks begin to form, a subpopulation of fibroblast and vascular smooth muscle cell progenitors from the epicardium undergo epithelial-to-mesenchymal transformation and enter the subepicardial space. These epicardial-derived mesenchymal cells then differentiate into vascular smooth muscle cells and perivascular fibroblasts that invest the endothelial networks of the subepicardium and myocardium.

Formation of the central coronary arteries occurs not by outgrowth of vessels from the aorta, but rather from ingrowth of vessels from an endothelial ring that forms at the base of the aorta. Strands from this peritruncal ring penetrate the aorta at all three cusps; however, strands to the posterior noncoronary cusp fail to form an ostium and regress. Mesenchymal cells recruited to invest the invading endothelial channels differentiate into smooth muscle after the coronary ostia are formed. As anterograde blood flow is established from the aorta, the coronary vascular network undergoes significant remodeling, including a severalfold increase in luminal diameter at the ostia. Although these insights into central coronary artery connection to the aorta have obvious implications for coronary arterial abnormalities in a variety of congenital heart defects, the signals governing these processes are unknown. Hopefully, as the molecular mechanisms underlying coronary vascular development are identified, the pathogenesis of abnormal coronary development in patients with congenital heart disease will be elucidated.

■ HUMAN GENETICS IN CONGENITAL HEART DISEASE

The majority of congenital heart defects are thought to result from interaction of genetic predisposition with environmental influences. In the past two decades, our understanding of the genetic contribution to congenital heart disease has advanced significantly. As illustrated in the previous sections, studies of cardiac development in model organisms have led to the discovery of many genes required for heart formation. Searching for mutations in these "candidate" genes in patients with congenital heart disease has yielded insight into the genetic basis of certain defects. In addition, molecular genetic analysis of families with documented Mendelian transmission of certain defects has led to the identification of disease-causing mutations in several cardiac transcription factors and signaling molecules. This section reviews what is currently known about the contribution of genetics to isolated cardiovascular malformations. The genetics of syndromic cardiovascular disease is discussed in Chapter 15. Research in this area is progressing rapidly, and the reader is referred to online public databases such as Online Mendelian Inheritance in Man (OMIM, http://www.ncbi.nlm.nih.gov/ omim) and Gene Reviews (http://www.ncbi.nlm.nih.gov/sites/ GeneTests/review?db=genetests) for more information.

Congenital heart disease most often occurs as an isolated defect rather than as part of a syndrome. Although the etiology of the majority of nonsyndromic congenital heart disease is likely multifactorial, recent studies have shown that mutations in single genes can result in specific forms of disease in some cases. However, the same mutation can result in different forms of congenital heart disease even within the same kindred, reinforcing the concept that additional genetic and/or environmental factors contribute to expression of the disease phenotype. These mutations often result in haploinsufficiency, although dominant-negative gain-of-function mutations are also observed. Table 1-1 lists single gene disorders and the defects with which they have been associated. The possible functional significance of these gene mutations, and thus their causal relationship with the associated defects, awaits further study.

The first discovery of single gene mutations resulting in nonsyndromic cardiac defects came from analysis of several families with autosomal dominant congenital heart disease consisting most commonly of atrial septal defect and atrioventricular conduction delay. There was evidence of progressive conduction disease on serial studies in some individuals, and there was a strong history of sudden death in these families. After linkage studies mapped the disease locus, mutations were found in the candidate gene *NKX2.5*. These mutations were found in all affected individuals, were absent in unaffected family members and other control samples, and were shown to alter the DNA-binding and/or transcriptional activation function(s) of the protein. Subsequent studies extended the association between *NKX2.5* mutations, congenital heart disease, and atrioventricular conduction disorders, while animal models have confirmed a role for Nkx2.5 in maintenance of the atrioventricular conduction system (see earlier text). Alterations in the *NKX2.5* coding region have also been found in a small proportion of patients with sporadic atrial septal defect, as well as other lesions, including ventricular septal defect, tetralogy of Fallot, and (very rarely) hypoplastic left heart syndrome. However, the functional significance of some of these mutations is unknown. Testing for *NKX2.5* mutations is available clinically and may be useful in cases of familial atrial septal defect to predict those at risk for progressive atrioventricular conduction disorders.

GATA4 and Tbx20 partner with Nkx2.5 to regulate expression of genes critical to myocardial differentiation and function, including the genes encoding the sarcomeric proteins myosin heavy chain (*MYH6*) and cardiac actin (*ACTC1*). Mutations in *GATA4, TBX20, MYH6,* and *ACTC1* have all been reported in patients with atrial septal defects. There were no associated conduction disorders. The *GATA4* mutations caused decreased DNA-binding affinity and transcriptional activity. One of the alterations disrupted the interaction between GATA4 and TBX5, the transcription factor that is mutated in individuals with atrial septal defects and Holt-Oram syndrome (Chapter 15). Subsequent studies have shown *GATA4* sequence alterations in a small percentage of sporadic cases of atrial septal defect, ventricular septal defect, tetralogy of Fallot, and atrioventricular septal defect. *TBX20* mutations have also been associated with ventricular septal defects and dilated cardiomyopathy. Mutations in *MYH6* and *ACTC1* are found in patients with various forms of cardiomyopathy (Chapter 9).

Analysis of several families with autosomal dominant aortic valve disease led to the discovery of mutations in the signaling molecule *NOTCH1* in individuals with bicuspid aortic valve and aortic stenosis. Affected family members, including several with trileaflet aortic valves, developed

■ **TABLE 1-1.** Single Gene Disorders Associated With Isolated CHD

Congenital Heart Defect	Gene(s)	Protein
Aortic stenosis/bicuspid aortic valve	NOTCH1	Signaling molecule
Atrial septal defect	NKX2.5 (with AV conduction disturbances)	Transcription factor
	GATA4	Transcription factor
	TBX20	Transcription factor
	MYH6	Cardiac muscle sarcomeric protein
	ACTC1	Cardiac muscle sarcomeric protein
Atrioventricular septal defect	CRELD1	Signaling molecule
	NKX2.5	Transcription factor
	GATA4	Transcription factor
	GDF1	Signaling molecule
	CFC1	Signaling molecule
Double-outlet right ventricle	CFC1	Signaling molecule
	GDF1	Signaling molecule
	NODAL	Signaling molecule
Supravalvar aortic stenosis	ELN	Structural protein
Tetralogy of Fallot	NKX2.5	Transcription factor
	JAG1	Transcription factor
	ZFPM2/FOG2	Transcription factor
	GATA4	Signaling molecule
	GDF1	Signaling molecule
	CFC1	Transcription factor
	FOXH1	Signaling molecule
	NODAL	
d-transposition of the great arteries	PROSIT240	Signaling molecule
	GDF1	Signaling molecule
	CFC1	Signaling molecule
	FOXH1	Transcription factor
	NODAL	Signaling molecule
Ventricular septal defect	GATA4	Transcription factor
	NKX2.5	Transcription factor
	TBX20	Transcription factor

severe valve calcification. Animal models confirmed that *Notch1* is highly expressed in the developing aortic valve, and may play a role in regulating calcium deposition. Further study is needed to understand the extent to which mutations in the Notch pathway contribute to aortic valve disease and other left-sided lesions. Mutations in the Notch ligand *JAGGED-1* underlie most cases of Alagille syndrome (Chapter 15), and are also associated with other defects including isolated pulmonary stenosis and tetralogy of Fallot.

■ THE FUTURE

The past decade has seen dramatic progress in elucidating the molecular mechanisms that control cardiac development. Sequence analysis of candidate genes identified in model systems as being important for aspects of heart development has complemented classical human genetic mapping approaches to start to unravel the genetic basis of congenital heart disease. However, the heterogeneity of congenital heart disease associated with single gene defects, as demonstrated for *NKX2.5* or *GATA4* mutations, makes mechanistic understanding of the effects of gene mutations challenging, and points to the importance of modifier genes, environmental factors, and genetic polymorphisms in determining the severity and type of disease. The availability of high throughput methods of detecting genetic sequence variants in candidate genes should facilitate analysis of multiple genes within pathways to determine additional regulators or modifiers of potential disease causing genes. In addition, improvements in tools and methods for hemodynamic manipulation of genetically favorable organisms such as mice should advance the important study of the interaction between environmental factors, including flow and pressure, and genetic pathways in the pathobiology of congenital heart disease. Advances in noninvasive in utero imaging of mice embryos are beginning to facilitate the analysis of functional, as well as structural, effects of various mutations upon the developing heart. Most importantly, ongoing collaborations between pediatric cardiologists, human geneticists, and development biologists are needed to expand the identification of genetic variants and to determine their contributions to the development of these defects. Such information is already impacting aspects of clinical pediatric cardiology. Clinical testing is increasingly available for many of the genetic alterations that underlie congenital heart disease, and information derived from those tests is impacting management and counseling of patients and their families. In the future, it is conceivable that it may also direct preventative and therapeutic approaches as well.

SUGGESTED READINGS

General

Bruneau BG. The developmental genetics of congenital heart disease. *Nature.* 2008;451(7181):943-948.

Buckingham M, Meilhac S, Zaffran S. Building the mammalian heart from two sources of myocardial cells. *Nat Rev Genet.* 2005; 6(11):826-835.

High FA, Epstein JA. The multifaceted role of notch in cardiac development and disease. *Nat Rev Genet.* 2008;9(1):49-61.

Hoogaars WM, Barnett P, Moorman AF, Christoffels VM. T-box factors determine cardiac design. *Cell Mol Life Sci.* 2007;64(6):646-660.

Hoover LL, Burton EG, Brooks BA, Kubalak SW. The expanding role for retinoid signaling in heart development. *ScientificWorldJournal.* 2008;8:194-211.

Olson EN. Gene regulatory networks in the evolution and development of the heart. *Science.* 2006;313(5795):1922-1927.

Srivastava D. Making or breaking the heart: from lineage determination to morphogenesis. *Cell.* 2006;126(6):1037-1048.

Thomas H, Vincent MC, Robert HA, Antoon FMM. Can recent insights into cardiac development improve our understanding of congenitally malformed hearts? *Clin Anat.* 2009;22(1):4-20.

Early Cardiogenesis

Brand T. Heart development: molecular insights into cardiac specification and early morphogenesis. *Dev Biol.* 2003;258(1):1-19.

Dunwoodie SL. Combinatorial signaling in the heart orchestrates cardiac induction, lineage specification and chamber formation. *Semin Cell Dev Biol.* 2007;18(1):54-66.

Tzahor E. Wnt/beta-catenin signaling and cardiogenesis: Timing does matter. *Dev Cell.* 2007;13(1):10-13.

Heart Field Patterning

Dyer LA, Kirby ML. The role of secondary heart field in cardiac development. *Dev Biol.* 2009;336(2):137-144.

Harvey RP, Meilhac SM, Buckingham ME. Landmarks and lineages in the developing heart. *Circ Res.* 2009; 104(11):1235-1237.

Rochais F, Mesbah K, Kelly RG. Signaling pathways controlling second heart field development. *Circ Res.* 2009; 104(8):933-942.

Cardiac Looping and Chamber Formation

Cai C-L, Zhou W, Yang L, et al. T-box genes coordinate regional rates of proliferation and regional specification during cardiogenesis. *Development.* 2005;132(10):2475-2487.

Christoffels VM, Burch JBE, Moorman AFM. Architectural plan for the heart: early patterning and delineation of the chambers and the nodes. *Trends Cardiovasc Med.* 2004; 14(8):301-307.

Zaffran S, Kelly RG, Meilhac SM, Buckingham ME, Brown NA. Right ventricular myocardium derives from the anterior heart field. *Circ Res.* 2004;95(3):261-268.

Myocardial Growth

Grego-Bessa J, Luna-Zurita L, del Monte G, et al. Notch signaling is essential for ventricular chamber development. *Dev Cell.* 2007;12(3):415-429.

McNally E, Dellefave L. Sarcomere mutations in cardiogenesis and ventricular noncompaction. *Trends Cardiovasc Med.* 2009;19(1):17-21.

Moorman AF, Christoffels VM. Cardiac chamber formation: development, genes, and evolution. *Physiol Rev.* 2003; 83(4):1223-1267.

Left-Right Asymmetry and Heart Development

Franco D, Campione M. The role of pitx2 during cardiac development: linking left-right signaling and congenital heart diseases. *Trends Cardiovasc Med.* 2003;13(4):157-163.

Palmer AR. Symmetry breaking and the evolution of development. *Science.* 2004;306(5697):828-833.

Ramsdell AF. Left-right asymmetry and congenital cardiac defects: getting to the heart of the matter in vertebrate left-right axis determination. *Dev Biol.* 2005;288(1):1-20.

Outflow Tract Development and the Cardiac Neural Crest

Baldini A. Dissecting contiguous gene defects: Tbx1. *Curr Opin Genet Dev.* 2005;15(3):279-284.

High F, Epstein JA. Signaling pathways regulating cardiac neural crest migration and differentiation. *Novartis Found Symp.* 2007;283:152-161; discussion 61-64, 238-241.

Hutson MR, Kirby ML. Model systems for the study of heart development and disease: cardiac neural crest and conotruncal malformations. *Semin Cell Dev Biol.* 2007; 18(1):101-110.

Xu H, Morishima M, Wylie JN, et al. Tbx1 has a dual role in the morphogenesis of the cardiac outflow tract. *Development.* 2004;131(13):3217-3227.

Cardiac Valve Formation

Armstrong EJ, Bischoff J. Heart valve development: endothelial cell signaling and differentiation. *Circ Res.* 2004;95(5):459-470.

Combs MD, Yutzey KE. Heart valve development: regulatory networks in development and disease. *Circ Res.* 2009; 105(5):408-421.

Cardiac Conduction System Development

Hatcher CJ, Basson CT. Specification of the cardiac conduction system by transcription factors. *Circ Res.* 2009;105(7): 620-630.

Mikawa T, Hurtado R. Development of the cardiac conduction system. *Semin Cell Dev Biol.* 2007;18(1):90-100.

Epicardial and Coronary Artery Development

Lavine KJ, Ornitz DM. Shared circuitry: developmental signaling cascades regulate both embryonic and adult coronary vasculature. *Circ Res.* 2009;104(2):159-169.

Tomanek RJ. Formation of the coronary vasculature during development. *Angiogenesis.* 2005;8(3):273-284.

Genetics of Human CHD

Benson DW. Genetic origins of pediatric heart disease. *Pediatr Cardiol.* 2010;31:422-429.

Garg V, Muth AN, Ransom JF, et al. Mutations in notch1 cause aortic valve disease. *Nature.* 2005;437(7056): 270-274.

Roessler E, Ouspenskaia MV, Karkera JD, et al. Reduced nodal signaling strength via mutation of several pathway members including foxh1 is linked to human heart defects and holoprosencephaly. *Am J Hum Genet.* 2008; 83(1):18-29.

Schott J-J, Benson DW, Basson CT, et al. Congenital heart disease caused by mutations in the transcription factor nkx2-5. *Science.* 1998;281(5373):108-111.

Regulation of Myocyte Contraction and Relaxation

■ INTRODUCTION

As described in Chapter 1, the developing heart undergoes a series of extremely complex processes during structural organogenesis. Considerable insight into the genetic control of these pathways has been gained in recent years. Of equal importance are the functional changes in cardiac contraction and relaxation that must accompany the morphological development of the cardiovascular system. However, much less is known about the genetic, molecular, and cellular processes that control cardiac contractile

function in the mammalian heart during embryonic development and fetal maturation.

Although age-related changes occur in the cardiac responses to virtually every pharmacological or physiological intervention, understanding of the underlying mechanisms is generally incomplete. In particular, there is relatively little known about fundamental mechanisms of excitation-contraction coupling and regulation of contractile function in the immature human heart. It is only by gaining a thorough understanding of the basic molecular and cellular processes governing contractile function that we can develop more rational and age-appropriate pharmacological strategies for fetal and neonatal patients.

This chapter will present current concepts of developmental aspects of myocyte contraction, relaxation, and excitation-contraction coupling that have been derived from animal models. Where appropriate, relevant data from human studies will be presented. In this manner, we can begin to form the scientific foundation for understanding the regulation of myocardial contractile function in infants and children. The list of suggested readings at the end of this chapter refers to several excellent monographs that provide a comprehensive and detailed overview of contractile function in the mature heart. In addition, several recent reviews are listed that provide additional information regarding developmental changes in cardiac ultrastructure, metabolism, electrophysiology, and responses to pathophysiological states. Integration of these myocellular changes into a larger perspective of developmental physiology and cardiac mechanics is presented in Chapter 3.

■ GENERAL OVERVIEW OF CELLULAR ASPECTS OF CARDIAC FUNCTION

Excitation, contraction, and relaxation of myocardial cells are mediated by complex ion transport processes and coordination of calcium delivery to and from the contractile proteins (Figure 2-1). At rest, active transport processes (mainly the sodium-potassium pump) maintain electrochemical gradients across the sarcolemmal membrane. Consequently, a resting membrane potential is established with the cell interior being negative relative to the extracellular space. Depolarization of the cardiac sarcolemmal membrane occurs largely due to the opening of sodium channels, which results in an influx of sodium and a rapid rise in membrane potential from negative to positive values. As described in more detail in the following discussion, this change in membrane potential is ultimately translated into an increase in intracellular cytosolic calcium, binding of calcium to the contractile protein complex in the myofibrils, and cell shortening (contraction). Relaxation occurs as the resting sarcolemmal membrane potential is reestablished, intracellular cytosolic calcium decreases, and calcium dissociates from the contractile protein complex.

These processes must be very tightly regulated to maintain calcium homeostasis and control of contraction and relaxation. During the past several years, it has become clear that many of the pathways and proteins involved in these processes undergo developmental regulation. Consequently significant age-related differences exist in the very fundamental mechanisms of cardiac contraction, relaxation, and regulation of contractile function.

Much of our knowledge regarding developmental aspects of cardiac contractile function is derived from animal models, especially chickens, rats, rabbits, and mice. A recurring problem in developmental cardiology relates to extrapolating animal studies to human physiology. However, it is clear that many events in human cardiac morphogenesis are comparable to those in other species and in many instances the results from animal and human studies are similar. Because cardiac development and maturation are controlled by genetic and epigenetic factors, there may be species-specific events that are unique for a given animal model. It is therefore useful to compare results from one or more animal models. Studies using human myocardium provide more relevant results, but the availability of tissue for these types of research is limited, especially for fetal and neonatal human hearts. We are therefore left extrapolating data obtained from animal models to the immature human heart.

■ STRUCTURAL COMPONENTS INVOLVED IN CONTRACTION AND RELAXATION

Changes in Myocyte Size and Morphology

In the human embryo, the elements required for rhythmic contraction and relaxation of the heart become functional by approximately 3 weeks after conception. The major functional units include the sarcolemmal membrane, sarcoplasmic reticulum, mitochondria, and contractile proteins. Each of these elements undergoes progressive development and maturation throughout embryonic, fetal, and early postnatal life. In the early embryo and fetus, the ultrastructural appearance and spatial arrangement of cellular structures are quite different compared to those of the fully mature heart.

Ventricular myocytes change considerably with regard to size, shape, and overall appearance during the transition from late fetus to the adult. In general, the perinatal maturation phase is largely characterized by addition of cellular structures and more precise spatial organization of the elements involved in contraction and relaxation. Newborn myocytes exhibit random orientation of myofibrils with incomplete sarcomeres. Myofibrils are frequently located in the subsarcolemmal region. Regularly scattered throughout the cell are ribosomes, rough endoplasmic

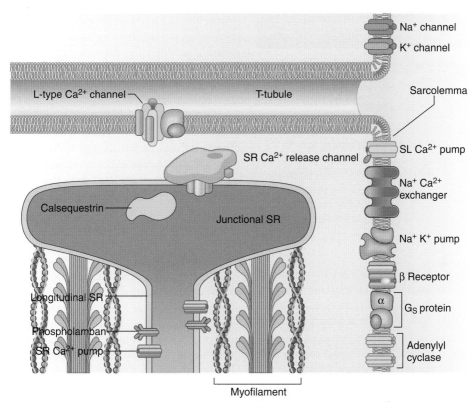

Na⁺ channel

K⁺ channel

L-type Ca²⁺ channel

T-tubule

Sarcolemma

SR Ca²⁺ release channel

SL Ca²⁺ pump

Calsequestrin

Junctional SR

Na⁺ Ca²⁺ exchanger

Na⁺ K⁺ pump

β Receptor

Longitudinal SR

α   Gₛ protein

Phospholamban

SR Ca²⁺ pump

Adenylyl cyclase

Myofilament

FIGURE 2-1. Schematic diagram of the major components involved in calcium transport, excitation-contraction coupling, contraction, and relaxation in mature mammalian ventricular myocytes. At rest, a negative membrane potential is maintained largely by the action of the sodium-potassium pumps. Contraction in adult myocytes (Figure 2-4A) is triggered by membrane depolarization (opening of sodium channels), which then promotes opening of voltage-dependent L-type calcium channels. The resulting influx of a relatively small amount of calcium causes the release of a large amount of calcium from the junctional sarcoplasmic reticulum by triggering the opening of specific sarcoplasmic reticulum calcium release channels. This process is termed calcium-induced calcium release. The central role of transverse-tubules (T-tubules) in providing the proper spatial orientation for close coupling of L-type calcium channel calcium influx to sarcoplasmic reticulum calcium release is depicted. The rise in cytosolic calcium results in calcium binding to troponin C, activation of the myofilaments and contraction. The predominant mechanism for lowering calcium to promote relaxation (Figure 2-4B) is the ATP-dependent reuptake of calcium into the longitudinal sarcoplasmic reticulum via the actions of sarcoplasmic reticulum calcium pumps, which are in turn regulated by the phosphorylation state of phospholamban. During steady state, the same amount of calcium that enters the cell is extruded, mainly by the sodium-calcium exchanger. The β-adrenergic receptor/G protein/adenylyl cyclase complex is illustrated to signify the central role of this system in regulating cardiac contraction and relaxation.

reticulum, and mitochondria. Nuclei are round and centrally located. Relative to cell volume, nuclear volume decreases steadily after birth, coincident with progressive cellular hypertrophy. The clusters of ribosomes, rough endoplasmic reticulum, and extensive Golgi apparatus are all consistent with active protein synthesis during rapid cell growth.

Although the general patterns are similar, the precise timing and temporal relationships of the ultrastructural changes vary from species to species. Table 2-1 summarizes

■ TABLE 2-1. Species Differences in Maturation of Ventricular Myocytes

Species	Appearance of T-tubules	Maturation of SR
Rat	21 d of age	1-11 d of age
Rabbit	8-10 d of age	–5-14 d of age
Hamster	16 d of age	1-30 d of age
Guinea pig	Complete at birth	Complete at birth
Dog	60 d of age	Postnatally
Human	32 wk gestation	First appearance at 30 wk gestation; functional maturation unknown

comparisons among various species for the timing of appearance and maturation of important elements involved in cardiac contraction and relaxation. The information presented in Table 2-1 is somewhat generalized because maturation is not uniform throughout the same heart within a given species. Furthermore, considerable variation in the morphologic appearance of myocytes can be found within the same heart.

An important change during postnatal development is a progressive decrease in surface area-to-volume ratio. This is due largely to a progressive increase in myocyte volume during postnatal development. Myocyte division (hyperplasia) is commonly observed during fetal growth and in the early newborn period. However, shortly after birth, continued growth of the heart is attributable largely to hypertrophy of existing myocytes, with relatively slow turnover and cell division. The mechanisms involved in this postnatal switch from hyperplastic to hypertrophic growth are incompletely defined at present. A number of laboratories are working to unravel the basis for this fundamental change in myocyte biology, since the implications for cardiac repair and regeneration are profound.

Sarcolemma and Transverse Tubules

The cell membrane in muscle cells is referred to as the sarcolemma or sarcolemmal membrane. In cardiac myocytes, the sarcolemmal membrane is well defined throughout fetal and postnatal development and the glycocalyx can be visualized quite early in cardiac development. Transverse tubules (T-tubules) are invaginations of the sarcolemma into the cell that allow the extracellular environment to extend into the inner cellular structures. In species with small ventricular myocytes (eg, birds and fish), the T-tubular system is generally not present, presumably because it is not required for efficient excitation-contraction coupling. However, in larger cells, a T-tubular system is necessary to allow transsarcolemmal fluxes to occur deep within the cell interior. The presence of T-tubules compensates for the increased cell volume by providing a mechanism for overcoming diffusional restrictions. The T-tubular system is therefore an integral component of contraction and relaxation processes in mammalian myocytes. This is the site of highest density of calcium channels (for the influx of calcium) and the area in which the sarcolemma is in close physical relationship with the sarcoplasmic reticulum (the source of activator calcium for myocellular contraction) (Figure 2-1).

In mammalian hearts, T-tubules are one of the last organelles to develop and generally do not appear until after birth. The time course of appearance of T-tubules varies among species (Table 2-1). The relatively constant ratio of cell area to volume during postnatal maturation, in the face of a rapidly lengthening cell, is a result of the concomitant development of T-tubules and an increase in cell surface area.

Sarcoplasmic Reticulum

Coincident with the progressive development and maturation of the T-tubule system is a change in the appearance and function of the sarcoplasmic reticulum. The sarcoplasmic reticulum is a specialized form of endoplasmic reticulum that is an essential component of contraction and relaxation in the mammalian heart. In mature cardiac myocytes, the sarcoplasmic reticulum stores, releases, and reaccumulates the majority of the calcium that is involved in contraction and relaxation.

The sarcoplasmic reticulum is composed of junctional and longitudinal elements (the longitudinal sarcoplasmic reticulum is also referred to as the free sarcoplasmic reticulum). Important maturational changes in the amount, appearance, and function of the sarcoplasmic reticulum are apparent during late fetal and early postnatal maturation. In the adult, sarcoplasmic reticulum membranes are well organized and prominently related to the thick filaments of myofibrils. The junctional sarcoplasmic reticulum is immediately adjacent to the T-tubules in structures termed dyads. It is this close physical relationship that is the central element in transduction of the changes in sarcolemmal membrane potential and calcium influx to the sarcoplasmic reticulum to trigger calcium release and contraction. This close spatial relationship between the junctional sarcoplasmic reticulum and the sarcolemma is observed in all mammalian species.

In mature myocytes, the junctional sarcoplasmic reticulum contains the sarcoplasmic reticulum calcium release channels. These channels (also known as ryanodine receptors because of their high-affinity binding to this neutral plant alkaloid) open during excitation-contraction coupling to allow discharge of stored calcium into the cytosol for contraction to occur. In addition, the junctional sarcoplasmic reticulum contains high concentrations of calsequestrin, a calcium-binding protein. This is the site of storage of most of the calcium that cycles through the sarcoplasmic reticulum to and from the contractile proteins with each sequence of contraction and relaxation. Triadin and junctin are smaller proteins contained in the junctional sarcoplasmic reticulum that appear to be important in maintaining the proper spatial relations between calsequestrin and the calcium release channel. Other structural proteins include FK-binding protein (also known as calstabin) that helps to stabilize the calcium release channels and promote coordinated calcium release.

Longitudinal sarcoplasmic reticulum contains the greatest density of the ATP-dependent calcium pumps involved in calcium reuptake into the sarcoplasmic reticulum. These proteins are termed SarcoEndoplasmic Reticulum Calcium ATPases, abbreviated as SERCA. The cardiac-specific isoform is SERCA2a. The reuptake of calcium into the sarcoplasmic reticulum by SERCA2a is modulated by a regulatory protein, phospholamban, which is in close physical relationship with SERCA2a. In the basal unphosphorylated state, phospholamban acts as a "brake" to inhibit SERCA2a activity and calcium reuptake into the sarcoplasmic reticulum. When phospholamban is phosphorylated (eg, in response to β-adrenergic stimulation), the inhibition is removed, SERCA2a activity increases, and relaxation is facilitated due to enhanced sarcoplasmic reticulum calcium reuptake.

In the late fetus and early newborn, peripheral subsarcolemmal couplings between the junctional sarcoplasmic reticulum and sarcolemma can be observed prior to the acquisition of a well-organized T-tubular system. However, as the cells enlarge and the T-tubular system develops, deeper internal couplings (dyads) are acquired. The volume and distribution of the sarcoplasmic reticulum increase during late fetal and early postnatal maturation. The timing of appearance of the sarcoplasmic reticulum

during development in several species is presented in Table 2-1. Each of the components of the mature sarcoplasmic reticulum undergoes developmental regulation and maturation (ryanodine receptors, SERCA2a, phospholamban, etc).

Contractile Elements

Sarcomeres

The sarcomere is the primary contractile unit of striated muscle. Contraction and relaxation of cardiac muscle depends upon the structural organization of contractile and modulatory proteins into filaments that repeatedly move back and forth past one another. Anchoring of the structural filaments combined with sliding of complementary filaments results in shortening and generation of force. In mature cardiac cells, the myofibrils are organized into sarcomeres, which are delineated at each end by Z-discs. The Z-disc is a complex group of proteins that links the myofilaments from opposing sarcomeres into a highly ordered network (Figure 2-2) (see following discussion).

The Z-discs contain projections toward the center of the sarcomere that are termed thin filaments and contain an abundance of actin. Thick filaments are polymers of myosin and titin, a very large structural protein. The thick filaments are arranged along the same long axis of the sarcomere and are interspersed among the thin filaments (Figure 2-2). I-bands are composed of thin filaments, troponin complexes, and tropomyosin. A bands are composed of overlapping thin and thick filaments. The dark M band in the center of the A band consists of thick filaments cross-linked to titin. Mutations in a variety of sarcomeric and Z-disc proteins are associated with both hypertrophic and dilated forms of familial cardiomyopathy (Chapter 9).

In early fetal life, sarcomeres can be observed in cardiac myocytes. However, the contractile apparatus remains relatively disorganized in the fetal and early newborn heart. Myofibrils initially are irregular and scattered about the interior of the cell and are arranged in the subsarcolemmal region around a large central mass of nuclei and mitochondria in immature cells. As maturation progresses, the myofibrils come to lie along the long axis of the cell. Progressive organization of the sarcomeres occurs even as contraction and relaxation are occurring.

A progressive increase in myofilament content and maturation of the sarcomeres is consistent across mammalian species, although the timing may vary. A developmental increase in the myofibrillar population with a more orderly arrangement of myofilaments during maturation

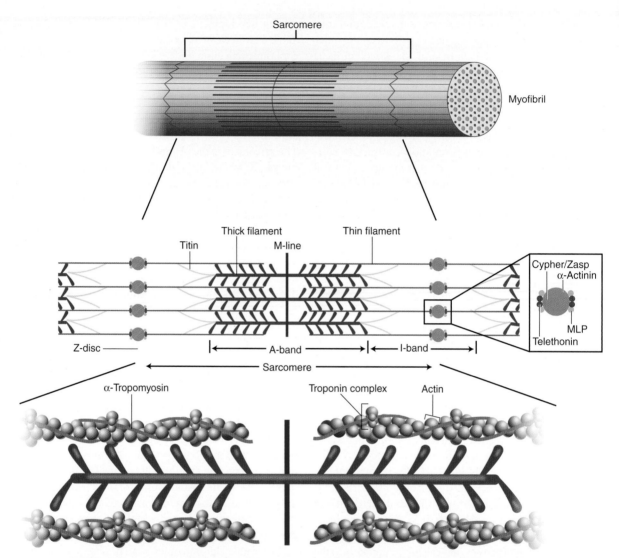

FIGURE 2-2. Schematic diagram showing arrangement of thick and thin filaments within the sarcomere. Thick filaments contain myosin, myosin-binding protein C, and titin. The tails of the myosin heavy chains are woven together to form the thick filament. The globular head projects outward to form crossbridges. The thin filaments include actin (which forms the backbone of the thin filament), the troponins, and tropomyosin. Tropomyosin binds to troponin T at multiple sites along the major groove of the actin filament and inhibits actin-myosin interaction. Troponin T binds the troponin complex to tropomyosin, troponin I inhibits interactions between actin and myosin, and troponin C binds calcium. The sarcomere, which lies between two Z-discs, is anchored by interactions between titin and actin with Z-disc proteins including LIM domain-binding protein 3 (cipher/ZASP), α-actinin, cardiac LIM domain protein (MLP) and telethonin. *Adapted from Mahony L. Development of myocardial structure and function. In: Allen HD, Driscoll DJ, Shaddy RE, Feltes TF, eds. Moss and Adams' Heart Disease in Infants, Children and Adolescents. 7th ed. Philadelphia, PA. Lippincott Williams & Wilkins; 2008:577.*

is often cited as the primary factor responsible for the increase in force generation observed during the late fetal and early newborn period in the mammalian heart. However, developmental changes in sarcomeric protein isoform expression also play an important role in maturational changes in force generation (see following discussion).

Myofilament Proteins

Myofilaments are composed predominantly of myosin and actin (approximately 80% of the total contractile protein content). Other less abundant components such as troponin and tropomyosin provide regulatory control and structural support (Figure 2-2).

Giant filament. An essential component of the structural foundation of the sarcomere is titin, the largest protein known in humans. Titin spans half of the sarcomere from the Z-disc at the end to the M-line at the center. The N-terminal ends of titin overlap within the Z-disc and the C-terminal ends overlap at the M-line to create a continuous filament system (so-called "giant" filament) that aligns the thick filaments within the myofibril.

Titin does more than simply connect the myofibrils. The segment of titin at the I-band contains serial spring elements that determine passive tension of the myocardium, thereby impacting late diastolic filling and resting sarcomere length. In addition, this extensible region provides elastic recoil that drives early diastolic filling.

Thick filaments. The predominant protein in thick filaments is myosin. Individual thick filaments contain several different polypeptides comprising a globular head and a tail section (Figure 2-2). Each of the approximately 300 myosin molecules per sarcomere is composed of two heavy chain myosin monomers and a stalk of four light chain monomers. The heavy chains form a large, bilobed globular head and contain its ATPase activity, essential to release the energy necessary for crossbridge formation. The light chains (essential and regulatory) form the long stalk of the thick filament, joined to the head by a flexible joint. It is the globular head that forms the crossbridge with the actin molecule, the ultimate step in sarcomere shortening.

An important protein associated with the thick filaments is myosin-binding protein C. This protein helps to stabilize thick filaments by forming transverse fibers that connect adjacent filaments near the center of the sarcomere. Other important structural proteins at the M-line include myomesin, M-protein, and obscurin, all of which appear to act with myosin-binding protein C to facilitate force transmission along the thick filaments.

Thin filaments. Each thin filament contains three major proteins: actin, tropomyosin, and troponin (Figure 2-2). It is the repetitive association and dissociation of actin with myosin that results in contraction and relaxation. Troponin is composed of three major subunits. The inhibitory subunit is termed troponin I (TnI), the calcium-binding subunit is troponin C (TnC) and the tropomyosin binding subunit is termed troponin T (TnT). These proteins are required in the final stages of activation of actin binding with myosin to form the actomyosin complex which initiates contraction.

Calcium plays an integral role in relaxation and contraction by binding to one of the troponin subunits, troponin C (TnC). Although there are several calcium-binding sites on TnC, attachment to the low-affinity site II is thought to be the trigger for crossbridge formation. Binding of calcium to this site removes the inhibition that the tropomyosin-troponin complex confers on the actin-myosin interaction and triggers force generation and contraction. The number of crossbridges formed contributes to the amount of force developed by the contracting myocyte and depends on the amount of calcium released by the sarcoplasmic reticulum and intrinsic properties of the contractile proteins such as calcium sensitivity. At a given calcium concentration, an increase in calcium sensitivity results in greater force, and a decrease in calcium sensitivity reduces force. Relaxation occurs as calcium dissociates from TnC and the proteins return to their resting conformational states.

Regulation of contraction and relaxation is very complex and cannot be explained simply by delivery of calcium to and removal from the contractile proteins. It is clear that an increase in cytosolic calcium is a necessary *trigger* for the onset of contraction, but the conformational changes in thin filament proteins are too rapid to limit force production. Furthermore, there is compelling evidence that cytosolic calcium peaks well before maximum force production is achieved and that calcium is nearly completely removed from the contractile elements before the onset of relaxation. These observations suggest that cooperative signaling and mechanical feedback through thick and thin filaments are critical determinants of contraction, force generation, and relaxation. In addition, there is a growing body of literature implicating post-translational modification of sarcomeric proteins (phosphorylation, nitrosylation, peroxidation) via various signaling pathways as important regulators of calcium sensitivity and crossbridge cycling rates. The relationships among the various myofilament proteins, cytoskeletal proteins, extracellular matrix, and signal transduction pathways are complex and not fully understood. However, it is clear that mutations or abnormalities in the function of many of these proteins can have profound effects on cardiac contractile function. Mutations in myofilament proteins are clearly associated with cardiomyopathy, which are more fully described in Chapter 9. As our understanding of intrinsic sarcomere function and regulation continues to expand, it is likely that new therapeutic approaches targeted at improving contractile function will be developed, but the implications for newborns with heart disease are not defined.

Isoform switching. Developmental changes in thick and thin protein isoforms impact on the ability of the sarcomere to contract and relax. Important age-related changes in regulatory processes include changes in myofibrillar ATPase activity (determined by differential expression of myosin isoforms), troponin regulatory proteins, and proteins involved in delivery of calcium to and removal from the contractile complex. In addition to developmental regulation, other factors may affect isoform expression. Hormonal changes, nutritional status, workload, and innervation all play an integrated role in regulating protein isoform expression in the developing heart.

Titin isoforms. Titin is encoded by a single gene, but differential splicing generates isoforms with different degrees of extensibility. Titin isoform expression is developmentally regulated. In general, fetal hearts express more compliant titin isoforms than those expressed in mature hearts, but the time course of these changes varies among different species; the physiologic impact in humans is not known.

Myosin isoforms. The cardiac myosin heavy chain (MHC) exists in two isoforms, α-MHC and β-MHC. Myosin containing two α chains (V1) has the highest ATPase activity. V2 contains an α and a β chain and exhibits intermediate ATPase activity. Myosin containing two β chains (V3) has the lowest ATPase activity. ATPase activity of the heavy chain correlates with velocity of shortening of the myofibril. Myosin heavy chain isoform expression changes during development, but these changes vary among different

species. The V3 isoform is most abundant in the ventricles of rats during fetal life and is replaced by V1 in the adult rat heart. In contrast, in the human ventricle, the V3 isoform predominates during fetal, neonatal, and adult life.

Actin isoforms. The backbone of the thin filaments is formed by polymerization of two strands of actin monomers. Actin is a relatively small globular protein encoded by a multigene family. Two isoforms, skeletal α-actin and cardiac α-actin, are present in striated muscle. These isoforms differ by only four amino acids, two of which are in the myosin binding region. During development, both actin isoforms are expressed in the human ventricle. In fetal and neonatal hearts, skeletal α-actin mRNA constitutes more than 80% of the total actin, but in the mature heart, the cardiac α-actin isoform comprises more than 60% of the total actin. The functional consequence of this isoform shift in the human heart is unknown.

Troponin isoforms. The troponin complex of the thin filament confers calcium sensitivity to the actin-myosin complex. TnC, the calcium-binding subunit, remains constant and does not exhibit isoform switching. In contrast, TnI and TnT both exist as multiple isoforms with variable expression during development.

Three isoforms of TnI have been identified that are the products of three separate genes. These isoforms are classified as the fast skeletal form (TnI-f), slow skeletal form (TnI-s), and the cardiac muscle form (TnI-c). A major difference of the cardiac isoform from the other two forms is that TnI-c (but not TnI-s) has a long internal sequence that becomes phosphorylated in response to adrenergic stimulation. Phosphorylation of TnI-c plays an important role in modulating contractile performance by effects on cooperative activation and mechanical feedback at the level of the sarcomeres.

Developmental changes in TnI isoform expression are proposed to at least partly explain changes in contractile function during perinatal maturation of the heart. In the human fetal heart, the predominant isoform is TnI-s, but TnI-c is detectable. The transition to TnI-c alone with the disappearance of TnI-s occurs by approximately 9 months of age after birth in the human heart. The extended postnatal time course of TnI isoform switching in humans is likely to affect inotropic responsiveness.

TnT plays a role in regulating myofibrillar ATPase activity and the responsiveness to calcium. Troponin T exists as multiple isoforms that appear to be products of a single gene that undergoes developmentally regulated alternative splicing. Expression patterns during development vary among species. Fetal human and rabbit hearts express four cardiac TnT isoforms, TnT_{1-4}. Expression of TnT_1 is highest in the fetal human heart and neonatal rabbit heart. The dominant isoform in adult rabbit myocardium is TnT_4 and in contrast, normal adult human hearts express only TnT_3. Isoform expression is affected by pathophysiological conditions, as well. Cardiac $cTnT_1$ and $cTnT_4$ are upregulated in failing human hearts harvested from transplant patients and in hearts from children with congestive heart failure. The level of expression of $cTnT_4$ is correlated with the severity of heart failure before surgery and with the duration of recovery. Changes in cardiac TnT isoform expression (both during development and in response to pathophysiological states) may contribute to changes in force development and to differences of myocardial sensitivity to acidosis.

Mitochondria

In immature myocardium, mitochondria are irregularly scattered about the cell. As the cells mature, mitochondrial size becomes more regular and mitochondria become centrally located and surrounded by myofilaments. During progressive myofibrillar organization, the mitochondria become distributed in a highly regular fashion along the myofilaments in order to meet the high energy requirements of active muscle.

In all mammalian species, a large increase in mitochondrial volume occurs during the postnatal period. In addition, the ultrastructural appearance of myocardial mitochondria changes during maturation. In the fetal heart, cristae are sparse and widely spaced. With progressive maturation of the heart during the postnatal period, the cristae become more densely packed.

These changes in mitochondrial appearance, position, and number reflect the increasing energy requirements following birth and parallel age-related changes in substrate utilization by the heart. Long-chain free fatty acids are the primary energy substrate in adult hearts. Activated free fatty acids are transported into the mitochondria and then are metabolized by β-oxidation, producing ATP. The enzyme carnitine palmitoyl coenzyme A transferase transports activated free fatty acids from the cytosol into the mitochondria. In immature hearts, the activity of this enzyme is decreased. As a result of these and other factors, the primary energy substrates in the immature heart are lactate and carbohydrates. It should be noted that these data are derived from animal studies and comparable information from fetal and neonatal human hearts is lacking. Abnormalities in mitochondrial substrate metabolism can result in cardiomyopathy (Chapter 9).

Cytoskeleton and Extracellular Matrix

It is increasingly evident that the cytoskeleton does much more than merely support the various components of the cardiac myocyte. The cytoskeleton provides the structural framework so that tension can be transmitted through the myocyte, but in addition, the cytoskeleton fosters the spatial arrangement of subcellular protein complexes that is required for proper intracellular signaling. Cytoskeletal structural proteins allow for communication between internal and external environments of the cell and are integrally involved in signal transduction and cell-to-cell signaling. The cytoskeleton determines cell size and organization and allows tension developed by the contractile proteins to be transmitted throughout the myocyte, to adjacent cells, and to the extracellular matrix. Mutations in several cytoskeletal proteins cause various form of cardiomyopathy (Chapter 9).

The ultrastructural appearance of immature myocytes suggests that the cytoskeletal structure is much less well organized compared with adult myocytes. Adult cells are compartmentalized by intermediate filaments that connect Z-discs to one another. The linking of adjacent sarcomeres organizes the cell and compartmentalizes sarcomeres with longitudinal sarcoplasmic reticulum, mitochondria, and microtubules. In contrast, immature myocytes contain central aggregations of nuclei and mitochondria. This results in an internal load against which the immature myofibrils contract. Consequently, the resting sarcomere length is shorter and sarcomere shortening is slower in immature cells. Thus, the relative disorganization of the cellular structures due to cytoskeletal immaturity may have an important impact upon the rate and amount of tension that an immature myocyte can generate.

The cytoskeleton is a much more dynamic structure than what was originally thought. Cytoskeletal proteins organize the co-localization of ion channels, signaling molecules, and messengers required for transduction of extracellular signals and mechanical stress. The cytoskeleton remodels during cell growth and in response to pathophysiologic signals such as systolic stress or diastolic stretch. Normal development and maturation of the heart and vasculature are critically dependent on proteins within the cytoskeleton and extracellular matrix. Developmental changes in the organization and location of intracellular organelles reflect changes in the composition and organization of the cytoskeleton.

Z-Discs

At each end of the sarcomere is the Z-disc that links the myofilaments from opposing sarcomeres into a tightly arranged compact lattice (Figure 2-2). A variety of proteins are localized to Z-discs, including α-actinin, telethonin (T-cap), nebulette, muscle LIM protein, filamin, and myotilin. Z-discs are crucial elements in the transmission of tension generated by individual sarcomeres along the length of the myofibril. In addition, Z-disc proteins serve as docking sites for transcription factors, calcium signaling proteins, and for a variety of kinases and phosphatases involved in regulation

of contractile function. Increasing evidence implicates the Z-disc and its associated components as sensing and transducing cellular mechanical signals into signals for cell growth, development, and remodeling (both electrical and mechanical).

Extramyofibrillar Cytoskeleton

The extramyofibrillar cytoskeleton is organized into three complimentary components, each playing related roles (Figure 2-3). Microfilaments, intermediate filaments, and microtubules make up the three major extramyofibrillar

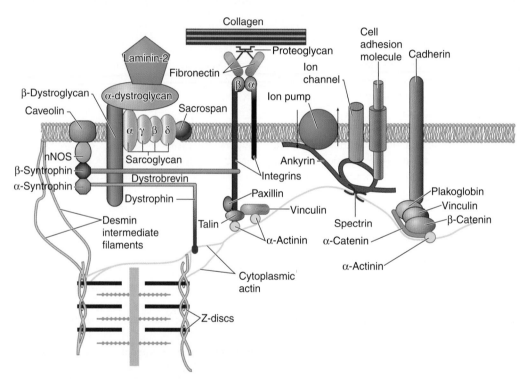

FIGURE 2-3. Cytoskeletal architecture of the cardiac myocyte. The dystrophin-sarcoglycan complex links the plasma membrane to cytoplasmic actin filaments. Integrins bind the cell to the extracellular matrix and are composed of α and β subunits that attach through various proteins (fibronectin, laminin, proteoglycans) to collagen. The intracellular part of the β subunit binds to cytoplasmic actin filaments through another protein complex that includes α-actinin, talin, vinculin, and paxillin. Ankyrin links membrane proteins such as ion pumps and channels together, thereby organizing interactions among proteins with related functions. Spectrin links ankyrin to the cytoplasmic actin filaments and is also associated with both costameres and intercalated discs at the sarcolemmal membrane. Cadherins mediate connection of cell-to-cell contacts in both desmosomes and fascia adherens. In the fascia adherens, cadherins link the cytoplasmic actin filaments of adjacent cells through vinculin, catenins, plakoglobin, and α-actinin. In addition to contributing to the structural integrity of the cell, many of these proteins are critically involved in cell signaling. *Adapted with permission from Mahony L. Development of myocardial structure and function. In: Allen HD, Driscoll DJ, Shaddy RE, Feltes TF, eds. Moss and Adams' Heart Disease in Infants, Children and Adolescents. 7th ed. Philadelphia, PA: Lippincott Williams & Wilkins; 2008:580.*

cytoskeletal components. Microfilaments are composed predominantly of actin and are found in the thin filaments of the sarcomere (sarcomeric actin) and in the cytosol (non-sarcomeric or cytoplasmic actin). Cytosolic microfilaments are localized mainly in the subsarcolemmal space and play an important role in linking the intracellular cytoskeleton with the extracellular matrix and adjacent myocytes.

Intermediate fibers form an intracellular network that helps to maintain the structural integrity of myocytes. These fibers are formed from polymers of desmin and link Z-discs together and to costameres, the sarcoplasmic reticulum, sarcolemmal and nuclear membranes. Stress-induced alterations of this network of intermediate fibers may mediate changes in gene expression.

Microtubules are formed from polymerized subunits of α and β tubulin that undergo continuous depolymerization and repolymerization. Stiffness of the cytoskeleton is moderated by the total amount of tubulin and the relative proportions in the polymerized state. Microtubules surround the nucleus and spread longitudinally throughout the cell. They serve to stabilize cell structure by anchoring subcellular organelles and are involved in the transmission of signals within and between cells.

Connections to Adjacent Cells and the Extracellular Matrix

The extracellular matrix surrounds myocardial cells and serves both structural and regulatory functions. The extracellular matrix is complex and exhibits a variety of components, including: (1) connective tissue, mainly elastin and various types of collagen; (2) a gel-like substance consisting of proteoglycans; (3) basement membrane proteins such as collagen, laminin, and fibronectin; and (4) other molecules such as cytokines, growth factors, and proteases. The extracellular matrix modulates cell migration, proliferation, adhesion, and cell-to-cell signaling, thereby playing a critical role in normal growth and development, as well as in pathological remodeling of the ventricles.

Intercalated discs connect myocytes at each end to adjacent myocytes and serve as important sites of force transmission between myocytes. Intercalated discs are complex structures that contain fascia adherens (analogous to adherens junctions in non-muscle cells), desmosomes, and gap junctions. A variety of proteins are involved in connecting cells both structurally and functionally by weaving together the various cytoskeletal elements.

The many protein complexes that link the myofibrils and membrane systems of the myocyte to the extracellular matrix are essential for stabilizing cell structure during the stresses of contraction and relaxation. Additionally, these protein complexes are involved in organizing and coordinating membrane signaling processes with the contractile systems. The various cytoskeletal networks within the myocyte and the extracellular matrix are linked through highly complex protein networks called costameres. These structures, which contain proteins including vinculin, talin, tensin, paxillin, and zyxin, encircle the lateral aspects of the myocyte perpendicular to its long axis forming a transmembrane physical attachment between the peripheral Z-discs and the extracellular matrix. Costameres thus anchor the myofibrils to the sarcolemma and transmit lateral contractile force from the sarcomere to the extracellular matrix and ultimately to neighboring myocytes. It appears that costameres play a role in converting mechanical stimuli to alterations in cell signaling and gene expression which can result in cell growth or hypertrophy.

Integrins are another essential component of the protein network responsible for transmission of force between myocytes and the extracellular matrix. Integrin molecules are heterodimers of various α and β subunits and found within the sarcolemmal membrane adjacent to costameres. The intracellular domain of integrin β subunits binds to actin microfilaments through costamere proteins and the extracellular portion of integrin interacts with various extracellular matrix proteins. Integrins are involved in signaling pathways mediated by several G proteins and protein kinases that modify interactions between the integrins and the extracellular matrix. These pathways are involved in both cell growth and apoptosis and play an essential role in pathophysiological conditions and in normal embryonic and fetal cardiovascular development.

The dystrophin glycoprotein complex also plays an important role in linking the intracellular cytoskeleton with the extracellular matrix. This complex binds actin microfilaments to the extracellular matrix thereby transmitting force to the extracellular matrix and providing another mechanism for signal transduction. Mutations in dystrophin cause muscular dystrophy and mutations in of the components of the dystrophin glycoprotein complex are present in patients with dilated cardiomyopathy.

Spectrin is another cytoskeletal protein that binds to actin and helps to coordinate membrane signaling systems with the contractile filaments. Spectrin is found in costameres, intercalated discs, and is a component of protein complexes related to the sarcoplasmic reticulum at the Z-discs. Ankyrins are adaptor proteins that bind to spectrin and also to a structurally diverse group of membrane proteins such as ion channels and pumps, calcium release channels, and cell adhesion molecules. In this manner, various proteins are physically linked together to foster interactions among proteins with related functions. Mutations in ankyrins are known to cause cardiac arrhythmias in humans and in murine models.

■ EXCITATION-CONTRACTION COUPLING

Central Role of the Sarcoplasmic Reticulum

Figure 2-4A illustrates the general features of excitation-contraction coupling and calcium transport during contraction in mature mammalian ventricular myocytes.

Depolarization of the sarcolemmal membrane promotes opening of voltage-dependent L-type calcium channels. This results in the influx of a relatively small amount of calcium, which alone is not sufficient to directly activate the contractile proteins. It is clear that contraction results from a much greater increase in intracellular calcium that results from release of a large amount of calcium from sarcoplasmic reticulum stores. The opening of specific sarcoplasmic reticulum calcium release channels (ryanodine receptors) is triggered by the influx of calcium across the sarcolemma through the L-type calcium channels. This process is known as calcium-induced calcium release.

The structural basis for calcium-induced calcium release is the co-localization of sarcolemmal L-type calcium

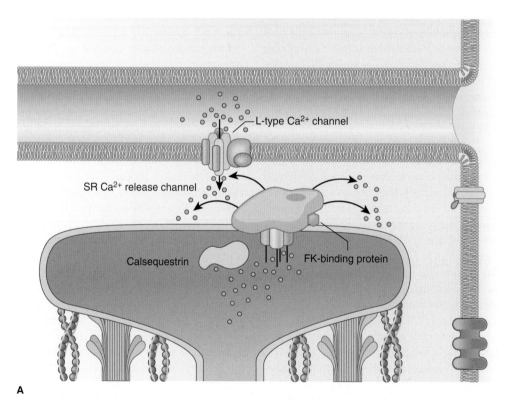

A

FIGURE 2-4. A. Schematic diagram of excitation-contraction coupling in mature mammalian ventricular myocytes. The close relationship between L-type calcium channels and sarcoplasmic reticulum calcium release channels is illustrated. Calcium (blue circles) entering the cell through L-type calcium channels (concentrated in the transverse tubules) triggers the opening of specific calcium release channels in the junctional sarcoplasmic reticulum. When this occurs, a large amount of calcium is released into the cytosol, resulting in contraction of the myofilaments. Sarcoplasmic reticulum calcium release channels are also known as ryanodine receptors. The major calcium-binding protein in the sarcoplasmic reticulum is calsequestrin. FK-binding proteins maintain stability of the sarcoplasmic reticulum calcium release channels and promote coordinated interaction among neighboring channels. See text for additional details.

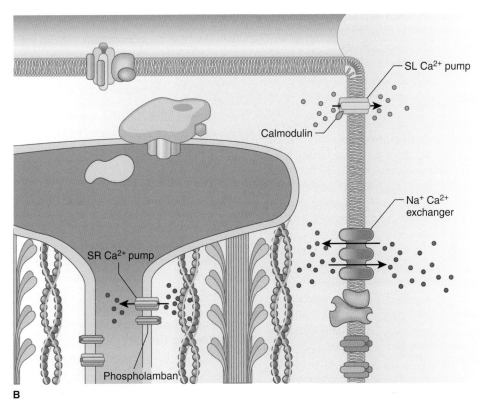

FIGURE 2-4. B. Schematic diagram of calcium transport pathways during relaxation in mature ventricular myocytes. In order for relaxation to occur, calcium must diffuse away from the myofilaments. This is achieved by removing calcium from the cytosol. Calcium reuptake into the longitudinal sarcoplasmic reticulum is the major pathway involved in relaxation in adult myocytes. The activity of the sarcoplasmic reticulum calcium pump is regulated by the phosphorylation state of phospholamban. In the dephosphorylated state, phospholamban acts to inhibit sarcoplasmic reticulum calcium pump activity. When phospholamban is phosphorylated by cAMP-dependent protein kinase or calcium-calmodulin kinase II, the inhibition is removed and sarcoplasmic reticulum calcium pump activity increases. During steady state, the small amount of calcium that enters the cell during depolarization is transported back out. This is achieved largely through the action of the sodium-calcium exchanger and to a lesser extent, the sarcolemmal calcium pump. See text for additional details.

channels (predominantly in the T-tubules) and junctional sarcoplasmic reticulum ryanodine receptors in the dyadic junction (Figure 2-4A). The close physical relationship of L-type calcium channels and ryanodine receptors (~10 nm) in this region allows a single or a small cluster of ryanodine receptors to open in response to a local, spatially restricted, microdomain of elevated calcium that results from the nearby influx of calcium through an L-type calcium channel. Localized, nonpropagating sarcoplasmic reticulum calcium release events (either evoked or spontaneously occurring) have been commonly termed "calcium sparks." It is the summation of these local release events that results in a global rise in intracellular calcium and activation of contraction. Modulation of the force of contraction is achieved primarily by regulation of the magnitude of the L-type calcium current. Evidence suggests that calcium-induced inactivation of ryanodine receptors is the primary mechanism for the beat-to-beat termination of calcium-induced calcium release. Contraction is terminated and relaxation occurs because of (1) a decrease in sarcoplasmic reticulum calcium release channel openings in conjunction with (2) the reuptake of cytosolic calcium back into the sarcoplasmic reticulum through calcium pumps (and to a much lesser extent, calcium extrusion from the cell via sodium-calcium exchange and sarcolemmal calcium pumps).

■ RELAXATION

In addition to providing the source of calcium for contraction, the sarcoplasmic reticulum plays a primary role in relaxation in the adult heart. After the rise in intracellular calcium that occurs after calcium release from the junctional sarcoplasmic reticulum, specific calcium pumps in the longitudinal sarcoplasmic reticulum sequester calcium back into the sarcoplasmic reticulum (Figure 2-4B). As cytosolic calcium declines, calcium dissociates from the contractile protein complex and relaxation occurs. Sarcoplasmic reticulum calcium pump activity is in turn regulated by the phosphorylation state of phospholamban, which provides another key mechanism for modulating contractile function.

During steady-state conditions, the amount of calcium that enters the myocyte from the extracellular space must be extruded during relaxation. This is achieved predominantly through the action of the sarcolemmal sodium-calcium exchanger. In addition to its role in relaxation, the exchanger can operate bidirectionally and transport calcium into the cell during depolarization. However, in mature myocytes, the major function of the exchanger is to extrude calcium during relaxation. In addition to the sodium-calcium exchanger, sarcolemmal calcium pumps (plasma membrane calcium-ATPase; PMCA) move calcium out of the cell, but their contribution to relaxation is relatively minor compared to the activities of SERCA2a and the exchanger.

■ CONTRACTION AND RELAXATION IN THE IMMATURE HEART

As described in the preceding discussion, the main components of the mature excitation-contraction coupling phenotype of calcium-induced calcium release include sarcolemmal L-type calcium channels (predominantly in the T-tubules) in close physical relation to junctional sarcoplasmic reticulum ryanodine receptors in the dyadic junction. These structural components are known to undergo developmental changes, which consequently impact significantly on the mechanisms of excitation-contraction coupling in the immature heart. Figure 2-5 summarizes the general developmental differences in calcium transport pathways in neonatal and adult ventricular myocytes.

Role of Developing Transverse Tubule System

In most species (such as rat, rabbit, dog, and hamster), T-tubules do not appear until approximately 2 weeks to 2 months after birth. In fully mature myocytes, calcium sparks occur along the T-tubules. Thus, the relative paucity of T-tubules may limit the close physical relation between sarcolemmal calcium channels and sarcoplasmic reticulum calcium release channels, resulting in functional isolation of the sarcoplasmic reticulum from participation in excitation-contraction coupling under physiological conditions. The developmental morphogenesis of T-tubules and the temporal relationship between the postnatal acquisition of T-tubules and the appearance of an adult excitation-contraction coupling phenotype remain to be determined in the human heart.

Diminished Role of the Sarcoplasmic Reticulum

Most of the calcium that cycles to and from the contractile proteins during contraction and relaxation is derived from sarcoplasmic reticulum release and reuptake in mature rabbit ventricular myocytes. In contrast, a large body of literature indicates that immature myocytes depend much less on sarcoplasmic reticulum calcium release. The profound differences between contraction and relaxation processes in the developing and mature heart are likely to be explained by fundamental developmental differences in the key cellular components involved in producing the mature excitation-contraction coupling phenotype, including the sarcoplasmic reticulum and T-tubules. The concept that the sarcoplasmic reticulum plays a lesser role in excitation-contraction coupling in the developing heart is supported by results from experiments employing ultrastructural, pharmacological, biochemical, electrophysiological, or molecular biological approaches.

Development of Sarcoplasmic Reticulum Calcium Release Channels

The sarcoplasmic reticulum calcium release channel (also known as the ryanodine receptor) is a homotetramer. To date, three different isoforms of the ryanodine receptor (RyR1, RyR2, RyR3) have been identified. RyR2, the so-called cardiac ryanodine receptor, is detected in the developing heart tube as early as embryonic day 8.5, whereas RyR3 increases around the time of

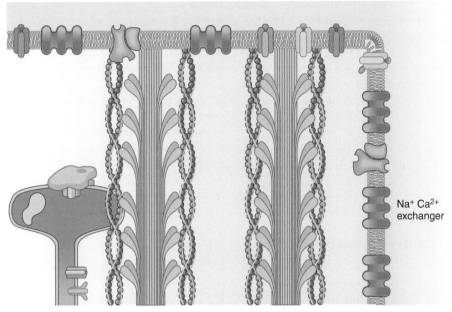

FIGURE 2-5. Schematic diagram of the major components involved in calcium regulation in fetal and neonatal ventricular myocytes. In contrast to adults (Figure 2-1), immature myocytes lack transverse tubules, are smaller in size, and have a greater surface area-to-volume ratio. Sarcoplasmic reticulum structures are underdeveloped and, as depicted, L-type calcium channels and sarcoplasmic reticulum calcium release channels are physically separated. Consequently, calcium-induced calcium release is diminished and immature myocytes are therefore much more reliant on transsarcolemmal calcium fluxes for contraction and relaxation. The sodium-calcium exchanger is the major transport pathway for providing calcium to and removal from the contractile proteins in fetal and neonatal myocytes. The subsarcolemmal location of the myofilaments facilitates these processes. See text for additional details.

birth. Both RyR2 density and mRNA level increase during the development, but RyR3 is only abundant in adult Purkinje cells.

In murine embryonic stem cell–derived cardiac precursor cells, ryanodine-sensitive calcium release is detected later (embryonic day 10) than when L-type calcium current proteins are expressed (embryonic day 7). Interestingly, the appearance of functional ryanodine receptors coincides with the initiation of contraction. Rapid application of caffeine opens ryanodine receptors and caffeine can induce calcium release in hearts isolated from mouse embryos as early as day 8.5. However, ryanodine or other sarcoplasmic reticulum calcium release inhibitors produce a greater negative inotropic effect in adult than in immature hearts. Whereas sarcoplasmic reticulum inhibition can largely abolish calcium transients or contraction in mature hearts, it only inhibits calcium transient or contraction in the immature heart by approximately 50% in rat, 30% in chicken and has almost no effect in rabbits. It

is also noteworthy that in RyR2 knockout mice, the heart still starts to spontaneously contract at embryonic day 9.5. However, severe morphological change in sarcoplasmic reticulum and mitochondria were detected at embryonic day 10 when the mice died. These results suggest that even though ryanodine receptor function may not play an important role in excitation-contraction coupling during early development, it might be crucial for calcium homeostasis during cardiogenesis.

Calcium Reuptake in the Immature Heart

The functional contribution of the sarcoplasmic reticulum to relaxation in the immature heart has received less attention compared to studies of the contribution of the sarcoplasmic reticulum to calcium for contraction. However, results from animal studies to date support the concept that in addition to a diminished role in providing calcium for contraction, the sarcoplasmic reticulum contributes relatively less to calcium reuptake during relaxation in immature ventricular myocytes. This conclusion is based primarily on studies involving pharmacological manipulation of sarcoplasmic reticulum reuptake that show relatively less impact on relaxation in the immature heart compared to adults. Results from experiments to assess relaxation when the sarcoplasmic reticulum is disabled indicate that the sodium-calcium exchanger is sufficient to promote normal relaxation in cardiac myocytes from newborn rabbit hearts. In addition, it appears that the other "slow" pathways (mitochondria and PMCA) are relatively more active in neonatal cells compared with adult cells. Taken together, these studies provide compelling evidence for a much lesser role of the sarcoplasmic reticulum in relaxation prior to cardiac maturation.

Transsarcolemmal Calcium Fluxes

As described earlier, under normal physiological conditions in adult ventricular myocytes, transsarcolemmal calcium influx does not participate directly in activating the myofilaments, but instead functions to trigger sarcoplasmic reticulum calcium release as the source of activator calcium. In contrast, morphological considerations in immature myocytes support the feasibility of transsarcolemmal calcium influx as a direct source of activator calcium for contractions (Figure 2-5). Despite a lack of T-tubules, fetal and newborn myocytes are relatively small and have a much higher cell surface area-to-volume ratio than adult myocytes. A high surface area-to-volume ratio and the subsarcolemmal position of myofibrils in fetal and newborn myocytes favor direct transsarcolemmal calcium delivery to (and from) the contractile proteins. Indeed, studies demonstrate that in the developing heart, transsarcolemmal entry of calcium may contribute substantially to the pool of activator calcium that produces contraction. The two major routes of calcium entry in the heart are calcium channels and the sodium-calcium exchanger.

Calcium Influx Through Calcium Channels

During normal excitation-contraction coupling in mature mammalian ventricular myocardium, the role of L-type calcium current is to trigger the opening of specific sarcoplasmic reticulum calcium release channels, thereby initiating calcium-induced calcium release (as described earlier). It is the calcium released from sarcoplasmic reticulum stores that serves as the source of activator calcium, and calcium influx via L-type calcium channels does not contribute directly to activation of the myofilaments. In developing myocardium, the comparatively

greater negative inotropic response to calcium channel blockers in a variety of species suggests a strong dependence upon L-type calcium channels for contraction. However, this is difficult to reconcile with electrophysiological studies which describe L-type calcium current density (compared with adults) to be smaller in neonatal rabbits, greater in rats and not different in humans. One possible explanation for the greater sensitivity of immature myocardium to the negative inotropic effects of L-type calcium channel blockers may be the greater depression of contractility from shortening of the action potential.

Ontogeny of Cardiac L-type Calcium Channels

L-type calcium channels are oligomeric complexes consisting of a pore-forming α_1 subunit along with an accessory β subunit and disulfide-linked α_2/δ subunits. At least six different genes for α_1 subunits (α_{1S}, α_{1A-E}), four for β subunits (β_{1-4}), and one for α_2/δ subunit have been identified by molecular cloning. In addition, alternative splicing may also add structural diversity to the multitude of L-type calcium channels. In cardiac myocytes, α_{1C} and β_2 subunits are preferentially expressed. Quantitative immunoblotting reveals that subunit expression is developmentally regulated. However, the functional implications of these observations remain to be determined.

Functional L-type calcium channels are observed in embryonic stem cell–derived cardiac precursor cells before the myocytes start to contract. The amplitude of L-type calcium current increased during myogenesis. Similarly, α_{1C}-subunit mRNA levels and the number of dihydropyridine binding sites increases during the perinatal period. Since there is a dramatic developmental change in cell size and membrane capacitance among different species, the density of the L-type calcium currents (ie, current amplitude normalized by cell capacitance) is either increased, decreased, or not changed with maturation.

In summary, L-type calcium channels are functionally mature during fetal stages. Thus, the physical separation of L-type calcium channels from the junctional sarcoplasmic reticulum might be responsible for the uncoupling of L-type calcium channels with sarcoplasmic reticulum calcium release channels in immature heart. This notion is supported by the observation that after birth, along with the development of T-tubules, up to threefold more abundant L-type calcium channels are located in T-tubules than in the peripheral sarcolemma, consistent with the postnatal maturation of cardiac excitation-contraction coupling.

Calcium Fluxes Through the Sodium-Calcium Exchanger

There is general agreement that the main functional role of the sodium-calcium exchanger in mature cardiac cells is to extrude calcium during relaxation. However, calcium entry via "reverse" sodium-calcium exchange clearly occurs in a variety of model systems.

Three genes (NCX1, NCX2, and NCX3) encode the mammalian sodium-calcium exchanger. NCX1 is primarily present in the heart. In embryonic mice, NCX1 expression is detected before the first heartbeat and initially appears in a heart-restricted pattern. It has been shown that targeted ablation of NCX1 is lethal during the embryonic period, apparently due to failure of the forming heart to begin beating. These studies suggest a primary role of the exchanger in supporting electrical excitability, contraction, and relaxation during cardiogenesis.

Sodium-calcium exchanger activity in sarcolemmal vesicles, sarcolemmal exchanger protein content, and steady-state mRNA levels are highest in late fetal and early newborn rabbits and declines postnatally to adult levels by 2 to 3 weeks of age. Immunohistochemical studies in intact myocytes confirm that exchanger protein expression is high at birth in rabbits and that the exchanger is homogeneously distributed over the cell surface. Increased expression of sodium-calcium exchanger message and protein in developing human hearts occurs in a pattern remarkably similar to that observed in rabbits.

The functional consequences of these developmental changes have been confirmed by convincing evidence demonstrating that sodium-calcium exchange alone is sufficient for generating contractions in newborn rabbit myocytes, but not in adult cells. Furthermore, when the sarcoplasmic reticulum is disabled, the sodium-calcium exchanger alone is sufficient for promoting normal relaxation in newborn myocytes, but not in adult cells. In addition, sodium-calcium exchanger current density is high at birth and declines during the first 3 weeks after birth in rabbit ventricular myocytes. Mathematical modeling studies suggested that calcium fluxes via sodium-calcium exchange during an action potential can account for the intracellular calcium transients and subsarcolemmal calcium gradients observed experimentally in newborn rabbit myocytes. These findings lend support to the concept that the sodium-calcium exchanger is a major route for sarcolemmal calcium entry and efflux in the immature heart.

Interestingly, during the first few weeks after birth, while the sodium-calcium exchanger is down-regulated, SERCA2a expression increases, consistent with a postnatal transition from the sarcolemma to the sarcoplasmic reticulum as the predominant source of activator calcium. The time course of the down-regulation of the sodium-calcium exchanger and upregulation of SERCA2a expression coincides with that of the postnatal acquisition of T-tubules. The relative roles of the various calcium transport pathways to contraction and relaxation in immature human myocytes remain to be elucidated. However, based upon evidence accumulated from various animal models, manipulation of sodium-calcium exchanger activity may represent a logical target for modulating contractility in the immature heart.

Initiation of the Heartbeat

As mammalian embryonic development proceeds, there comes a critical time at which a functional circulation must be established for the embryo to survive. This requires the developing heart to begin to function as a rhythmic pump. Early embryonic cardiac myocytes are small and do not have the cellular components and architecture observed in mature myocytes. Even so, mature ventricular myocytes are not spontaneously active and rely on transmission of electrical signals from the pacemaker cells in the sinoatrial node. Thus, questions arise as to how does the embryonic heart begin to beat and what triggers this phenomenon?

The mechanisms involved in establishing the heartbeat have been clarified in recent years. Two distinct mechanisms were proposed in the past. Originally, it was thought that because the sarcoplasmic reticulum is sparse and underdeveloped in embryonic myocytes, spontaneous depolarization of the sarcolemmal membrane triggers calcium influx through voltage-activated calcium channels. Subsequently, an opposing concept proposed that spontaneous sarcoplasmic reticulum calcium oscillations drive contractions and electrical activity. Leaking of sarcoplasmic reticulum calcium into the cytosol would activate the sodium-calcium exchanger to generate action potentials. Recent experimental evidence suggests that both pathways can be involved separately to generate action potentials and global calcium transients. During spontaneous sarcoplasmic reticulum calcium oscillations, the sodium-calcium exchanger extrudes calcium and triggers an action potential, which then promotes calcium influx and restoration of the sarcoplasmic reticulum calcium store so that the process can be repeated. It appears that inositol 1,4,5-trisphosphate may play an important role in this process. Conversely, if the action potential occurs sponta-neously, it can result in a global whole cell calcium tran-sient, as well. Having both mechanisms available allows embryonic cardiomyocytes to contract without requiring physical connections to other myocytes, enabling cell migration. However, in this manner, embryonic cells can also synchronize their electrical activity and form coordi-nated contractions with other myocytes.

Although we have a better understanding of how the embryonic heart begins to beat, the question of why the embryonic heart begins to beat rhythmically is perhaps less clear. The mammalian embryonic heart begins to beat before tissues need to be perfused with blood (and indeed, before the blood cells have formed). Recently, clues have been provided from studies of zebra fish and mice that indicate that a beating heart is necessary for normal vascu-lar development and for development of the hematopoi-etic system. Shear stress from fluid flowing through the devel-oping vascular bed stimulates the expression of hematopoi-etic stem cells. It appears that nitric oxide is a critical signal for this process. The mechanisms that signal to the embryo that it is time to establish the circulation remain elusive.

Modulation of Calcium Transients in the Immature Heart

In mature ventricular myocytes, graded control of sar-coplasmic reticulum calcium release and contraction amplitude is achieved largely by changes in the magnitude of L-type calcium current, by virtue of its role in triggering sarcoplasmic reticulum calcium release (as briefly reviewed in the preceding discussion). Under physiologi-cally relevant conditions, L-type calcium current is regu-lated by membrane potential and phosphorylation state. The evidence accumulated to date suggests that coupling of L-type calcium current with sarcoplasmic reticulum cal-cium release *does not* control contraction amplitude in immature myocytes. However, since contraction in imma-ture myocytes is not an all-or-none phenomenon, there must be alternative mechanisms for exerting graded con-trol of contraction amplitude in developing cells. If these overall concepts are correct, then graded control of intra-cellular calcium concentration and contraction amplitude are predicted to be achieved in immature myocytes pre-dominantly by factors that modulate sodium-calcium exchanger activity. Sodium-calcium exchanger activity may be influenced by a number of factors, but the extent and duration of membrane depolarization and the transsarcolemmal gradients of sodium and calcium are the

primary determinants of sodium-calcium exchanger activ-ity. β-Adrenergic stimulation by isoproterenol stimulates the sodium-calcium exchanger in guinea pig ventricular myocytes. However, these results are controversial and it is presently not known whether this is a relevant mechanism, nor if it occurs in immature cardiac myocytes. Nevertheless, based upon what is already known, control of contractile function in the immature heart is undoubtedly substan-tially different from the mechanisms operative in the fully mature heart. Additional studies will be necessary to deter-mine the effects of other factors noted earlier that may play a role in regulating sodium-calcium exchanger activity.

Action Potential

During a normal action potential, the magnitude of calcium entry is a complex function of the time and voltage dependence of L-type calcium channels and sodium-cal-cium exchanger activity. Action potential configuration changes during cardiac maturation in every mammalian species examined, although the perinatal pattern of change varies by species. The molecular basis for developmental changes in the action potential may be related to age-related differences in the transient outward current, but since the pattern of postnatal change differs among various species, the underlying mechanisms are likely to be species dependent. Regardless of the etiology of action potential variation, the important implication is that age-appropriate and species-specific action potentials should be considered as the most relevant driving ionic force for experimental studies of excitation-contraction coupling during develop-ment. Furthermore, a greater dependency on the sodium-calcium exchanger as the source of activator calcium (as may exist in immature myocardium) predicts that graded control of calcium influx (and hence, the force of contrac-tion) can be achieved by subtle changes in action potential duration and/or configuration. Although this has been con-firmed in animal studies, the relationship between action potential configuration and contractile function in the immature human heart remains to be determined.

Changes in Intracellular Sodium

It is known that cardiac sarcolemmal sodium pump activ-ity changes during development in a variety of different species. Results from these studies are generally consistent in demonstrating that sodium pump activity is higher in the neonate compared to the adult within the same species (including humans). It is clear that in adult myocytes, minor variations in intracellular sodium concentration can lead to substantial changes in intracellular calcium concentration, and hence, contraction amplitude. This relationship is determined by effects on sodium-calcium exchange activity. If the sodium-calcium exchanger plays a greater role during excitation-contraction coupling in the fetus and neonate, then sodium may be an even more important regulator of contraction in these age groups. Basal sodium concentration in quiescent ventricular myocytes has been reported to not differ significantly among immature rabbits from 3 to 21 days of age. However, additional work is necessary to determine the responses to physiological and pharmacological manipulation and to relate changes in intracellular sodium to contractile function, especially in the immature heart.

β-Adrenergic Stimulation

Driven by sympathetic neurotransmitters and adrenal hormones, β-adrenergic activation regulates virtually all major constituents of the cardiac excitation-contraction coupling cascade, for example, L-type calcium channels, ryanodine receptors, sodium-calcium exchanger, phospholamban and contractile proteins. These effects are mainly mediated via the classic stimulatory G protein (G_s)–adenylyl cyclase–cAMP–protein kinase A signaling cascade (Figure 2-6) with subsequent phosphorylation of the target proteins by protein kinase A. The overall results of β-adrenergic stimulation in the mature heart include increases in contractile force generation, enhanced relaxation, and increases in heart rate and conduction velocity. The effects on contractile function are due to increased calcium influx through L-type calcium channels to provide a greater trigger for sarcoplasmic reticulum calcium release. Enhanced relaxation results from more rapid dissociation of calcium from the contractile proteins (due to phosphorylation of TnI) and increased reuptake into the

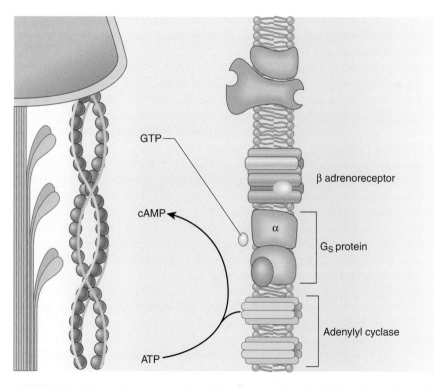

FIGURE 2-6. Schematic representation of the β-adrenergic signaling pathway. When a β-agonist binds to the β-adrenergic receptor (β adrenoreceptor), the conformational change promotes displacement of GDP by GTP and dissociation of the stimulatory G protein (G_s) complex into the α and βγ subunits. The result is activation of adenylyl cyclase and formation of cAMP, which then activates cAMP-dependent protein kinase (protein kinase A). The major substrates for protein kinase A that are involved in regulation of contraction and relaxation include L-type calcium channels, sarcoplasmic reticulum calcium release channel complex, phospholamban, troponin I, and the sodium-potassium pump. See text for additional details.

sarcoplasmic reticulum resulting from phosphorylation of phospholamban (in the phosphorylated state, the inhibitory effect of phospholamban on SERCA2a activity is reduced).

It is well known that β-adrenergic agonists also exert qualitatively similar responses in immature hearts. However, since these proteins and pathways for calcium transport are less important in the immature heart, alternative cellular and molecular mechanisms may be involved. As described earlier, evidence from animal studies is consistent with the sodium-calcium exchanger functioning as the major calcium transport protein in the immature heart. Until recently, β-adrenergic stimulation was thought to modulate the sodium-calcium exchanger in frog myocytes but not in mammalian cardiac myocytes. The nonselective β-adrenergic agonist isoproterenol enhances both inward and outward sodium-calcium exchange currents in adult guinea pig myocytes. In addition, the sodium-calcium exchanger response to isoproterenol is mimicked by the adenylyl cyclase activator forskolin and can be completely inhibited by a β-adrenergic antagonist or protein kinase A inhibitor. Regulation of sodium-calcium exchanger activity by protein kinase A appears to be isoform-specific. Although the cardiac-specific isoform of *NCX1* gene contains consensus protein kinase A phosphorylation sites within the large intracellular loop, whether the exchanger or some unidentified regulatory protein is phosphorylated under physiologically relevant conditions in vivo is not known. Furthermore, other laboratories have not been able to replicate some of these results and the potential role of β-adrenergic agonists in modulating the sodium-calcium exchanger remains in dispute.

In addition to the possibility that immature cardiac myocytes might possess qualitatively and quantitatively different sodium-calcium exchanger proteins, β-adrenergic signaling changes dramatically during development. Even though β-adrenergic receptors are detected in early fetal hearts long before postnatal sympathetic innervation, the response of L-type calcium current amplitude, calcium transients and cell contractions to β-adrenergic stimulation only becomes evident during late gestation. This is due to uncoupling of the receptor from downstream signaling during early gestation. Furthermore, the signal transduction pathways of β-adrenergic receptor in the immature heart might not be identical to that in mature heart. For example, the sensitivity of neonatal cardiac myocytes to β-adrenergic receptor agonists is much higher as compared to that of adult cardiac myocytes. The

β-adrenergic receptor is coupled to the arachidonic acid pathway in fetal chick ventricular myocytes. More surprisingly, repeated β-adrenergic receptor stimulation *sensitizes* the β-adrenergic signaling pathway in neonatal rat cardiac myocytes, which is in sharp contrast to the agonist-induced desensitization in adult cardiac myocytes.

Several studies have shown that immature myocytes exhibit positive inotropic and chronotropic responses to selective β_2-adrenergic receptor agonists, whereas the effects are minimal in mature cells. A recent study in neonatal rabbit ventricular myocytes provided evidence that this difference is attributable to developmental differences in the effects of a β_2-adrenergic receptor agonist on L-type calcium currents (current was stimulated in neonatal cells, but unchanged in mature myocytes). Furthermore, the response in newborns was not dependent upon activation of protein kinase A, suggesting alternative and as yet undefined pathways may be involved. These and other lines of evidence suggest that the responses to β-adrenergic stimulation in the immature heart may be mediated by much different mechanisms compared to those in the adult heart.

Cyclic Nucleotide Phosphodiesterases

A family of phosphodiesterase (PDE) enzymes mediates hydrolysis of cAMP and cGMP. Mammalian phosphodiesterases comprise a superfamily of 21 different genes that with alternative splicing encode at least 50 different protein products. These various proteins are grouped into 11 isoenzyme categories (PDE1 through PDE11) based on sequence, enzymatic properties, and sensitivity to various inhibitors. These isoenzymes exhibit different specificities for cAMP and cGMP and are differentially expressed in a variety of tissues. Even within cardiac ventricular myocytes, different phosphodiesterases are expressed in various cytosolic or membrane compartments. The isoform that initially commanded most of the interest in the heart was PDE3 because it is localized predominantly to the sarcoplasmic reticulum and plays a major role in regulation of phosphorylation state of phospholamban. It is this isoform that is the target of selective phosphodiesterase inhibitors such as amrinone and milrinone that are designed to increase contractility. However, PDE3 and other isoforms undergo developmental changes in expression and activity. In most animals species that have been studied, PDE3 activity is absent or markedly diminished at birth. Consequently, PDE3 inhibitors may have relatively little effect on the inotropic or lusitropic state in immature mammalian myocardium. However, in the clinical setting, milrinone improves hemodynamics in human infants, especially following cardiac surgery. This observation suggests that either PDE3 is expressed at birth in humans or that the favorable responses result from a decrease in afterload in response to milrinone (vasodilation).

Subsequently, other phosphodiesterase isoenzymes have garnered interest among cardiac biologists. PDE4 regulates β-adrenergic signaling and excitation-contraction coupling in mature rat heart and PDE5 modulates cardiac stress responses. The role of these isoenzymes in the immature heart has yet to be defined. More recently, PDE1 has been shown to regulate hypertrophic responses in both neonatal and adult rat myocytes.

Calcium-Calmodulin–Dependent Protein Kinase

Another important mechanism for regulating contractile function involves calcium-calmodulin–dependent protein kinase II (CaMKII). CaMKII is a serine/threonine kinase that is encoded by four separate genes. Alternative splicing produces at least 24 different proteins. Cardiac tissue expresses CaMKIIδC, which is involved in regulating contractility, relaxation, and heart rate. In addition, mammalian hearts express CaMKIIδB, which regulates nuclear function and gene expression. In cardiac myocytes, CaMKIIδC is activated in the presence of calcium and calmodulin. Calmodulin is a ubiquitous calcium-binding protein involved in a variety of cellular functions. CaMKII-δC in turn regulates contractile function by phosphorylating phospholamban and the ryanodine receptor complex. The effect of phosphorylating phospholamban is similar to that described earlier for protein kinase A-mediated phospholamban phosphorylation (relief of the inhibition of SERCA2a-mediated calcium uptake into the sarcoplasmic reticulum), resulting in positive lusitropic and inotropic effects. It is thought that this pathway may predominate in the basal unstimulated state, whereas the protein kinase A pathway may assume a greater role in regulating contractile function during β-adrenergic stimulation. Recent evidence indicates that CaMKIIδC-mediated phosphorylation may be involved in modulating ryanodine receptor activity, thereby providing another level of regulatory control of contractile function. When intracellular calcium is high, activation of CaMKIIδC may decrease ryanodine receptor openings, thereby down-regulating sarcoplasmic reticulum calcium release. Phosphorylation of phospholamban by CaMKIIδC would further help to reduce cytosolic calcium by enhancing reuptake into the sarcoplasmic reticulum. However, controversy

exists regarding the effects of calmodulin alone and that of CaMKIIδC-mediated phosphorylation on ryanodine receptor gating and sensitivity to calcium-induced calcium release. Additional experimental work is necessary to clearly define the roles of calmodulin and CaMKII in excitation-contraction coupling and the regulation of contractile function. Lastly, relatively little is known regarding potential age-related changes in CaMKII pathways, but evidence indicates that CaMKII expression is developmentally regulated in embryonic, fetal, and newborn rats. The functional implications of these changes in expression remain to be determined.

Phosphatases

As described in the preceding discussion, the phosphorylation state of regulatory proteins involved in excitation-contraction coupling plays a major role in modulating contractile function. Once a target protein is phosphorylated by protein kinase A or CaMKII, the effect will persist until the protein is dephosphorylated. This action is catalyzed by a family of phosphatases that specifically remove the phosphate group and return the protein to the native basal state. Thus, modulation of phosphatase activity or expression has a major influence on the regulation of cardiac contractile function.

Two major groups of serine/threonine phosphatases have been described, based upon substrate specificity and sensitivity to inhibitors. These are classified as protein phosphatase type 1 (PP1) and type 2 (PP2). There are at least four isoforms of PP1, termed PP1α, PP1β, PP1γ1, and PP1γ2. These isoforms are encoded by distinct genes, but share roughly 90% amino acid identity, diverging mainly at the C- and N-terminal ends of the protein. Type 2 phosphatases are classified as PP2A, PP2B, and PP2C, each with different structures, substrate specificities and regulation. PP2A exists as a heterotrimer in the cytosol with two regulatory subunits and a catalytic subunit. The catalytic subunit has two isoforms, PP2Aα and PP2Aβ.

The predominant phosphatase isoforms in mammalian cardiac tissue are PP1 and PP2A. Relatively less attention has been directed toward developmental regulation and expression of protein phosphatase isoforms in the heart. However, recent studies in rabbit myocardium showed that steady-state mRNA levels of PP1α, PP1β, and PP2Aα were much higher in newborns compared to adults. In addition, protein levels of PP1 and PP2A were also higher in newborn hearts and that PP1 was membrane bound and PP2A was found in soluble fractions. These findings are consistent with previous studies demonstrating a greater effect of inhibitors of PP1 and PP2A on increasing L-type calcium current in newborn myocytes compared to adult cells. Taken together, these results suggest that L-type calcium channels in the newborn heart are relatively dephosphory-lated, compared to adults. Strategies targeted at moderating the activity of cardiac PP1 and PP2A might prove to be useful approaches to increasing contractility in the immature heart, but additional studies are necessary.

■ EXCITATION-CONTRACTION COUPLING IN MODELS OF CONGENITAL HEART DISEASE

Although studies of congenital heart disease in animal models focus predominantly on various aspects of structural malformations, a few investigators have studied excitation-contraction coupling and calcium transport in chick and mouse models of cardiac neural crest abnormalities. These models are associated with conotruncal malformations such as persistent truncus arteriosus. Cardiac myocytes isolated from these animals demonstrate abnormal calcium transient kinetics and differences in the cellular processes involved in excitation-contraction coupling. At present, it is not known whether these changes represent primary defects or if they are secondary to hemodynamic influences related to the structural malformation. Regardless of the mechanism(s), these studies demonstrate the important link between cardiac structure and cellular function. Although much work remains to be done, it is tempting to speculate that there may be fundamental abnormalities in cardiac excitation-contraction coupling and regulation of contractile function that are not only attributable to immaturity, but also result directly from the underlying structural malformations.

■ EXCITATION-CONTRACTION COUPLING IN IMMATURE HUMAN HEART

Much of our current understanding of developmental changes in excitation-contraction coupling is based upon results from animal experiments (particularly rabbits). Few reports describe excitation-contraction coupling in immature human myocardium. Action potential duration was shorter in atrial muscle from young patients (2-22 months old) compared to adults (30-67 years). In contrast, more recent studies using freshly dissociated single atrial myocytes from infants demonstrated much slower early repolarization and a longer action potential compared to adult cells.

A few investigators have compared L-type calcium current in cardiac myocytes isolated from infants and children to adult cells or from infants compared with young children. A consistent finding has been that current amplitude, normalized for differences in cell size, does not differ among the different age groups. However, it is important to consider the effects of age-related changes in action potential configuration and controversy exists regarding developmental differences (or lack thereof) in L-type calcium current density in humans. For example, a more recent study in atrial cells demonstrated a 50% lower peak L-type calcium current in infant myocytes compared to adult cells.

Results from a single study using atrial myocytes from young children (3 days to 4 years of age) suggested that either L-type calcium current or caffeine can trigger sarcoplasmic reticulum calcium release and evoke a calcium transient. The relationships between developmental changes in action potential configuration, excitation-contraction coupling, and calcium transients in the human heart remain to be determined. Data are lacking on changes in cellular mechanisms and calcium regulatory proteins in myocytes isolated from human newborns. Thus, it is necessary to perform more direct and detailed studies to fully define mechanisms of normal excitation-contraction coupling, contraction, and relaxation in the immature human heart.

The results reviewed in the preceding discussion suggest that entirely new approaches are necessary when considering the fundamental mechanisms of calcium regulation in the immature heart. It seems inappropriate to extrapolate from adults, since the molecular and cellular basis for excitation-contraction coupling is vastly different in immature mammalian myocardial cells. Admittedly, most of the foundation for our current understanding of calcium regulation and cardiac contraction during human development is derived from animal studies. However, it is clear that many of the findings derived from immature animal models correlate with clinical observations in premature and term newborns, infants, and children. Infants born at 26 to 28 weeks gestation represent a much earlier phase of development than many of the mammalian fetal/newborn animal models that are known to exhibit profound immaturity of contractile function and inotropic responsiveness. Although infants and children with cardiac dysfunction represent a heterogeneous group, a common feature of all of these children is that the scientific foundation for understanding (and therefore, manipulating) their cardiac contractile function is markedly deficient.

SUGGESTED READINGS

General Aspects of Cardiac Functional Development

Anderson PAW. The heart and development. *Semin Perinatol.* 1996;20:482-509.

Mahony L. Development of myocardial structure and function. In: Allen HD, Driscoll DJ, Shaddy RE, Feltes TF, eds. *Moss and Adams' Heart Disease in Infants, Children and Adolescents.* 7th ed. Philadelphia, PA: Lippincott Williams & Wilkins; 2008:573-591.

Polin R, Fox W, Abman S, eds. *Fetal and Neonatal Physiology.* 3rd ed. Philadelphia, PA: Saunders Elsevier; 2004: Section XIII, Fetal and neonatal cardiovascular physiology.

Excitation-Contraction Coupling

Bers DM. *Excitation-Contraction Coupling and Cardiac Contractile Force.* 2nd ed. Dordrecht, The Netherlands: Kluwer Academic Publishers; 2001.

Cheng H, Lederer WJ. Calcium sparks. *Physiol Rev.* 2008; 88:1491-1545.

Hinken AC, Solaro RJ. A dominant role of cardiac molecular motors in the intrinsic regulation of ventricular ejection and relaxation. *Physiology.* 2007;22:73-80.

Moss RL, Razumova M, Fitzsimons DP. Myosin crossbridge activation of cardiac thin filaments: implications for myocardial function in health and disease. *Circ Res.* 2004;94: 1290-1300.

Developmental Aspects of Excitation-Contraction Coupling

Brillantes A-MB, Bezprozvannaya S, Marks AR. Developmental and tissue-specific regulation of rabbit skeletal and cardiac muscle calcium channels involved in excitation-contraction coupling. *Circ Res.* 1994;75:503-510.

Haddock PS, Coetzee WA, Cho E, et al. Sub-cellular $[Ca^{2+}]_i$ gradients during excitation-contraction coupling in newborn rabbit ventricular myocytes. *Circ Res.* 1999; 85:415-427.

Kim H, Kim D, Lee I, et al. Human fetal heart development after mid-term: morphometry and ultrastructural study. *J Mol Cell Cardiol.* 1992;24:949-965.

Wagner MB, Wang Y, Kumar R, et al. Calcium transients in infant human atrial myocytes. *Pediatr Res.* 2005;57:28-34.

Ziman AP, Gomez-Viquez NL, Bloch RJ, Lederer WJ. Excitation-contraction coupling changes during postnatal cardiac development. *J Mol Cell Cardiol.* 2010;48(2):379-386.

Sodium-Calcium Exchanger

Haddock PS, Coetzee WA, Artman M. Na^+/Ca^{2+} exchange current and contractions measured under Cl--free conditions in developing rabbit hearts. *Am J Physiol.* 1997;273:H837-H846.

Philipson KD, Nicoll DA. Sodium-calcium exchange: a molecular perspective. *Annu Rev Physiol.* 2000;62:111-133.

Qu YX, Ghatpande A, El Sherif N, et al. Gene expression of Na^+/Ca^{2+} exchanger during development in human heart. *Cardiovasc Res.* 2000;45:866-873.

Wakimoto K, Kobayashi K, Kuro-o M, et al. Targeted disruption of $Na^+/Ca2^+$ exchanger gene leads to cardiomyocyte apoptosis and defects in heartbeat. *J Biol Chem.* 2000; 275:36991-36998.

Developmental Aspects of β-Adrenergic Signaling

Collis L, Srivastava S, Coetzee WA, Artman M. β_2-Adrenergic receptor agonists stimulate L-type calcium current independent of PKA in newborn rabbit ventricular myocytes. *Am J Physiol Heart Circ Physiol.* 2007;293:H2826-H2835.

Kumar R, Joyner RW. Expression of protein phosphatases during postnatal development of rabbit heart. *Mol Cell Biochem* 2003;245:91-98.

Kuznetsov V, Pak E, Robinson RB, et al. β_2-Adrenergic receptor actions in neonatal and adult rat ventricular myocytes. *Circ Res.* 1995;76:40-52.

Maltsev VA, Ji GJ, Wobus AM, et al. Establishment of β-adrenergic modulation of L-type Ca^{2+} current in the early stages of cardiomyocyte development. *Circ Res.* 1999; 84: 136-145.

Perinatal Cardiovascular Physiology

■ INTRODUCTION

A comprehensive understanding of fetal cardiovascular physiology and of the changes that occur at birth is essential for developing a systematic approach to the diagnosis and treatment of a newborn with congenital heart disease. The fetus with complex congenital heart disease is rarely symptomatic, yet many newborn infants with the same defects are critically ill within hours or days after birth. In addition, specific cardiovascular abnormalities are associated with specific cardiac defects, and knowledge of such associations assists the clinician in the evaluation, diagnosis, and treatment of the critically ill newborn. This chapter reviews important physiologic aspects of the fetal circulation, how the fetal circulation can be monitored for hemodynamic stability, and the changes in circulatory physiology which occur at birth.

■ FETAL CARDIOVASCULAR PHYSIOLOGY

Essential Facts of Fetal Cardiovascular Function: An Overview

Four essential facts about the fetal circulation upon which to base an understanding of fetal cardiovascular physiology and its impact on congenital heart defects are listed here and discussed further in the following text.

1. **The right and left ventricles perform the same tasks in the fetus as they do postnatally.** Much has been written about the differences between the fetal and postnatal circulations. Most particularly, the case is frequently made that the former is a circulation in parallel, with the ventricles sharing the tasks of ejecting blood of similar oxygen content for oxygen uptake and delivery, while the latter is a circulation in series, with the right

ventricle ejecting poorly oxygenated blood to the lungs for oxygen uptake and the left ventricle ejecting more highly oxygenated blood to the highly metabolic organs for oxygen delivery. However, the fetal ventricles actually perform their normal postnatal tasks quite efficiently, achieving this by remarkable venous and intracardiac flow patterns, and central shunts that are unique to the fetal circulation.

2. **Only one ventricle is required for cardiovascular stability in the fetus.** Despite the separation of functions in the normal fetus, in the absence of two normal ventricles, in most instances the single functional ventricle is able to take over the function of the other ventricle to maintain a normal hemodynamic status in the fetus.

3. **The right ventricle, not the left, is the dominant ventricle in the fetus.** Postnatally, the left ventricle is dominant (has a greater mass) because it ejects an equal amount of blood as the right ventricle but does so under higher pressure. In the normal fetus, the right ventricle is dominant because it ejects blood at the same pressure as the left ventricle, but it ejects more blood.

4. **After embryogenesis, the size and orientation of a cardiovascular structure (cardiac chamber, valve, or blood vessel) is determined by the flow pattern and volume of blood passing through it.** Genetic and environmental determinants affect embryogenesis and can cause abnormal development of cardiac and vascular structures. These primary abnormalities may alter blood flow throughout fetal life which in turn may cause further abnormalities of structure and function. These secondary flow-determined abnormalities are often the dominant pathophysiologic processes that the cardiologist must correct when treating the newborn with congenital heart disease.

Tasks of the Fetal Ventricles

In the fetus, there are central shunts, or vascular communications, between the major vascular beds (systemic, pulmonary, and placental circulations) and the two sides of the heart (Figure 3-1). The ductus venosus joins the placental venous return to the systemic venous return, the ductus arteriosus connects the pulmonary arterial circulation directly to the systemic arterial circulation, the umbilical artery joins the systemic arterial circulation with the placental arterial circulation, and the foramen ovale joins the left and right sides of the heart. Many investigators argue that these shunts create a parallel circuit such that

the left and right ventricles perform the same tasks, receiving the same venous return and ejecting into the same vascular beds. This would be dramatically different than the postnatal state, in which the two ventricles perform very different tasks. However, careful analysis of fetal blood flow patterns indicates that the two fetal ventricles do not function in a completely parallel fashion and in fact, they are very efficient at performing their postnatal tasks. Fetal blood flow patterns permit the efficient distribution of poorly oxygenated blood to the right ventricle which is directed to the placenta for oxygen uptake, and well-oxygenated blood to the left ventricle for delivery to the highly metabolic organs (Figure 3-1). To understand this phenomenon it is necessary to understand venous blood flow patterns to the heart and arterial patterns to the various vascular beds.

The fetal central venous system can be divided roughly into six components: (1) the superior vena cava, which receives upper body blood flow; (2) the coronary sinus, which receives myocardial flow; (3) the ductus venosus, which receives most of the placental blood flow from the umbilical vein; (4) the inferior vena cava below the hepatic veins, which receives lower body flow; (5) the hepatic veins, which receive portal venous and hepatic arterial flow; and (6) the pulmonary veins, which receive pulmonary blood flow. The approximate percentage of total venous return from each of these components is presented in Figure 3-2.

Almost all of the blood flowing through the superior vena cava and coronary sinus returns to the right ventricle (Figure 3-3). The superior vena cava courses anteriorly and inferiorly as it enters the right atrium. The anatomy of the sinus venosus and of the eustachian valve promotes streaming so that almost all of the flow from the superior vena cava crosses the tricuspid valve into the right ventricle. Similarly, the coronary sinus enters the right atrium just above the medial aspect of the tricuspid valve annulus. The position of the coronary sinus ostium directs flow across the tricuspid valve into the right ventricle. Most of the superior vena caval blood is derived from the brain with lesser amounts from the upper extremities, and thus the blood is poorly oxygenated (Figure 3-4). Similarly, the coronary sinus blood is derived from the myocardium, and thus it is even more desaturated (Figure 3-4). Consequently, almost all of the poorly oxygenated blood from these two venous compartments enters the right ventricle.

The lower inferior vena cava joins with the right and left hepatic veins and the ductus venosus near the right

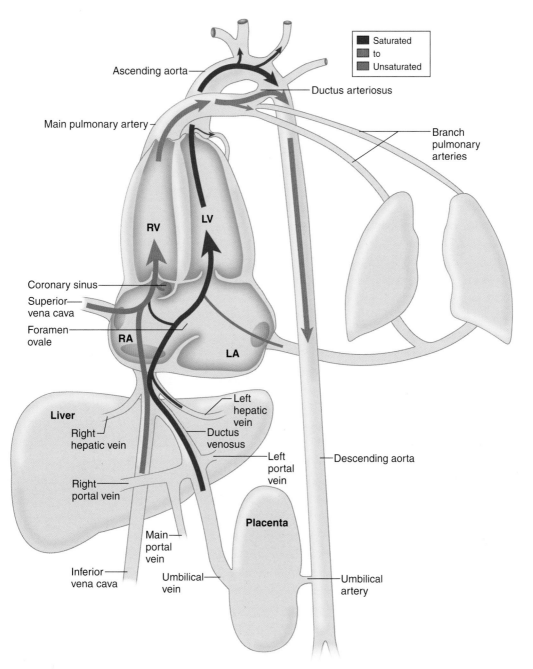

FIGURE 3-1. Fetal circulation, showing blood flow patterns throughout the central blood vessels and cardiac chambers. Poorly oxygenated blood streams through the right ventricle to the placenta and lower body, and well-oxygenated blood streams through the left ventricle to the heart and brain.

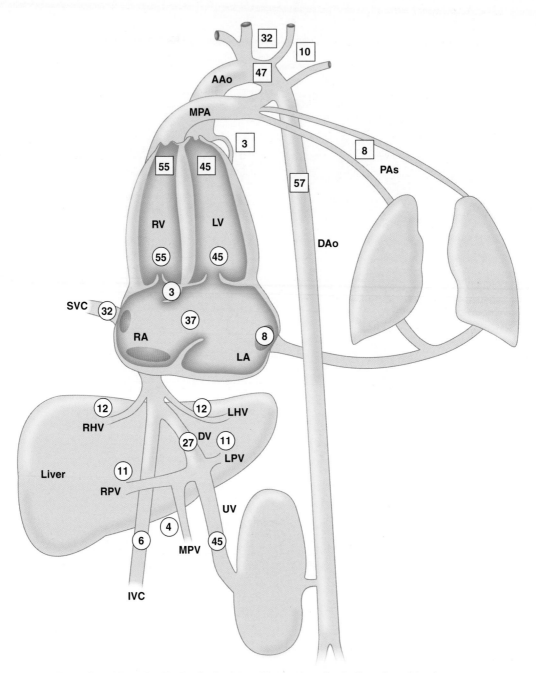

FIGURE 3-2. Blood flow distribution in the fetus. The percent distribution of combined venous return is represented in circles, and the percent distribution of combined ventricular output is represented in squares. These numbers represent estimates for human fetal blood flow distribution and are derived from sheep and human data. Abbreviations: AAo, ascending aorta; DAo, descending aorta; DV, ductus venosus; IVC, inferior vena cava; LA, left atrium; LHV, left hepatic vein; LPV, left portal vein; LV, left ventricle; MPA, main pulmonary artery; MPV, main portal vein; PAs, branch pulmonary arteries; RA, right atrium; RHV, right hepatic vein; RPV, right portal vein; RV, right ventricle; SVC, superior vena cava; UV, umbilical vein.

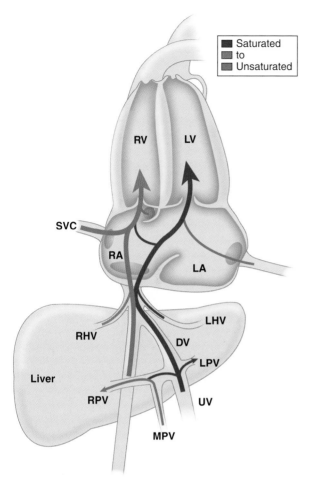

FIGURE 3-3. Venous blood flow patterns within the central veins and cardiac chambers. Umbilical venous blood primarily flows to the ductus venosus and left portal vein, whereas splanchnic venous blood passes via the main portal vein primarily toward the right portal vein. Subsequently, the well-oxygenated blood from the ductus venosus and left portal vein flows preferentially via the foramen ovale to the left ventricle. Blood from the inferior and superior vena cavae, the coronary sinus, and the right portal vein flows preferentially across the tricuspid valve to the right ventricle. See legend to Figure 3-2 for definitions of the abbreviations.

atrium to form the upper portion of the inferior vena cava, which delivers all of the venous return from the lower body and placenta to the heart (Figure 3-3). Although these venous systems join to form a single connection with the right atrium, the upper inferior vena cava is relatively short and exhibits fascinating streaming patterns. These patterns allow for the efficient distribution of the different venous systems to the two ventricles. The lower inferior vena cava carries blood from the lower body which, although not as desaturated as that of the upper body or coronary sinus, is much more desaturated than umbilical venous blood (Figure 3-4). This blood courses along the lateral wall of the upper inferior vena cava. It remains separate from the other sources of blood except for that from the right hepatic veins, which also enter the lateral wall of the upper inferior vena cava. The right hepatic veins primarily receive poorly saturated portal sinus blood from the splanchnic circulation and from the right hepatic arteries (Figure 3-4). The lower body and right hepatic vein streams join and course into the right atrium along the inferior margin of the eustachian valve, which directs most of that flow, along with that of the superior vena cava, across the tricuspid valve into the right ventricle.

Conversely, although umbilical venous blood is also delivered to the upper inferior vena cava, its course into the heart is quite different. The umbilical vein enters the portal sinus. From there, umbilical venous blood splits into the ductus venosus (60% of umbilical venous blood) and the left portal venous streams (Figure 3-3). Ductus venosus blood is entirely derived from the umbilical vein and is thus highly saturated (Figure 3-4). Left portal venous blood is mostly derived from the umbilical vein but joins with hepatic arterial flow in the left lobe of the liver to exit via the left hepatic vein. Because hepatic arterial blood represents only a small portion of hepatic blood flow, it does not appreciably decrease the saturation exiting the liver via the left hepatic veins. Blood from both the ductus venosus and the left hepatic vein enter the upper inferior vena cava along its medial margin, opposite that of the lower body and right hepatic venous blood. These two highly oxygenated streams flow together into the right atrium along the superior margin of the eustachian valve, and are directed by that structure toward the foramen ovale. The foramen acts as a windsock, directing blood into the body of the left atrium and then across the mitral valve into the left ventricle (Figure 3-3).

Lastly, pulmonary venous blood returns to the left atrium directly. Because the lungs are not very metabolically active in utero, this blood is not as desaturated as superior vena caval return. Moreover, this relatively poorly saturated blood passing to the left ventricle represents only 8% of combined venous return (Figure 3-2) and thus does not appreciably decrease left ventricular oxygen saturation.

The result of these circulatory patterns is that the right ventricle receives almost all of the blood with the lowest

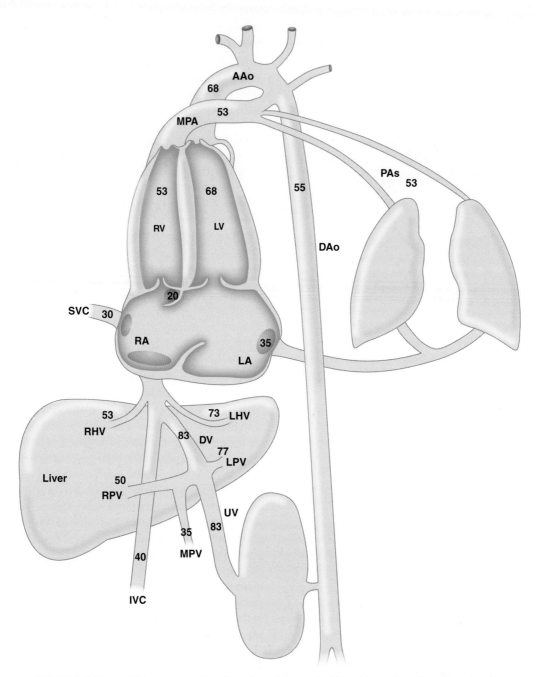

FIGURE 3-4. Hemoglobin oxygen saturations in various central blood vessels and cardiac chambers. These numbers are approximations derived from fetal sheep data. See legend to Figure 3-2 for definitions of the abbreviations.

oxygen saturation (venous return from the superior vena cava, coronary sinus, lower body, and right hepatic veins). Conversely, the left ventricle receives most of its blood from the ductus venosus and the left hepatic vein, the two sources of the most highly saturated umbilical venous blood. The oxygen saturation of blood in the left ventricle is estimated to be about 28% higher than that in the right ventricle. This difference is not significantly different from that in the postnatal state.

In order for the ventricles to accomplish their tasks efficiently, the left ventricle must not only receive more highly oxygenated blood but must deliver the majority of its blood to the highly metabolic organs, while the right ventricle must deliver the majority of its blood to the placenta for oxygen uptake (Figure 3-2). The most highly metabolic organs in the fetus are the heart, brain, and adrenal glands. Although the adrenal glands use a great deal of oxygen per gram of tissue, they are small and thus receive only a very small portion (<1%) of combined ventricular output. The heart and the brain receive all of their blood from the left ventricle. Approximately 7% of left ventricular output is delivered to the heart via the coronary arteries, and 55% is delivered to the brain via the carotid and vertebral arteries. Of the remaining left ventricular output, 15% is delivered to the upper extremities and only 23% is delivered across the aortic isthmus to the descending aorta. Note that the aortic isthmus is very narrow in the fetus because of its low flow. The relative narrow isthmus functions as a resistor, providing further evidence that the ventricles do not eject blood in parallel.

Thus, only a small portion of left ventricular output joins that of the right ventricle in the descending aorta. In contrast, the descending aorta receives most of the output of the right ventricle. The right ventricle delivers its output according to the relative resistances of the pulmonary, systemic, and placental vascular beds. In the fetal circulation, the resistance to blood flow in the pulmonary vascular bed is extremely high, much more so than that of the systemic and placental vascular beds. Thus, only a very small percentage of fetal right ventricular output (15%, or 8% of combined ventricular output) is delivered to the lungs. The remainder crosses the ductus arteriosus into the descending aorta. Of that flow, approximately one-third is delivered to the lower body and two-thirds to the placenta for oxygen uptake. Thus, the majority of the relatively desaturated right ventricular output goes to the placenta for oxygen uptake and most of the remainder goes to organs of low metabolic activity. The majority of highly

saturated left ventricular output is delivered to the highly metabolic heart and brain. Thus, the ventricles perform their tasks in an efficient manner, albeit somewhat less so than in the postnatal state.

The efficiency of the circulatory system is apparent from analysis of the proportion of available oxygen that is actually used by the fetus. Fractional extraction of oxygen is defined as the fraction of oxygen removed by the organism from the blood that is delivered to the organs by the arterial system. In the postnatal state, only 25% to 30% of available oxygen is extracted from blood. Thus, there is a large oxygen reserve for extraction during stress, even without an increase in cardiac output. In the fetus, despite the lower oxygen saturation of blood delivered to the fetal body, only about 30% of oxygen is extracted, leaving the fetus with almost the same oxygen extraction reserve. This reserve is achieved in part by the remarkable fetal blood flow pathways described earlier.

One Ventricle Can Maintain Cardiovascular Stability

The central mixing of left and right ventricular output somewhat decreases the efficiency of oxygen delivery, but this inefficiency is advantageous to the fetus with congenital heart disease when one or the other ventricle is underdeveloped. Because central shunts allow both ventricles to eject into all three vascular beds, only one ventricle is necessary for cardiovascular stability.

This fact can be most readily demonstrated in the fetus with only one functional ventricle. Many infants with congenital heart disease have hypoplasia of one atrioventricular valve, usually in association with atresia of the corresponding semilunar valve. The physiology of the fetus with one of the more common defects, hypoplastic left heart syndrome, is instructive in understanding the impact of congenital heart disease on fetal cardiovascular physiology (Figure 3-5). All venous return (except the very small amount of blood which passes through the pulmonary circulation) enters the right atrium normally. Rather than crossing the foramen ovale to the left atrium, the ductus venosus and left hepatic venous blood cross the tricuspid valve with the rest of the systemic venous return. Pulmonary venous return, instead of crossing the mitral valve, crosses the foramen ovale in a left-to-right direction and then enters the right ventricle. Thus, the right ventricle receives all of the venous return. As is normally the case, the right ventricle ejects its blood into the main pulmonary artery and about 8% enters the pulmonary

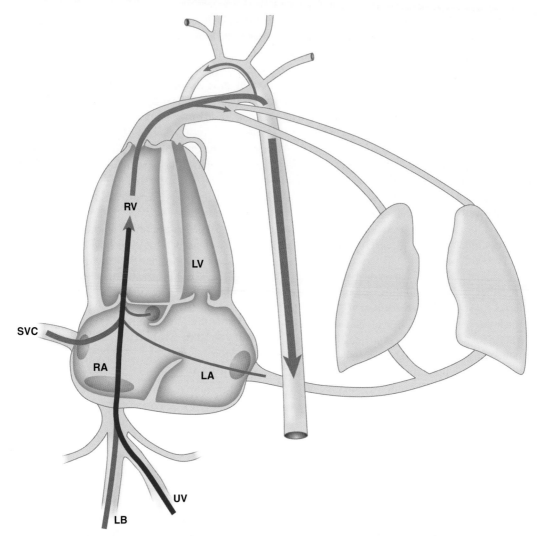

FIGURE 3-5. Hypoplastic left heart syndrome. Blood flow patterns show that all of the venous return is directed across the tricuspid valve to the right ventricle because of reversal of blood flow across the foramen ovale. The right ventricle is able to supply blood to all vascular beds, ejecting blood to the upper body and heart by reverse flow across the aortic isthmus. Note that the ascending aorta is markedly hypoplastic because it only receives coronary blood flow. LB represents blood flow from the lower body, consisting of splanchnic and lower limb venous return. See legend to Figure 3-2 for the definitions of the other abbreviations.

circulation. The remaining 92% crosses the ductus arteriosus to the descending aorta. Because the aortic valve is atretic, blood flow from the ductus arteriosus not only passes down the descending aorta to the lower body and placenta, but also passes retrograde, up the aortic isthmus and arch to supply the upper body and heart. In this way,

blood flow to all tissues of the body is preserved and the fetus usually grows normally. Only when the foramen ovale is restrictive, which occurs infrequently, do the fetal blood flow patterns in hypoplastic left heart syndrome have a deleterious effect on the developing fetus and even then, those effects are usually not clinically evident until after birth.

Right Ventricular Dominance

Although the left and right ventricles eject the same output in the mature circulation, the left ventricle generates a much higher pressure. Consequently, its mass greatly exceeds that of the right ventricle. Because of the greater mass and wall stress, the left ventricle is less compliant than the right ventricle. The decreased compliance and greater ejection pressure causes the left ventricle to exert a direct effect on the filling and ejection of the right ventricle (much more so than the right exerts on the left). Thus, the left ventricle is considered the dominant ventricle in the mature circulation.

In the fetus, however, the relationship between the left and right ventricles is quite different. The peak systolic pressure in the two ventricles is the same because they eject into the same vascular beds. In addition, the fetal ventricles do not eject the same volume of blood. The right ventricle ejects 55% of the combined output of the ventricles. The mass of the right ventricle is therefore somewhat greater than that of the left, and the diastolic and systolic interactions are reversed, though not as pronounced as in the mature circulation. The fetal right ventricle is thought to significantly constrain left ventricular filling and is considered the dominant ventricle. This constraint of left ventricular filling may contribute to the underdevelopment of the fetal left ventricle in conditions in which the right ventricle receives even more of the combined venous return, such as total anomalous pulmonary venous connection. In this lesion, pulmonary venous blood returns to the right atrium, not the left, and that blood is directed across the tricuspid valve. Despite the fact that this represents only a small amount of combined venous return, the left ventricle is diminutive at birth. Similarly, the right ventricle is even more dominant than normal in the fetus with coarctation of the aorta. Contrary to the postnatal circulation in which this obstruction is imposed on the left ventricle, in the fetus the right ventricle is exposed to the effects of the coarctation because far more blood crosses the ductus arteriosus from the right ventricle than crosses the aortic isthmus from the left ventricle. Consequently, that load increases the constraint of the right ventricle on the left ventricle. Echocardiography of a fetus with coarctation of the aorta demonstrates a marked discrepancy in ventricular size. The fetal echocardiographer must carefully evaluate the aortic arch whenever the right ventricle appears more dominant than normal.

Blood Flow Effects on Cardiac and Vascular Structure

The primary defect in cardiac structure occurs during embryogenesis in most forms of congenital heart disease. These abnormalities of embryogenesis are discussed in detail in Chapter 1. Once the primary defect is established, however, secondary alterations in the structure and size of various cardiac chambers, blood vessels, or shunts occur. These secondary changes result from abnormalities in the amount and direction of blood flow through the fetal cardiac and vascular structures and are important determinants of the presentation of neonates with congenital heart disease. For example, the primary event in the fetus with hypoplastic left heart syndrome likely is inadequate development of the aortic valve. Once this occurs, several secondary abnormalities develop. Normally, somewhat over one-third of venous return passes through the foramen ovale from the right atrium to the left atrium and left ventricle. In hypoplastic left heart syndrome, the diminutive or atretic aortic valve limits the amount of forward flow across the mitral valve, and both that valve and the left ventricle do not develop normally. This obstruction to forward flow inhibits the normal flow of blood from right-to-left across the foramen ovale. If the aortic valve is completely atretic, foramen ovale flow reverses and becomes left-to-right, as the small amount of pulmonary venous blood decompresses into the right atrium (Figure 3-5). Thus, the foramen ovale may be quite small and abnormally configured, which is of great consequence after birth when pulmonary blood flow increases markedly. The large postnatal increase in left atrial venous return must cross the small foramen ovale, which may result in obstruction to pulmonary venous drainage. This is often associated with markedly increased left atrial pressures and secondary pulmonary edema.

Abnormal flow patterns also affect the development of the ascending aorta and aortic arch. Normally, the ascending aorta receives 45% of fetal combined ventricular output (Figure 3-2). Because the aortic arch and ascending aorta are perfused in a retrograde manner via the ductus arteriosus (Figure 3-5), there is separation of the blood flow from the ductus arteriosus into a stream that courses inferiorly to the lower body and placenta, and a stream that passes superiorly into the aortic arch. This divergence of blood flow within the aorta may cause a shelf to develop between the aortic isthmus and descending aorta, leading to coarctation of the aorta that is manifest after birth. In addition, most of the blood coursing superiorly in the aorta is delivered to the upper body. Only the very small volume of blood eventually perfusing the coronary arteries courses in a retrograde manner down the ascending aorta which causes the ascending aorta to be hypoplastic in this syndrome.

The secondary alterations in cardiac and vascular structures are extremely important in congenital heart disease. Some are serious problems, and may require urgent therapy in the newborn to ensure survival. Others may be of no hemodynamic significance, but may lead to a specific diagnosis because they cannot occur in the presence of the other potential defects under consideration (this is discussed in greater detail with examples of specific associations in Chapters 6 to 8). For these reasons, it is always important to consider normal and abnormal physiology and blood flow patterns when evaluating the newborn with suspected congenital heart disease. If associated defects are defined which can or cannot occur for each diagnosis under consideration, the differential diagnosis can be narrowed.

Vascular Ultrasonographic Evaluation of Hemodynamic Stability

The use of fetal echocardiography in the diagnosis of congenital heart disease and fetal cardiac dysfunction is discussed in Chapter 4. This section will briefly review how fetal vascular ultrasonography can be used to evaluate metabolic stability. Over the years, many of the findings regarding blood flow distribution and flow mechanics described in fetal sheep have been corroborated in the human by echocardiography, and normal blood flow patterns in all major vessels and vascular beds have been described. The fetal ultrasonographer is now able to use this information to determine when there is a disturbance in cardiovascular dynamics, which can lead to the diagnosis, prognosis, and treatment of specific pathophysiologic processes.

Inadequate placental oxygen uptake leads to fetal hypoxemia, inadequate substrate delivery, and fetal growth retardation. Anemia, primary ventricular dysfunction, and arrhythmias also cause metabolic decompensation in the fetus. In all of these situations, blood flow patterns are disturbed in both the arterial and venous circulations. On the arterial side, compensatory mechanisms are initiated by arterial chemoreceptors and other signals, which lead to redistribution of blood flow to the cerebral and myocardial vascular beds. This is associated with specific changes in arterial waveforms. As metabolic decompensation progresses, significant alterations in fetal venous waveforms

appear. It is hypothesized that when arterial blood flow is maximally redistributed and is no longer able to maintain sufficient oxygen delivery, fetal heart failure ensues, at which time characteristic changes in venous flow waveforms occur. The progression of these changes reflects the progression of heart failure, and can be used as a scoring system for fetal cardiovascular instability.

On the arterial side, hypoxemia, growth retardation, or decreased ventricular output lead to increased resistance in the lower body and fetal placenta vascular beds. This is demonstrated by a reduction in peak systolic velocity in the descending aorta and umbilical artery, and an even greater reduction in end-diastolic velocity, leading to increased pulsatility (Figure 3-6). The pulsatility index is calculated to quantify this change:

$$\frac{S - D}{M}$$

where S is the peak systolic velocity, D is end-diastolic velocity, and M is the mean velocity across the cardiac cycle. Conversely, end-diastolic velocities increase in the cerebral and myocardial circulations, leading to a reduction in the pulsatility index. These findings demonstrate the "brain and heart sparing" effects of metabolic stress on the fetus.

On the venous side, blood flow patterns reproducibly change as afterload increases and the heart begins to fail. The veins typically interrogated are the inferior vena cava, the ductus venosus, and the umbilical vein within the umbilical cord. The blood flow patterns are very different from each other, and sequential changes in them reflect the progression of hemodynamic instability.

The normal flow signal in the inferior vena cava shows the largest forward wave in ventricular systole (S), a somewhat lower forward wave during peak forward flow across the tricuspid valve during diastole (D), and a relatively small backward wave during atrial systole (a). A pulsatility index for veins has been calculated as

$$\frac{S - a}{D}$$

but it is not used routinely. Another index used in describing the flow patterns is $|a|/S$. More distal from the heart, the negative 'a' wave no longer exists—within the ductus venosus, end-diastolic flow (just after atrial contraction) the 'a' wave is usually positive. In addition, the two forward waves become of a more similar size and eventually merge

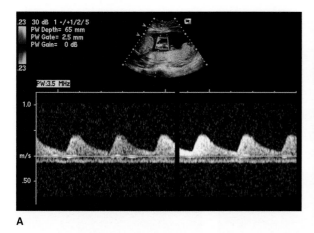

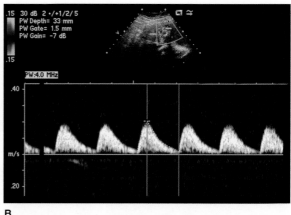

FIGURE 3-6. Umbilical arterial blood flow patterns by Doppler ultrasonography in normal and stressed fetuses. A. Normal pattern with forward flow throughout systole and diastole. **B.** Stressed pattern showing decreased systolic velocity and a significantly more decreased diastolic velocity, so that the pulsatility index is increased. Note that the velocity scale is reduced compared to A.

into one wave. In the umbilical vein in the cord, the flow pattern varies only minimally, showing a continuous forward flow pattern that undulates only slightly. Thus, the farther a vein is from the heart, the less the pulsatility is in the normal fetus (Figure 3-7).

If a fetus develops increased afterload and eventually heart failure, pulsatility increases in the proximal veins and extends more distally. The first sign of decompensation is an exaggeration of the negative 'a' wave in the inferior vena cava, which is less than 7% of the forward flow area normally. Subsequently, there is increased pulsatility in the ductus venosus, with the development of 'a' wave reversal as a late event. Increases in |a|/S have been shown to correlate with the severity of growth retardation and of hydrops fetalis. The finding of atrial pulsations in the umbilical vein in the cord represents the end-stage heart failure. This finding has been called "diastolic block" and it is a strong predictor of perinatal mortality. When the umbilical vein demonstrates a pattern similar to the inferior vena cava (the "double venous pulsation"), fetal death is usually imminent (Figure 3-7).

■ TRANSITIONAL CIRCULATION

Essential Facts of the Transition to the Postnatal Circulation

At birth, there are rapid and profound changes in cardiovascular function and blood flow patterns as the newborn adapts to a new circulation in which oxygen exchange occurs in the lungs, the placenta is removed from the circulation, and thermoregulation becomes necessary. For the newborn to remain hemodynamically and metabolically stable during the first few minutes of postnatal life, **three critical adaptations** must occur:

1. **Pulmonary blood flow increases dramatically**, to about 20 times that of pulmonary blood flow in the fetus.

2. **Central blood flow patterns are significantly altered**. The central shunts (the ductus venosus, the foramen ovale, the umbilical artery, and the ductus arteriosus) are abolished, and blood flow through the cardiac chambers and great vessels is converted to a circulation in series.

3. **Combined ventricular output increases greatly**, to meet the newly increased energy requirements imposed by the work of breathing and thermoregulation.

As with fetal cardiovascular physiology, much of the information on these changes is derived from studies in fetal sheep, in which the animals were instrumented chronically in utero. The independent effects of ventilation, oxygenation, umbilical cord occlusion, and thermoregulation on cardiovascular function have been ascertained. It is important to understand each of these effects, not only to understand how a fetus normally adapts to the postnatal environment, but also what stresses

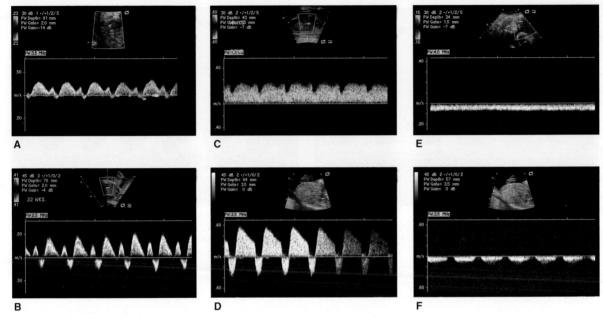

FIGURE 3-7. Venous blood flow patterns by Doppler ultrasonography in normal and stressed fetuses.
A shows the normal venous waveform in the inferior vena cava, with positive systolic and early diastolic waves followed by a very small negative 'a' wave during atrial systole; **B** represents the stressed fetus, with a much larger negative 'a' wave; **C** shows the normal venous waveform in the ductus venosus, showing pulsatility but no negative waves; **D** represents the stressed fetus, showing 'a' wave reversal; **E** shows the normal waveform in the umbilical vein, consisting of a low-velocity wave with little pulsatility; **F** represents the stressed fetus, with the umbilical venous waveform demonstrating significant pulsatility.

are imposed upon the fetus with congenital heart disease as it copes with a new environment.

Increase in Pulmonary Blood Flow

Much of the change in the circulation occurs in the first few minutes after birth (Figure 3-8). Subsequently, more subtle and gradual changes occur during the next several weeks after birth.

The initial circulatory changes occur as the fetus is delivered and takes its first breaths. There is an immediate and dramatic increase in pulmonary blood flow to levels approximating 20 times resting fetal levels. Although oxygen is a potent pulmonary vasodilator, ventilation with low concentrations of oxygen is capable of inducing approximately two-thirds of the decrease in pulmonary vascular resistance and increase in pulmonary blood flow that are observed at birth. In fact, rhythmic ventilation is not required, as similar changes can be induced by inflating the lungs with a syringe containing nitrogen gas. The

decrease in pulmonary vascular resistance induced by ventilation alone may in part be caused by a direct effect, as changes in surface tension at the alveolar air-liquid interface reduce perivascular tissue pressures.

However, alterations in the metabolic milieu of the distal vasculature are also likely to be very important effectors. Prostaglandin metabolites have significant effects on pulmonary tone. Prostacyclin, a potent pulmonary vascular dilator, is produced in the lungs by distention or mechanical stimulation. Leukotriene metabolites affect the pulmonary vascular significantly, and are thought to mediate hypoxic pulmonary vasoconstriction in the adult. Interestingly, the leukotriene blocker, FPL 57231, increases pulmonary blood flow to a remarkably similar extent as does ventilation with gas containing concentrations of nitrogen and oxygen present during fetal life. Other metabolically active substances, such as bradykinins, angiotensin II, and histamine, may play some role in the normal postnatal pulmonary vasodilation.

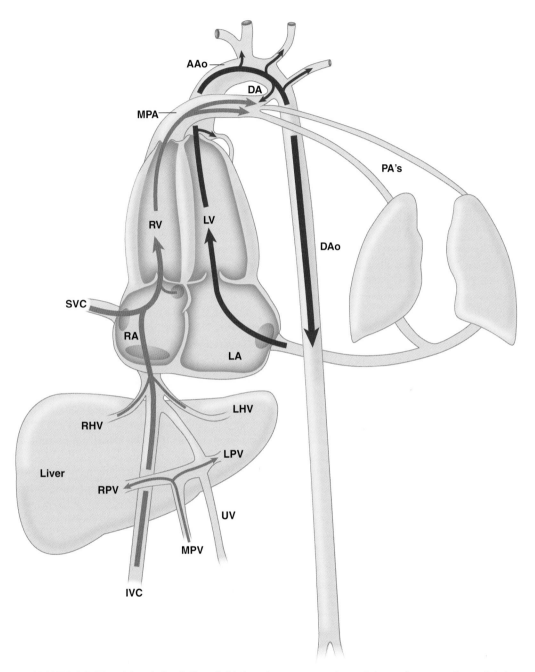

FIGURE 3-8. Transitional circulation. At birth, pulmonary vascular resistance decreases immediately. This increases pulmonary blood flow above systemic levels by abolishing the right-to-left ductal shunt and creating a small left-to-right ductal shunt. The increased left atrial return in turn abolishes the right-to-left shunt across the foramen ovale. Blood flow through the umbilical vein ceases with loss of the placental circulation, which then stops flow through the ductus venosus (although both remain patent for several days). DA indicates ductus arteriosus. See legend to Figure 3-2 for the definitions of the other abbreviations.

Oxygen is capable of further decreasing pulmonary vascular resistance and increasing pulmonary blood flow to levels seen in the immediate postnatal period. Thereafter, remodeling of the pulmonary vascular bed occurs over the next several weeks, as the muscularity of the proximal arteriolar bed decreases and the muscularity of the most distal bed increases. These changes decrease pulmonary vascular resistance to mature levels within 1 to 2 months after birth and transfer control of pulmonary vascular tone to local metabolites present in the distal pulmonary bed.

Changes in Central Blood Flow Patterns

Concomitant with the dramatic increase in pulmonary blood flow, changes in central blood flow patterns occur (Figure 3-8). These changes create a circulation in which the right and left ventricles must function efficiently in series (a condition that is not possible in many forms of congenital heart disease).

Umbilical arterial flow ceases as soon as the infant is separated from the placenta by the clamping of the umbilical cord. With the associated loss of umbilical venous flow, ductus venosus flow markedly decreases. Anatomic closure of the ductus venosus is probably delayed for several hours or days, as demonstrated by the ability to pass a catheter through the umbilical vein and ductus venosus in newborn infants. Thereafter, the ductus venosus is no longer patent because of the absence of flow, and possibly, the effects of prostaglandin metabolites and sympathetic stimulation.

Flow through the other central shunts, the foramen ovale and ductus arteriosus, is abolished primarily by the decrease in pulmonary vascular resistance with a simultaneous large increase in pulmonary blood flow, and secondarily by the increase in systemic arterial oxygen tension. The foramen ovale is the central shunt within the fetal heart that allows for right-to-left flow of over one-third of combined venous return to enter the left atrium and left ventricle. This shunt is maintained in the fetus by the tenfold greater venous return directly to the right atrium as compared to the left. The floor of the foramen ovale consists of a flap, or windsock, of tissue that protrudes into the left atrium. At birth, the amount of pulmonary venous return directly to the left atrium increases dramatically. This causes the flap to be displaced toward the right atrium, effectively abolishing the right-to-left shunt immediately after birth. Left atrial pressure usually exceeds that of the right and it is frequently possible to

demonstrate a very small left-to-right shunt through the foramen ovale in newborn infants. This physiologically normal flow through the foramen ovale cannot be distinguished from a small secundum atrial septal defect, so newborns with small atrial shunts should not be thought to have congenital heart disease. Because the foramen ovale is only functionally closed from a right-to-left direction because of the pressure differential between the left and right atria, a right-to-left shunt can occur when a newborn infant cries and increases thoracic impedance to right ventricular output, which in turn may cause a transient increase in right atrial pressure. Infants with this transient desaturation must be distinguished from those with cyanotic heart disease who may present with duskiness only with crying or feeding. Although not apparently cyanotic at rest, infants with cyanotic congenital heart disease show some desaturation by pulse oximetry at all times, whereas the normal newborn has normal saturations at rest.

The last central shunt to close after birth is the ductus arteriosus. Unlike the other three shunts, flow through the ductus arteriosus does not cease immediately but does so over the first 12 to 48 hours of life. During fetal life, a large volume of blood flows through the ductus arteriosus in a right-to-left direction. Although the right-to-left shunt is abolished immediately at birth because of the large decrease in pulmonary vascular resistance, a small left-to-right shunt occurs, thereby increasing pulmonary blood flow to levels exceeding systemic blood flow. Closure of the ductus arteriosus is initiated by oxygen, to which the mature newborn ductus is very responsive. Other factors that play a role in the decrease in pulmonary vascular resistance, such as bradykinin, catecholamines, and arachidonic acid metabolites, may contribute to ductus arteriosus closure. Arachidonic acid metabolites are particularly important agents in controlling ductus tone and this explains the efficacy of using prostaglandin E_1 to maintain patency of the ductus arteriosus in newborn infants with critical congenital heart defects.

The last major change in central blood flow patterns is the change from right ventricular dominance to left ventricular dominance. Although the left ventricle is dominant in the mature circulation because it pumps at higher pressure, in the transitional circulation it not only pumps at higher pressure but it also ejects more blood. Right ventricular systolic pressure decreases in the newborn infant because pulmonary vascular resistance falls and the ductus arteriosus begins to constrict. The reversal of flow in the ductus arteriosus is caused not only by the very rapid and large decrease in pulmonary vascular resistance but also by an increase in systemic vascular resistance. Systemic vascular resistance increases because the very compliant placental vascular bed is removed from the systemic circulation and because local systemic vascular beds such as those in the myocardium and the brain constrict in response to the increase in oxygen tension. The combination of the large decrease in pulmonary vascular resistance and increase in systemic vascular resistance causes all of the output of the right ventricle to flow to the pulmonary vascular bed, and for some of the output of the left ventricle to cross the ductus arteriosus into the lungs.

Although the placenta is physically removed from the newborn circulation very soon after birth, placental blood flow is nearly completely abolished even before it is removed because placental flow is exquisitely sensitive to oxygen. As the systemic vascular bed constricts while the pulmonary vascular bed dilates, the lungs, which receive less than 10% of the combined ventricular output during much of fetal life, receive significantly more than half immediately after birth. The pulmonary veins return about 55% to 60% of total venous blood to the heart, which flows almost exclusively to the left ventricle. The left ventricle not only ejects under higher pressure, but it also receives more blood than the right ventricle. Thus both the filling pressure and systolic pressure are greater in the left than in the right ventricle, which removes the constraint of the right ventricle on left ventricular function that exists in the fetus. This allows the left ventricle to increase its output greatly, another important component of the cardiovascular transition at birth.

Increase in Combined Ventricular Output

The third important change in cardiovascular status at birth is the near tripling of left ventricular output, required because of the large increase in oxygen demand. In the fetus, systemic arterial oxygen levels are very low, averaging about 20 to 25 torr. However, oxygen demand is similarly low and the oxygen dissociation curve is shifted to the left, allowing for a considerable amount of oxygen to be taken up by hemoglobin in the placenta despite the low oxygen tension. Thus, the fractional extraction of oxygen, which is perhaps the best indication of the reserve that exists to respond to periods of stress, is approximately 30% (similar to the postnatal state).

Birth is associated with two new major metabolic requirements that mandate a large increase in oxygen delivery. Respiratory work uses about 30% of the oxygen consumed by the newborn. In addition, thermoregulation can require almost as much oxygen. Thus, oxygen consumption nearly triples at birth. Moreover, the left ventricle, which primarily supplies oxygen to the heart, brain, and upper body before birth, must supply oxygen to the entire body immediately after birth. Consequently, left ventricular output must increase nearly threefold if fractional extraction remains unchanged. The increase in left ventricular output occurs because of increases in heart rate and stroke volume.

It has been of great interest to investigators that the left ventricle can greatly increase its output after birth, yet its ability to increase output in the fetus is very limited. The fetal left ventricle can eject, at most, only 50% more blood in response to alterations in load, heart rate, or contractility. In contrast the left ventricle at birth is capable of increasing its output nearly threefold but contractility does not increase. Results from a variety of studies indicate that the primary reason that the left ventricle is able to increase output is because, as discussed earlier, filling and contraction of the left ventricle are no longer constrained by right ventricle after birth. Other contributing factors include increased β-adrenergic receptor activity in association with thyroid hormone and cortisol surges in the perinatal period, and an improved relationship between preload and afterload.

SUGGESTED READINGS

Fetal Cardiovascular Physiology

Allan L, Hornberger LK, Sharland G. *Textbook of Fetal Cardiology*. London, United Kingdom: Greenwich Medical Media Limited; 2000.

Anderson DF, Bissonnette JM, Faber JJ, et al. Central shunt flows and pressures in the mature fetal lamb. *Am J Physiol* 1981;241:H60-H66.

Brown DL, Durfee SM, Hornberger LK. Ventricular discrepancy as a sonographic sign of coarctation of the fetal aorta: how reliable is it? *J Ultrasound Med.* 1997;16(2):95-99.

Burggren W, Johansen K, Alfred Benzon Foundation. Cardiovascular Shunts: Phylogenetic, Ontogenetic and Clinical Aspects: Proceedings of the Alfred Benzon Symposium 21 held at the premises of the Royal Danish Academy of Sciences and Letters, Copenhagen, 17-21 June 1984. Copenhagen, Munksgaard, New York, Raven Press, 1985.

Edelstone DI, Rudolph AM. Preferential streaming of ductus venosus blood to the brain and heart in fetal lambs. *Am J Physiol.* 1979;237(6):H724-H729.

Edelstone DI, Rudolph AM, Heymann MA. Liver and ductus venosus blood flows in fetal lambs in utero. *Circ Res.* 1978;42(3):426-433.

Fisher DJ, Heymann MA, Rudolph AM. Myocardial oxygen and carbohydrate consumption in fetal lambs in utero and in adult sheep. *Am J Physiol.* 1980;238(3):H399-405.

Garg V, Muth AN, Ransom JF, Schluterman MK, Barnes R, King IN, et al. Mutations in NOTCH1 cause aortic valve disease. *Nature.* 2005;437(7056):270-274.

Gluckman PD, Heymann MA, eds. *Pediatrics and Perinatology: The Scientific Basis.* 2nd ed. London, United Kingdom: Oxford University Press, New York, NY: Arnold; 1996.

Hornberger LK, Bromley B, Lichter E, Benacerraf BR. Development of severe aortic stenosis and left ventricular dysfunction with endocardial fibroelastosis in a second trimester fetus. *J Ultrasound Med.* 1996;15(9):651-654.

Hornberger LK, Need L, Benacerraf BR. Development of significant left and right ventricular hypoplasia in the second and third trimester fetus. *J Ultrasound Med.* 1996; 15(9):655-659.

Kleinman CS, Glickstein JS, Shaw R. Fetal echocardiography and fetal cardiology. In: HD Allen, DJ Driscoll, RE Shaddy, TF Feltes. *Moss and Adams'. Heart Disease in Infants, Children, and Adolescents Including the Fetus and Young Adult.* 7th ed. vol. 1, Philadelphia, PA: Lippincott Williams & Wilkins; 2008: Chapter 28.

Polin RA, Fox WW, eds. *Fetal and Neonatal Physiology.* Philadelphia, PA: Saunders; 1992.

Srivastava D, Gottlieb PD, Olson EN. Molecular mechanisms of ventricular hypoplasia. *Cold Spring Harb Symp Quant Biol.* 2002;67:121-125.

Vascular Ultrasonography in the Fetus

Groenenberg IA, Wladimiroff JW, Hop WC. Fetal cardiac and peripheral arterial flow velocity waveforms in intrauterine growth retardation. *Circulation.* 1989;80(6):1711-1717.

Hecher K, Campbell S, Doyle P, Harrington K, Nicolaides K. Assessment of fetal compromise by Doppler ultrasound investigation of the fetal circulation. Arterial, intracardiac, and venous blood flow velocity studies. *Circulation.* 1995; 91(1):129-138.

Huhta JC. Fetal congestive heart failure. *Semin Fetal Neonatal Med.* 2005;10(6):542-552.

Krapp M, Gembruch U, Baumann P. Venous blood flow pattern suggesting tachycardia-induced 'cardiomyopathy' in the fetus. *Ultrasound Obstet Gynecol.* 1997;10(1):32-40.

Rychik J. Fetal cardiovascular physiology. *Pediatr Cardiol.* 2004;25(3):201-209.

Postnatal Cardiovascular Physiology

Cassidy SC, Chan DP, Allen HD. Left ventricular systolic function, arterial elastance, and ventricular-vascular coupling: A developmental study in piglets. *Pediatr Res.* 1997;42(3):273-281.

Katz AM. *Physiology of the Heart.* 2nd ed. New York, NY: Raven Press; 1992.

Little WC, Cheng CP. Left ventricular-arterial coupling in conscious dogs. *Am J Physiol.* 1991;261(1 Pt 2):H70-H76.

Ross J, Jr. Afterload mismatch and preload reserve: a conceptual framework for the analysis of ventricular function. *Prog Cardiovasc Dis.* 1976;28:255-264.

Rudolph AM. *Congenital Diseases of the Heart: Clinical-Physiological Considerations.* 3rd ed. Chichester, West Sussex, United Kingdom: Wiley-Blackwell; 2009.

Rudolph AM, Iwamoto HS, Teitel DF. Circulatory changes at birth. *J Perinat Med.* 1988;1(9):9-21.

Teitel DF, Iwamoto HS, Rudolph AM. Changes in the pulmonary circulation during birth-related events. *Pediatr Res.* 1987;27(4 Pt 1):372-378, 1990.

Teitel DF, Iwamoto HS, Rudolph AM. Effects of birth-related events on central blood flow patterns. *Pediatr Res.* 1987;22(5):557-566.

Teitel D, Rudolph AM. Perinatal oxygen delivery and cardiac function. *Adv Pediatr.* 1985;32:321.

Prenatal Evaluation and Management

■ INTRODUCTION

Evaluation of a fetus for structural or functional heart disease is commonplace, as the application of clinical fetal ultrasound has become widespread in modern obstetrical practice. Furthermore, our current understanding of the genetic basis for congenital heart defects prompts screening in patients who otherwise might not have been referred for evaluation in the past. It is important to understand the uses and limitations of fetal echocardiography to optimally utilize this technology and to provide appropriate counseling to parents. The purpose of this chapter is to provide a brief overview of fetal cardiology that can be used as a foundation for understanding selected aspects of fetal heart disease. More comprehensive references on fetal cardiology and, in particular fetal echocardiography, are listed at the end of this chapter.

■ FETAL ECHOCARDIOGRAPHY

Fetal echocardiography is the primary method for diagnosing fetal cardiovascular disease and monitoring progression and management of the disease process. This chapter will provide a succinct overview of fetal echocardiography to provide basic information about its indications and limitations, and will discuss how to apply findings from a fetal echocardiogram to the patient. Additional information about the application of echocardiography to assess cardiac and vascular function in the fetus is presented in Chapter 3.

A complete fetal echocardiogram is similar in scope to a postnatal transthoracic echocardiogram. Cardiac and great vessel anatomy and relationships, cardiac function, blood flow patterns, and cardiac rhythm are all assessed. A wide range of cardiovascular diseases can be detected and defined in the fetus, including simple and complex cardiovascular structural malformations, cardiomyopathies, tumors, and arrhythmias. Newer techniques of three- and four-dimensional echocardiography are being applied in many centers, but at present, the role of these modalities in improving detection, management, and follow-up requires additional research.

If indicated (see subsequent discussion), the first fetal echocardiogram is generally performed around 18- to 20 weeks gestation using a standard transabdominal approach. In some centers, transvaginal fetal echocardiography is offered as early as 11 weeks gestation. However, controversy exists regarding the usefulness of early transvaginal ultrasound and it is not widely used at present. Transabdominal studies performed at around 18 to 20 weeks gestation provide excellent resolution of the cardiovascular structures and are sufficiently early in gestation so that elective termination can be considered if the family so desires.

Indications

As discussed in Chapter 15, the incidence of congenital cardiovascular malformations in the United States is around 10 per 1000 live births. The incidence of structural cardiovascular malformations in all pregnancies is not known precisely, but it is most certainly higher for at least three reasons: (1) severe structural or functional cardiovascular malformations may not permit survival of the fetus; (2) some mothers elect to terminate the pregnancy if an extracardiac malformation or chromosomal abnormality is detected; and (3) the structural defect may be subtle or even nonexistent in the fetus, and may manifest only after birth when the circulation transitions to the postnatal state. In all three situations, the presence of a congenital cardiovascular malformation may go unrecognized.

Because a complete diagnostic fetal echocardiogram is time-consuming and labor-intensive, fetal echocardiography is not well suited for routine screening of all pregnant women. Therefore, it is important to develop a strategy for appropriate targeted referrals for fetal echocardiography. The general indications for fetal echocardiography can be considered as primarily maternal, familial, or fetal. These indications are categorized and listed in Table 4-1.

Maternal Indications

Congenital heart disease in the mother clearly increases the risk of a structural cardiovascular malformation in the fetus. However, the incremental increase in risk appears to vary depending upon the type of maternal heart disease. For example, a mother with an atrioventricular septal defect has a 10% to 12% risk of having a fetus with some type of congenital cardiovascular malformation. In contrast, a mother with tetralogy of Fallot (not associated with a microdeletion of chromosome 22q11) has only about a 2% risk of having an infant with heart disease. Given the autosomal dominant pattern of inheritance of some forms of long QT syndrome (LQTS), a mother with confirmed LQTS will have a 50% chance of the fetus having LQTS.

■ **TABLE 4-1.** Indications for Fetal Echocardiography

Maternal Indications
- Maternal congenital cardiovascular malformation
- Exposure to known cardiovascular teratogen (anticonvulsants, alcohol, rubella, etc)
- Metabolic disorder (diabetes mellitus, phenylketonuria)
- Connective tissue disease
- Maternal anxiety[a]
- Advanced maternal age[a]

Family Indications
- Previous child or fetus with congenital cardiovascular malformation
- Paternal congenital cardiovascular malformation
- Family history of genetic syndrome (especially DiGeorge and related syndromes, Holt-Oram, Noonan, Marfan, Williams, long QT Syndrome)
- Family history of malformation syndrome
- Family history of other birth defects

Fetal Indications
- Suspected structural cardiovascular malformation on obstetrical ultrasound
- Extracardiac malformation
- Chromosomal abnormality
- Twin-to-twin transfusion syndrome
- Hydrops fetalis
- Arrhythmia
- Increased nuchal translucency

[a]These are relative indications without proven utility.

Despite considerable progress, the complex genetics and inheritance of congenital cardiovascular malformations remains incompletely understood (Chapter 15). In the past, the situation was even more unclear because many children with congenital heart disease did not survive to reproductive age and fetal echocardiography was not available. As more women with congenital cardiovascular malformations survive into adulthood and have children, the relationship between maternal congenital heart disease and the risk to offspring will become much better defined. In concert with the ability to define the incidence of heart defects using fetal echocardiography, continued advances in the genetics of congenital cardiovascular malformations will enhance our understanding of the risks of recurrence and lead to improved fetal screening.

In addition to congenital heart disease in the mother, other maternal factors may predispose the fetus to be at risk for congenital heart disease. Maternal exposure to known cardiovascular teratogens can affect the developing cardiovascular system. Maternal viral infections may be associated with structural malformations (eg, rubella and patent ductus arteriosus or pulmonary artery stenosis) or cardiomyopathy (eg, parvovirus or Coxsackievirus). Other recognized teratogens include anticonvulsants, alcohol, and retinoic acid, among others.

Diabetes mellitus is the most common maternal metabolic disorder that is associated with an increased risk of fetal cardiovascular malformations. It is estimated that the presence of maternal diabetes increases the risk of structural congenital heart disease by two- to fivefold. In addition, transient hypertrophic cardiomyopathy at birth is common in this population. Maternal phenylketonuria is associated with an increased risk of tetralogy of Fallot, left heart obstructive lesions, and ventricular septal defects.

The presence of a connective tissue disorder in the mother is associated with fetal atrioventricular block and cardiomyopathy. Specific maternal antibodies, anti-SSA/Ro and anti-SSB/La, have been implicated in the development of fetal atrioventricular block and cardiomyopathy, but the precise cellular and molecular mechanisms are not entirely clear. Maternal connective tissue disease should prompt an evaluation for autoantibodies and fetal monitoring for the presence or development of atrioventricular block and cardiomyopathy. The corollary is that if an infant is born with congenital complete atrioventricular block, the mother should be evaluated for the presence of subclinical connective tissue disease. Over half of previously asymptomatic mothers are found to have laboratory evidence of connective tissue disease or later present with clinical findings. The most common disease found is Sjögren syndrome, followed by systemic lupus erythematosus.

Maternal anxiety and advanced maternal age are relative indications for fetal echocardiography. A normal fetal echocardiogram may be reassuring to a mother who, for whatever reason, is overly concerned about the possible presence of fetal heart disease. The value of fetal echocardiography in the setting of advanced maternal age (especially if amniocentesis is refused) has not been proven.

Family Indications

The risk of recurrence of congenital cardiovascular malformations in subsequent siblings is related to the genetic basis of the particular defect or to other underlying maternal factors (see preceding discussion). In general, the risk of recurrence is approximately two to five times greater than in the unaffected population. However, this figure may be much higher if there is underlying maternal disease that has already affected a previous fetus or if a known autosomal-dominant single gene defect is present. In most cases of recurrent congenital cardiovascular malformations, the same defect recurs. However, even in the case of families with confirmed single gene defects, the penetrance and phenotypic expression may be quite variable (Chapter 15). The presence of other forms of birth defects in previous children is also associated with a higher incidence of cardiovascular malformations.

Fetal Indications

Obstetrical ultrasound evaluation is routine and commonplace. However, a routine obstetrical ultrasound evaluation does not constitute a complete fetal echocardiogram. Every obstetrical ultrasound evaluation should include an attempt to obtain a four-chamber view of the fetal heart (Figure 4-1). A normal four-chamber screen is helpful in excluding many serious major structural congenital heart defects, but a number of malformations may

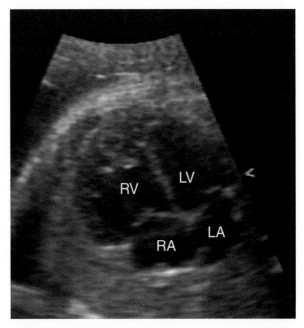

FIGURE 4-1. Normal four-chamber view. This echocardiographic image was obtained in a normal fetus at 29 weeks gestation. Abbreviations: LA, left atrium; LV, left ventricle; RA, right atrium; RV, right ventricle.

be missed (see section "Limitations"). In an effort to improve the utility of a routine obstetrical ultrasound as a screen for fetal cardiovascular malformations, some authorities recommend using the outflow tract views as an alternative or in addition to the four-chamber screen. Although perhaps technically slightly more difficult to obtain, the outflow tract views will detect a greater percentage of serious cardiovascular malformations. It is estimated that the four-chamber view is abnormal in about one in 500 pregnancies and in about 60% of fetuses with major structural cardiovascular malformations. An abnormal four-chamber view or outflow tract screen should prompt referral for a complete fetal echocardiogram. In addition, detection of specific cardiovascular malformations or extracardiac malformations constitutes an indication for a complete fetal echocardiogram. Extracardiac anomalies that have a high association with cardiovascular malformations include omphalocele, diaphragmatic hernia, duodenal atresia, tracheoesophageal fistula, cystic hygroma, and single umbilical artery. Many chromosomal abnormalities (eg, trisomy 21) are associated with congenital cardiovascular malformations. If the karyotype analysis from amniocentesis is abnormal, fetal echocardiography should be performed. Lastly, nuchal translucency is being used with increasing frequency as a screening test for congenital heart disease. By itself, increased nuchal translucency is of only moderate specificity, but when associated with tricuspid insufficiency or an abnormal flow pattern in the ductus venosus, the likelihood of congenital heart disease is high. In addition, the greater the nuchal translucency, the more likely congenital heart disease is present. Currently, many perinatologists use a nuchal translucency greater than the 95th percentile as an indication for fetal echocardiography.

Twin pregnancies are characterized by an increased incidence of fetal complications, especially in monozygotic twins. Most monochorionic twins share blood supply through vascular anastomoses in the placenta. In 10% to 20% of monozygous twin pregnancies, this shared blood supply is unequal and results in twin-to-twin transfusion syndrome. Severe twin-to-twin transfusion syndrome produces asymmetrical fetal growth and if untreated, results in death of one or both fetuses in over 80% of cases, especially if this condition is noted before 28 weeks gestation. Cardiovascular compromise is common in the recipient twin. Fetal echocardiographic findings include ventricular hypertrophy and dilation, tricuspid regurgitation, and, less commonly, mitral regurgitation. The prevalence

of pulmonary stenosis is fourfold greater in twin-to-twin transfusion syndrome than in twin pregnancies without evidence of twin-to-twin transfusion syndrome. It has been proposed that progressive right ventricular hypertrophy and severe tricuspid regurgitation result in decreased flow across the pulmonary valve with resulting acquired pulmonary stenosis (or atresia in severe cases). A variety of treatments have been used for twin-to-twin transfusion syndrome, including selective feticide, serial amnioreduction, septostomy of the intertwin membrane, and endoscopic laser photocoagulation. Selective endoscopic laser photocoagulation of anastomotic vessels is currently the primary treatment in many centers and should be considered when twin-to-twin transfusion syndrome is diagnosed, regardless of the initial severity.

Hydrops fetalis is a serious fetal condition defined as abnormal fluid accumulation in two or more fetal compartments. Fluid may collect in the pleural, pericardial, and/or abdominal cavities. Excess fluid often collects in the skin, as well. In some cases there is placental edema and/or polyhydramnios. Fetal ultrasound is invaluable in diagnosing, assessing severity, and monitoring treatment in cases of hydrops fetalis. Hydrops fetalis has many causes (Table 4-2), most of which are not related to primary cardiovascular abnormalities. The most common overall cause of hydrops fetalis is severe anemia, which can be due to a variety of conditions. In the past, if the fetus was not anemic, the etiology of hydrops fetalis was often undefined (idiopathic), but more recently the list of conditions that can cause hydrops has expanded. With greater accuracy in diagnosis, for example, it has become clear that a number of genetic abnormalities and inborn errors of metabolism (especially lysosomal storage diseases) can cause hydrops fetalis. A cause is now identified in approximately 75% cases of nonimmune hydrops fetalis. A primary cardiovascular abnormality is attributed to roughly 20% to 25% of cases of nonimmune hydrops fetalis. Most of those cases are secondary to tachy- or bradyarrhythmias, but structural cardiovascular defects can also cause hydrops fetalis. Figure 4-2 illustrates an example of echocardiographic findings in a fetus with hydrops and large pericardial and pleural effusions associated with complex cardiovascular structural abnormalities.

Decreased systemic perfusion leading to hydrops fetalis affects the fetus only when the pathophysiological process impacts both ventricles. A common example is sustained supraventricular tachycardia, which may present in utero with biventricular failure. The ability of the fetal heart to

■ TABLE 4-2. Causes of Hydrops Fetalis

Hematologic causes
- Isoimmunization (hemolytic disease; Rh most common)
- Other hemolytic disorders
- Disorders of red cell production
- Fetal hemorrhage

Cardiovascular causes
- Nonstructural abnormalities
  - Tachyarrhythmias
  - Complete atrioventricular block
  - Myocarditis
  - Cardiomyopathies
- Structural abnormalities
  - Hypoplastic left heart syndrome
  - Coarctation of the aorta
  - Arteriovenous malformation (including within the placenta)
  - Highly vascularized tumors (most commonly hemangiomas)
  - Heterotaxy syndromes
  - Atrioventricular septal defects
  - Cardiac tumors
  - Ebstein anomaly
  - Tetralogy of Fallot with absent pulmonary valve

Infectious causes
- Parvovirus (B19V)
- Toxoplasmosis
- Cytomegalovirus
- Herpes simplex
- Hepatitis B
- Syphilis
- *Listeria monocytogenes*

Inborn errors of metabolism (partial listing)
- Glycogen storage disease, type IV
- Lysosomal storage diseases
- Thyroid disorders

Genetic syndromes (partial listing)
- Achondrogenesis
- Arthrogryposis
- Prune-belly syndrome (Eagle-Barrett syndrome)
- Noonan syndrome
- Smith-Lemli-Opitz syndrome
- Tuberous sclerosis

Chromosomal abnormalities (partial listing)
- Trisomy syndromes (trisomy 13, 15, 18, or 21)
- Turner syndrome
- Beckwith-Wiedemann syndrome

Intrathoracic tumors or masses
- Mediastinal teratoma
- Rhabdomyoma
- Bronchopulmonary sequestration
- Cystic adenomatoid malformation of the lung
- Diaphragmatic hernia

Abdominal tumors or masses
- Polycystic kidneys
- Neuroblastoma
- Hepatic tumor (hepatoblastoma or mesenchymal hamartoma)

Other conditions
- Placental abnormalities
- Cystic hygroma
- Intussusception
- Teratoma

increase output in response to stress is very limited compared to that of the newborn heart. As discussed in Chapter 3, the fetal ventricles cannot readily increase end-diastolic volume or preload. This limitation in ability to increase preload, in the presence of an already low afterload and high-contractile state, does not allow the fetal heart to increase its output with stress. Consequently, decompensation occurs in response to any process that causes dysfunction of both ventricles. Structural defects that may be associated with hydrops fetalis include heterotaxy syndromes (particularly with associated complete atrioventricular block), atrioventricular septal defects, and hypoplastic left heart syndromes. Isolated defects that cause hydrops often are associated with severe tricuspid or mitral regurgitation, which increase atrial filling pressures, which in turn leads to fluid accumulation. Additional information regarding the use of fetal echocardiography to assess fetal cardiac and vascular function is presented in Chapter 3.

Fetal cardiac arrhythmias typically present as an abnormal fetal heart rate or irregular rhythm that is noted during a routine prenatal examination. Fetal arrhythmias are noted in approximately 2% of all pregnancies. In the majority of cases (roughly 90%), the arrhythmia is transient, self-limited, and does not require any intervention. A sustained fetal heart rate below 100 or above 180 beats/min should be considered abnormal and warrants further investigation. During fetal heart rate monitoring, a gradual increase or decrease in heart rate is suggestive of

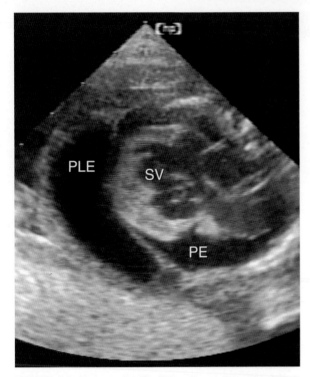

FIGURE 4-2. Hydrops fetalis. This echocardiographic image was obtained at 21 weeks gestation in a fetus with single ventricle, pulmonary stenosis with dilation of the main pulmonary artery, severe tricuspid regurgitation, and markedly depressed systolic contractile function. Ultrasound imaging demonstrated fluid collections in the pleural, pericardial, and abdominal cavities. Abbreviations: PE, pericardial effusion; PLE, pleural effusion; SV, single ventricle.

normal fetal heart rate acceleration, especially if the rate remains below 200 beats/min.

Abrupt onset and termination of an accelerated heart rate is highly suggestive of fetal supraventricular tachycardia. Fetal supraventricular tachycardia is most commonly due to atrioventricular reentrant tachycardia and less commonly to atrial flutter. Atrial ectopic tachycardia and permanent junctional reciprocating tachycardia are unusual but must be considered in the differential diagnosis. Intrauterine ventricular tachycardia and atrial fibrillation are quite rare. Chapter 10 presents additional details about arrhythmia mechanisms and pathophysiology.

Fetal tachycardia is not always due to an abnormal cardiac rhythm. Fetal distress and chorioamnionitis are also associated with increased fetal heart rate (although the rate is usually less than 200 beats/min). Fetal tachycardia due to a primary arrhythmia may follow an unpredictable course. Some fetuses will tolerate brief periods of tachycardia quite well and do not need therapy. The major determinants of the effect of supraventricular tachycardia on the fetus are the duration and frequency of the episodes, and the rate of the tachycardia. Frequent and/or sustained tachycardia carries a high risk of hydrops fetalis. Once a fetus with an arrhythmia becomes hydropic, the mortality is quite high and intervention must not be delayed (see following text).

Fetal bradycardia is defined as a heart rate less than 100 beats/min. Figure 4-3 is an example of complete atrioventricular block with a slow ventricular rate in a 26-week gestation fetus with heterotaxy syndrome and a two-chambered heart (the mother did not have evidence of connective tissue disease). Other causes of fetal bradycardia include frequent blocked premature atrial contractions and long QT syndrome. In general, premature atrial contractions are benign and resolve with time. In contrast, long QT syndrome and complete atrioventricular block are serious conditions that require careful monitoring and further investigation.

Premature atrial contractions are relatively common and most often are benign. Only about 0.5% (or less) of fetuses with isolated premature atrial contractions will develop sustained supraventricular tachycardia. Thus, reassurance can be offered, but it is generally recommended that the fetal heart rate be monitored weekly for several weeks to exclude a sustained arrhythmia. If sustained elevations of fetal heart rate are noted, then referral for further evaluation is indicated.

Fetal heart rate monitoring and fetal echocardiography are commonly used to diagnose fetal arrhythmias, but these methods have limitations. Simple auscultation or Doppler assessment of the fetal heart rate is useful for diagnosing tachycardia, bradycardia, and irregular rhythms, but the mechanism is left undetermined. Fetal electrocardiography can often provide additional insight into the mechanism for the arrhythmia, but sometimes the diagnosis is obscure. Direct recording of the fetal electrocardiogram (ECG) noninvasively is difficult because interference from the higher amplitude signals from the mother. Fetal electrocardiography is most commonly applied during labor when a scalp electrode can be placed.

More advanced recording techniques include electronic signal processing to isolate the fetal ECG and magnetocardiography. The fetal magnetocardiogram is a recording of

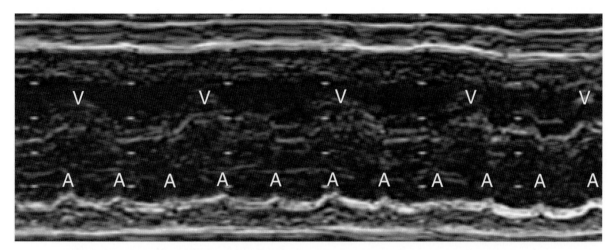

FIGURE 4-3. Complete atrioventricular block. This M-mode tracing was obtained at 26 weeks gestation in a fetus with heterotaxy syndrome and a two-chambered heart. The atrial activity (detected by movement of the atrial wall) was unrelated to the opening and closing of the atrioventricular valve). The atrial rate was approximately 105 beats/min and the ventricular rate was approximately 45 beats/min. Abbreviations: A, atrial contraction; V, ventricular contraction.

the magnetic field that is generated by the electrical activity of the fetal heart. Fetal magnetocardiography is noninvasive and can provide high-quality signals that have been useful for diagnosing various types of fetal arrhythmias. The major limitation of this technique is that the fetal magnetic signal is very weak, requiring expensive and sophisticated magnetic field sensors and specially isolated rooms to house the equipment. This technique is available in only a few centers worldwide.

Limitations of Fetal Echocardiography

Despite its enormous utility and overall accuracy, limitations do exist. The foramen ovale and ductus arteriosus are open in the normal fetus and it is impossible to predict whether these communications will close postnatally. Thus, an atrial septal defect or persistent patent ductus arteriosus cannot be diagnosed in the fetus. It can be difficult to diagnose coarctation of the aorta in the fetus because the ductus arteriosus delivers the majority of blood flow to the lower body and placenta (Chapter 8 and Figure 8-1). The area of coarctation is typically just proximal to the insertion of the ductus arteriosus into the descending aorta and it is normally narrow because of the limited flow that passes through this area from the aortic isthmus. The presence of a posterior shelf narrowing the

area further and leading to a postnatal coarctation can be difficult to appreciate. Occasionally, the coarctation site is directly opposite the insertion of the ductus arteriosus on the posterior wall of the aorta. In this situation the right ventricle may be ejecting against the obstruction. This leads to the finding of right ventricular dilation and hypertrophy in the fetus, a finding that should lead to the presumptive diagnosis of coarctation of the aorta if the pulmonary valve is normal.

In addition, small ventricular septal defects or mild stenosis of the atrioventricular or semilunar valves may be undetected during a fetal echocardiogram. Because of the small size and limited flow within the pulmonary veins, fetal echocardiography cannot completely exclude partial anomalous pulmonary venous connection or pulmonary vein stenosis. Some fetal abnormalities may not be entirely obvious at the initial fetal echocardiogram at around 18 weeks gestation, but the severity progresses as gestation proceeds. Examples include right and left heart obstructive lesions, cardiomyopathies, atrioventricular valve regurgitation, and arrhythmias.

Counseling Families

Perhaps the most important aspect of fetal echocardiography is related to the appropriate communication of results and information to the mother and family. Discussing a normal study is relatively easy and straightforward. Even so, it is important to provide an overview of the potential limitations of a "normal" fetal echocardiogram.

Much more difficult is the discussion that must follow the detection of significant structural or functional cardiovascular disease in the fetus. Unfortunately, relatively little attention and training is devoted to this critically important aspect of fetal cardiology. In many cases, the parents are already suspecting that there may be some problem with the fetus since they have been referred for advanced testing. It is best to discuss the results in an environment other than the examination room, if possible. The overall objective is to provide accurate information about the diagnosis, pathophysiology, prognosis, and options that are available. Specific details are dependent upon the precision and certainty of the diagnosis, the gestational stage, anticipated prenatal and postnatal course, surgical outcomes (if surgery is an option), and the presence or absence of underlying extracardiac anomalies and/or known genetic syndromes. If the diagnosis is incomplete or uncertain, then a follow-up examination within a few days is imperative. A complete and accurate diagnosis is essential for proper counseling.

The counselor must have sufficient knowledge and experience to provide accurate up-to-date information regarding the long-term prognosis for the specific cardiovascular abnormality. Information must be presented in a clear and comprehensible manner that encourages a dialog so that the counselor can ascertain the parent's level of understanding. The use of diagrams and written materials is helpful. Frequently, the family is overwhelmed at the time of initial diagnosis and a follow-up session within a few days may be beneficial. It is inappropriate to withhold information or to use vague euphemisms in a misguided attempt to protect the family. In especially complex cases (eg, maternal disease, genetic syndromes) it is helpful to enlist the aid of perinatologists and genetic counselors, for example, to provide accurate information about the anticipated outcome and prognosis.

If the problem is severe and detected early enough, termination of the pregnancy may be considered. The role of the counselor should be to help the family make the decision that is best for them and then to support the family in their decision. Whichever route the parents choose will change the course of their lives and it is imperative that they be as comfortable and confident as possible with their decision.

■ TRANSPORT

It is beyond the scope of this book to review guidelines and procedures for fetal or neonatal transport, but it is important to be mindful of a few general principles. A newborn infant with significant congenital heart disease may represent the most challenging and unstable type of patient to transport to a tertiary center for more definitive care. It is essential to have a fully equipped neonatal transport ambulance and experienced practitioners. In general, experienced nursing personnel and a respiratory therapist are required. Critically ill infants often require more than one caregiver in order to appropriately monitor and manage the baby during transport. If ductus-dependent congenital heart disease is suspected, an infusion of prostaglandin E_1 should be initiated immediately. Delaying administration of prostaglandin E_1 can be life threatening and unless there are extenuating circumstances, it is not necessary to wait for transport to a tertiary care center to begin an infusion. The most serious side effect is apnea, so it is imperative that appropriately skilled personnel and supplies for managing the airway and ventilation are immediately available.

With increasing use of fetal echocardiography, more infants with structural congenital heart disease are being diagnosed prenatally. Because of the inherent difficulties associated with transporting a critically ill newborn with unstable cardiovascular physiology as described in the preceding discussion, serious consideration should be given to transporting the mother to the tertiary center prior to delivery. Although not yet convincingly proven, it is logical to expect that anticipation, parental education, preparation, and delivery at tertiary care center will result in improved care and outcomes for infants diagnosed prenatally with structural or functional heart disease.

■ MEDICAL THERAPY FOR THE FETUS

General Principles

Drug therapy for the fetus represents an especially complex and challenging problem. This is probably the only case in which the patient is treated with drugs that have been taken by another individual and is exposed to drug metabolites that have been formed by someone else. Factors that contribute to the difficulties in developing effective drug therapy for the fetus are outlined in Table 4-3.

Virtually all maternally ingested drugs cross the placenta to the fetus, primarily by passive diffusion. The rate

■ **TABLE 4-3.** Difficulties Related to Providing Effective Fetal Drug Therapy

- Maternal drug metabolism and clearance are affected by pregnancy and change during gestation.
- Fetal drug distribution, metabolism, and excretion are variable and change during gestation.
- Fetal circulatory patterns and blood flow distribution are unique.
- Fetal monitoring and sampling are difficult.

and extent of transfer varies depending on the concentration gradient of the free drug. Maternal, placental, and fetal factors interact to influence the relative distribution and free drug concentrations in the various compartments. The major determinants of placental transfer include extent of protein binding, relative degrees of lipid and water solubility, molecular weight of the drug, maternal drug clearance, and placental function (placental blood flow and metabolism). The physicochemical properties of the drug will remain constant, but drug transfer may vary because of changes in maternal drug clearance or in placental blood flow and metabolism.

Although additional complexity exists, the general principles governing drug responses in newborns also apply to the fetus. Fetal drug responses are related to drug concentration at the receptor (pharmacokinetic principles) and drug receptor-effector interactions with subsequent biochemical and/or physiological effects (pharmacodynamic principles). However, pharmacokinetics and pharmacodynamics in the fetus are exceedingly difficult to study, especially in humans. Drug therapy in the human fetus is generally extrapolated from experiments in other species or case reports, and it is difficult to generalize or predict drug responses at various gestational ages in the human fetus. In addition to unique circulatory patterns, fetal drug distribution is affected by lower fetal protein binding, higher percentage of total body weight as water in the fetus, and age-dependent changes in relative organ weights and metabolic capacity.

As in older children and adults, most fetal drug metabolism occurs in the liver. A unique property of the fetus is that the fetal adrenal gland participates in drug metabolism to a much greater degree than in infants and older children. Although fetal hepatic metabolic activity is relatively low and intrinsic drug clearance is generally reduced,

the more rapid maternal and placental clearance of most drugs diminishes the impact of impaired fetal drug clearance. Therefore, drug concentration at fetal receptor sites is determined largely by maternal and placental clearance, rather than by fetal drug clearance.

Treatment of Fetal Arrhythmias

Supraventricular Tachycardia

Management of intrauterine arrhythmias remains a therapeutic challenge and requires a combined approach with input from pediatric cardiologists, perinatologists, adult cardiologists, and neonatologists. There are basically three options when a fetal arrhythmia is detected: (1) no intervention except for heightened and frequent monitoring, (2) drug therapy, or (3) delivery and treatment (if necessary) of the neonate. The prognosis and success of medical therapy for fetal arrhythmias are worse in the presence of hydrops fetalis. Decisions must be made jointly to develop the most effective approach to therapy for each patient. Gestational age, duration, and frequency of episodic supraventricular tachycardia, the presence or absence of hydrops fetalis, and the presence of associated structural heart disease all influence the therapeutic approach. For example, a fetus presenting at 38 weeks gestation with sustained supraventricular tachycardia and mild hydrops fetalis should be treated by urgent delivery and management of the arrhythmia after birth. Conversely, a 26-week gestation fetus with supraventricular tachycardia and no evidence of hydrops fetalis should be monitored closely with consideration of drug therapy if there are sustained or prolonged episodes of tachycardia. If a fetus with supraventricular tachycardia and significant hydrops fetalis is thought to be nonviable because of extreme prematurity, then aggressive intrauterine therapy is indicated in an effort to maintain sinus rhythm and promote resolution of fetal hydrops. In this case, therapy can be continued until elective delivery closer to term.

Currently, the most common indication for fetal cardiovascular drug therapy is intrauterine supraventricular tachycardia. The mainstay of diagnosis and monitoring efficacy remains fetal echocardiography. Although techniques are under development for recording the fetal ECG, these are cumbersome, labor-intensive, and limited to use at a handful of centers at present. A combination of two-dimensional, Doppler, and M-mode echocardiography can generally provide sufficient information to determine the fetal atrial and ventricular rates and insights into the mechanism of the tachyarrhythmia.

In general, most supraventricular tachycardias in newborn infants are relatively easy to control medically. In contrast, management of fetal arrhythmias is less likely to be successful. Difficulties in controlling fetal arrhythmias are largely related to the inability to maintain a sufficiently high drug concentration in the mother to provide an effective concentration in the fetus. At present, the drugs most commonly used for controlling fetal supraventricular tachycardia are digoxin, sotalol, and flecainide (generally in that order of priority). Amiodarone is reserved as a last choice agent due to unreliable placental transfer and the potential for thyroid toxicity in the fetus. Other drugs and drug combinations have been used, including procainamide, propafenone, and digoxin plus verapamil, but with variable, and generally, much less success.

Maternal drug toxicity often limits the successful use of antiarrhythmic agents for treating fetal supraventricular tachycardia. Many of these drugs have toxic effects, including proarrhythmia. Maternal toxicity is common because high maternal doses are often necessary to ensure adequate transplacental passage of the drug to the fetus. It is helpful to involve adult cardiologists experienced with the use of these drugs to help follow the mother and to monitor for adverse maternal effects.

Direct drug administration to the fetus via the umbilical vein, intraperitoneal administration or fetal intramuscular injection is possible and has the advantage of bypassing the maternal and placental components. Drugs that have been reportedly administered by these routes include adenosine, propafenone, digoxin, amiodarone, and flecainide. However, in most instances the experience is limited and specific details are lacking. Although some centers may advocate these approaches as the preferred method (especially for cases of hydrops fetalis), they are technically more demanding, may incur greater risk to the fetus, and are generally reserved for selected high-risk situations.

Bradycardia

Fetal bradycardia is defined as a ventricular rate less than 100 beats/min. Transient episodes of slowing of the heart rate that last less than a minute or two are common and benign, especially during the first and second trimesters. These brief episodes are attributed to sinus bradycardia and do not require any special intervention. However, a prolonged or persistent decrease in heart rate may be due to pathological conditions that cause sinus bradycardia such as fetal hypoxia, congenital sinus node dysfunction (rare), or long QT syndrome. Atrial bigeminy

or trigeminy with blocked premature beats may result in a low average heart rate, but these conditions are generally benign and resolve spontaneously. It is important to differentiate blocked premature beats from second- or third-degree atrioventricular block.

Although rare (occurring in 1 in 15,000-22,000 live births), third-degree or complete atrioventricular block is irreversible and potentially life threatening. Complete atrioventricular block is associated with structural cardiovascular malformations in about 50% of fetuses. The most common structural malformation is heterotaxy syndrome with left atrial isomerism, occurring in nearly 70% of cases. The remainder of fetuses with complete atrioventricular block and structural heart disease generally have some form of discordant atrioventricular and ventriculoarterial connections, although hypoplastic right heart syndrome, ventricular septal defect, and tetralogy of Fallot have all been associated with complete atrioventricular block, albeit infrequently. Fetal diagnosis of left atrial isomerism should prompt careful evaluation and follow-up in anticipation of atrioventricular block, and likewise, in utero diagnosis of complete atrioventricular block requires a thorough structural evaluation. Fetal complete atrioventricular block in the setting of heterotaxy syndrome has a poor prognosis, with combined fetal and neonatal survival rates of 20% or less. Direct pacing of the fetal heart has been reported in only a few isolated cases and is without long-term success. Additional technical improvements and new approaches are necessary for fetal cardiac pacing to become a reasonable option. Thus, treatment at present is limited to maternal administration of beta-sympathomimetic agents such as salbutamol or terbutaline. These drugs have been shown to increase fetal heart rate by 10% to 20%, but it is not clear that there is any beneficial impact on overall fetal mortality. However, if hydrops fetalis develops in this setting, it seems prudent to attempt drug therapy and if no benefit is seen, then delivery of the infant should be considered.

In the remaining 50% of cases without structural heart disease, complete atrioventricular block is attributed to transplacental passage of maternal IgG antibodies (anti-SSA/Ro or anti-SSB/La) in the setting of maternal connective tissue diseases, most commonly systemic lupus erythematosus or Sjögren syndrome. The incidence of congenital complete atrioventricular block in first pregnancies among mothers with connective tissue disorders is around 2% and increases to up to 18% for recurrent pregnancies. It is thought that the maternal antibodies promote inflammation of the developing conduction system and myocardium, resulting in atrioventricular block and myocardial dysfunction. However, the mere presence of anti-SSA/Ro or anti-SSB/La in the mother does not necessarily mean that the fetus will develop atrioventricular block. Indeed, the minority of pregnancies in this situation result in fetal atrioventricular block. Atrioventricular block generally occurs after 18-weeks gestation, peaks around 20 to 24 weeks, and almost always occurs before 30 to 32 weeks. In general, the prognosis for autoimmune-mediated complete atrioventricular block is better than that in the setting of structural heart disease, but still carries an overall fetal/neonatal mortality rate of approximately 25%.

Given the proposed pathogenesis of atrioventricular block (inflammation of the developing conduction system), it seems logical that the administration of anti-inflammatory agents to the mother might prevent or ameliorate atrioventricular block in the fetus. Given the low incidence, it has been difficult to resolve this issue and considerable controversy exists regarding the efficacy of such agents administered to the mother. There have been a small number of case studies of maternal plasma exchange or administration of immunoglobulins or azathioprine, but the numbers are too small to allow meaningful conclusions.

Administration of steroids to the mother has been performed more commonly in this setting, but considerable controversy persists. Despite this, analysis of the results from studies of maternal steroid therapy for fetal atrioventricular block reveals several consistent findings. First, fluorinated corticosteroids, such as dexamethasone or betamethasone, must be administered since these are only minimally metabolized by the placenta (in contrast to prednisone which is largely inactivated by placental metabolism and exhibits poor transfer to the fetus). Second, there is a general consensus that complete atrioventricular block is irreversible and steroid therapy is not effective in reversing this condition. Third, progression to complete atrioventricular block can be very rapid and occur within 1 week following a normal fetal echocardiogram.

Lastly, the major area of remaining controversy surrounds the potential efficacy of steroids in preventing progression of first- or second-degree atrioventricular block to complete atrioventricular block. There is some evidence, based on a limited number of cases, that if prolongation of the PR interval (first-degree atrioventricular block) is detected in the fetus, then maternal steroid therapy limits

progression to complete atrioventricular block. Measurement of fetal PR interval by conventional Doppler techniques may not be sufficiently accurate and it is likely that larger trials using fetal ECG recording or measuring spectral tissue Doppler-derived atrioventricular intervals will be necessary to resolve this issue. Given the potential adverse effects (both short and long term) of steroid therapy on the fetus, careful consideration to this form of therapy is necessary. However, the risk of therapy must be balanced against the high mortality and morbidity associated with congenital complete atrioventricular block. Given the existing information, if a prolonged PR interval is diagnosed in the fetus of a mother with anti-SSA/Ro or anti-SSB/La antibodies, it seems reasonable to initiate steroid therapy.

■ FETAL INTERVENTIONAL CATHETERIZATION

During the past few decades, with the advent of more widespread use of fetal echocardiography, we have gained additional insights into the natural progression of various cardiovascular malformations detected in utero. It is clear that some conditions such as severe aortic stenosis and severe pulmonary stenosis can progress to hypoplastic left heart syndrome and hypoplastic right heart syndrome, respectively. As both of these conditions continue to carry relatively high postnatal morbidity and mortality, it is reasonable to consider fetal intervention in an effort to promote ventricular growth and preserve a biventricular circulation after birth. Similarly, an intact interatrial septum or a severely restrictive foramen ovale complicating d-transposition of the great arteries or hypoplastic left heart syndrome is associated with poor fetal and neonatal outcomes because of compromised fetal circulation and injury to the developing pulmonary vascular bed. This is another situation in which fetal intervention might be anticipated to improve long-term outcomes.

Fetal intervention for aortic or pulmonary valve stenosis or an obstructed atrial septum remains controversial and is limited to only a few centers worldwide. The risks to the fetus and the mother must be considered, especially if maternal general anesthesia is utilized as the intervention has the potential for jeopardizing two lives. In addition, as the neonatal management of these conditions improves (both surgical and catheter-based interventions), there must be a compelling evidence that fetal intervention is highly likely to be superior to conventional postnatal intervention alone to justify the risk to mother and fetus. Unfortunately, there are no randomized controlled trials upon which to judge the efficacy of fetal interventional catheterization. Furthermore, the ability to predict which fetus with aortic or pulmonary stenosis will progress to a functional univentricular circulation is imprecise.

It is beyond the scope of this textbook to describe specific technical details of fetal interventional cardiac catheterization, but a team approach is necessary. Following either local or general anesthesia for the mother, the maternal fetal high-risk obstetrician uses ultrasound guidance and aseptic technique to introduce a long needle through the maternal abdomen and uterus into the fetal chest. An anesthetic agent (generally fentanyl) is administered to the fetus (intramuscularly, intravenously, or into a cardiac chamber) and some centers administer a muscle relaxant, as well. Alignment of the needle along the right or left ventricular outflow tract is essential, at which point a guide wire is introduced, over which a balloon catheter can be advanced. The balloon is positioned across the aortic or pulmonary valve and inflated and deflated, much like when conventional balloon valvuloplasty is performed in neonates or infants. In cases of an atretic pulmonary valve, the valve can be perforated with a needle, followed by balloon dilation. Similar techniques are used to create an opening in an intact atrial septum.

The degree of success from these approaches is debatable and extends beyond simply achieving technical success (crossing the valve and inflating the balloon successfully). Success must be measured by favorable biventricular morphology and function, a normal or near normal pulmonary vascular bed, and in the longer term, improved functional and neurodevelopmental outcomes. At present, this is an evolving field and much remains to be learned regarding patient selection, timing of intervention, and long-term outcomes before firm recommendations can be made. Additional details regarding short-term outcomes and technical aspects are provided in publications listed at the end of this chapter.

SUGGESTED READINGS

General Aspects of Fetal Cardiology and Echocardiography

Allan L, Hornberger LK, Sharland G. *Textbook of Fetal Cardiology*. London, United Kingdom: Greenwich Medical Media; 2000.

Allan LD, Cook AC, Huggon IC. *Fetal Echocardiography: A Practical Guide*. New York, NY: Cambridge University Press; 2009.

Chiappa EM, Cook AC, Botta G, Silverman NH. *Echocardiographic Anatomy in the Fetus*. London, United Kingdom: Springer; 2009.

Clur SA, Ottenkamp J, Bilardo CM. The nuchal translucency and the fetal heart: a literature review. *Prenat Diagn*. 2009; 29(8):739-748.

Drose, JA. *Fetal Echocardiography*. St. Louis, MO: Saunders; 2010.

Habli M, Lim FY, Crombleholme T. Twin-to-twin transfusion syndrome: a comprehensive update. *Clin Perinatol*. 2009;36:391-416.

Jone P-N, Schowengerdt KO. Prenatal diagnosis of congenital heart disease. *Pediatr Clin North Am*. 2009;56(3):709-715.

Sklansky MS, Berman DP, Pruetz JD, Chang R-KR. Prenatal screening for major congenital heart disease. *J Ultrasound Med*. 2009;28:889-899.

Turan S, Turan O, Baschat AA. Three- and four-dimensional fetal echocardiography. *Fetal Diagn Ther*. 2009;25:361-372.

Yagel S, Gembruch U, Silverman NH, eds. *Fetal Cardiology: Embryology, Genetics, Physiology, Echocardiographic Evaluation, Diagnosis and Perinatal Management of Cardiac Disease*. London, United Kingdom: Informa Healthcare; 2008.

Diagnosis and Management of Fetal Arrhythmias

Api O, Carvalho JS. Fetal dysrhythmias. *Best Pract Res Clin Obstet Gynaecol*. 2008;22(1):31-48.

Jaeggi ET, Friedberg MK. Diagnosis and management of fetal bradyarrhythmias. *PACE*. 2008;31:S50-S53.

Jaeggi ET, Nii M. Fetal brady- and tachyarrhythmias: new and accepted diagnostic and treatment methods. *Semin Fetal Neonatal Med*. 2005;10:504-514.

Li Z, Strasburger JF, Cuneo BF, Gotteiner NL, Wakai RT. Giant fetal magnetocardiogram P waves in congenital atrioventricular block. *Circulation*. 2004;110:2097-2101.

Lopes LM, Tavares GMP, Damiano AP, et al. Perinatal outcomes of fetal atrioventricular block: one-hundred-sixteen cases from a single institution. *Circulation*. 2008;118: 1268-1275.

Maeno Y, Hirose A, Kanbe T, Hori D. Fetal arrhythmia: prenatal diagnosis and perinatal management. *J Obstet Gynaecol Res*. 2009;35(4):623-629.

Mevorach D, Elchalal U, Rein AJJT. Prevention of complete heart block in children of mothers with anti-SSA/Ro and anti-SSB/La autoantibodies: detection and treatment of first-degree atrioventricular block. *Curr Opin Rheumatol*. 2009;21:478-482.

Strasburger JF, Cheulkar B, Wichman HJ. Perinatal arrhythmias: diagnosis and management. *Clin Perinatol*. 2007; 34:627-652.

Fetal Interventional Catheterization

Gardiner HM. The case for fetal cardiac intervention. *Heart.* 2009;95:1648-1652.

Matsui H, Gardiner H. Fetal intervention for cardiac disease: The cutting edge of perinatal care. *Semin Fetal Neonatal Med.* 2007;12:482-489.

McElhinney DB, Marshall AC, Wilkins-Huag LE, et al. Predictors of technical success and postnatal biventricular outcome after in utero aortic valvuloplasty for aortic stenosis with evolving hypoplastic left heart syndrome. *Circulation.* 2009;120:1482-1490.

Pavlovic M, Acharya G, Huhta JC. Controversies of fetal cardiac intervention. *Early Hum Devel.* 2008;84:149-153.

Turner CGB, Tworetzky W, Wilkins-Huag LE, Jennings RW. Cardiac anomalies in the fetus. *Clin Perinatol.* 2009; 36:439-449.

Tworetzky W, McElhinney DB, Marx GR, et al. In utero valvuloplasty for pulmonary atresia with hypoplastic right ventricle: techniques and outcomes. *Pediatrics.* 2009; 124:e510-e518.

Initial Evaluation of the Newborn With Suspected Cardiovascular Disease

■ INTRODUCTION

Critical Congenital Heart Disease: Extent of the Problem

Congenital heart disease occurs in about 1% of live births (excluding bicuspid aortic valve and hemodynamically insignificant lesions such as small atrial and ventricular septal defects). Critical congenital heart disease consists of a group of defects which will result in death or severe morbidity if unrecognized in early infancy. Such defects often depend on patency of the ductus arteriosus to maintain either pulmonary or systemic blood flow. Signs of rapidly progressive heart failure and cardiovascular collapse develop as the ductus arteriosus constricts during the first few days after birth. It is important to recognize that a newborn with critical congenital heart disease may show little evidence of cardiovascular compromise on physical examination in the first 24 to 48 hours of life. Cardiovascular instability may not occur until after the infant is discharged from the hospital.

Approximately 4,300,000 children were born in the United States in 2006, which means that about 43,000 infants were born with heart defects. Of all such infants, almost one-third are predicted to have critical heart disease, defined as a heart defect that is likely to cause death within 2 months of age if undiagnosed. Thus, it is estimated that over 14,000 infants are born with critical congenital heart disease in the United States each year. Diagnosis before the onset of cardiovascular decompensation is essential for optimal outcome. However, of those not diagnosed as a fetus, about 70% of infants with critical heart disease are not diagnosed before 2 days of age and about 20% are discharged from hospital undiagnosed. This leads to severe morbidity and mortality in many hundreds of newborns each year in the United States alone, at a large social and economic cost. Thus, it is incumbent upon all physicians and other health care professionals who care for newborns to rigorously evaluate every newborn for the possibility of critical heart disease. Furthermore, if there is any indication that such disease might exist, the infant must be referred for further evaluation without delay.

Presentation of Congenital Heart Disease: An Overview

The evaluation of the infant to exclude critical heart disease should focus on the three cardinal signs of neonatal cardiovascular distress: **cyanosis**, **decreased systemic perfusion**, and **tachypnea**. Cyanosis may be appreciated by careful visual inspection and pulse oximetry, decreased systemic perfusion is identified by examination of the extremities, and tachypnea is noted by observing the respiratory rate and pattern. The presence of a congenital heart defect (or less commonly, a cardiomyopathy or arrhythmia) must be considered in the differential diagnosis of any infant with one or more of these findings. A cyanotic infant likely has underlying heart disease, and almost certainly does in the absence of significant respiratory distress. An infant with decreased systemic perfusion may be septic or have a primary metabolic abnormality, but about one-half of such infants have symptomatic heart disease. An infant who has tachypnea without either cyanosis or decreased perfusion usually has primary parenchymal or extraparenchymal lung disease but may have a primary cardiac defect. A thoughtful and rational approach to the differential diagnosis of all three of these signs is important for prompt recognition and appropriate management. Moreover, the clinician must be cognizant of the fact that the transition from a fetal to a mature postnatal circulation does not occur immediately but rather over the first several days or weeks of life, so that serial evaluations are necessary, each as rigorous as the first.

Each cardinal sign of neonatal heart disease can be attributed to one of at least two pathophysiologic causes:

Cyanosis
1. Decreased pulmonary blood flow
2. Normal to increased pulmonary blood flow but with a transposed aorta, for example, simple d-transposition of the great arteries

Decreased systemic perfusion
1. Obstruction of the left heart (inflow or outflow)
2. Cardiac dysfunction without obstruction (primary cardiomyopathy or secondary dysfunction)

Tachypnea (due to excessive pulmonary blood flow)
1. Exclusive left-to-right shunt
2. Dominant left-to-right shunt with a lesser right-to-left shunt

The cardiac defects in each hemodynamic category are discussed in Chapters 6 (cyanosis), 7 (tachypnea), and 8 (decreased systemic perfusion). This chapter will describe the general approach to the cardiovascular evaluation of the newborn, including history, physical examination, and ancillary tests. The information obtained from each step of the evaluation should lead in a logical progression, from recognizing the primary sign, defining the underlying pathophysiologic process, and eventually determining the specific diagnosis. The latter is rarely important at the initial evaluation. Understanding the pathophysiologic process allows effective initiation of therapy and stabilization of the patient. The specific diagnosis is usually only important to implement the definitive therapeutic plan.

From these considerations a focused and rational approach to the newborn with symptomatic congenital heart disease can be developed. Admittedly, this approach is imperfect; some lesions are complex with overlapping manifestations (eg, an infant with hypoplastic left heart syndrome who has decreased systemic perfusion may also be tachypneic and mildly cyanotic). However, even in the most complex cases, one of the major signs usually predominates and provides a clue to the most likely category of disease. The concepts described in this and other chapters emphasize the importance of a simple, clear, logical, and stepwise approach to the evaluation and treatment of each infant with heart disease.

■ HISTORY

The prenatal evaluation of the newborn for congenital heart disease is reviewed in Chapter 4, including the evaluation of the fetus with a family history of congenital heart disease or a genetic syndrome which is associated with heart disease. In the absence of such a history, aspects of the immediate perinatal history that suggest heart disease as the cause of a postnatal problem probably can best be considered in the negative. That is, the more benign the perinatal history, the more likely that a problem causing symptoms is cardiac in origin. It is often not until the signs become manifest over the first hours, days, or weeks of life, that the history becomes significant.

Cyanosis is caused by either congenital heart disease, pulmonary hypertension of the newborn, or intra- or extraparenchymal lung disease. The primary differential diagnosis of congenital heart disease is persistent pulmonary hypertension of the newborn. The cyanotic infant with primary parenchymal lung disease usually has severe respiratory distress requiring mechanical ventilation and has an abnormal chest radiograph. The infant with pulmonary hypertension may only have mild or moderate respiratory distress, and a perinatal history of birth asphyxia, with or without meconium aspiration. Additionally, the infant may be small for gestational age, or the mother may have taken nonsteroidal anti-inflammatory medications over the weeks prior to birth, which can cause intrauterine constriction of the ductus arteriosus and subsequent pulmonary hypertension.

The infant with cyanotic heart disease typically has a benign birth history with a normal or nearly normal Apgar score. The ductus arteriosus usually maintains adequate blood flow and mixing immediately after birth and cyanosis is not readily apparent. It is not until hours or days after birth that the infant becomes cyanotic, frequently during feeding or crying. The increased physical effort associated with feeding or crying increases oxygen consumption and decreases pulmonary blood flow, resulting in cyanosis. Despite the presence of cyanosis, a history of respiratory distress is usually not obtained. The chemoreceptor response to hypoxemia is intact so that mild tachypnea often occurs but respiratory distress (eg, retractions, nasal flaring, grunting) is usually absent because ventilation is normal. Early discharge to home of newborn infants is increasingly common. It is thus important to recognize even mild cyanosis on the first or second day of life because progression to severe hypoxemia may not occur until after discharge. If there is any question, then pulse oximetry should be performed to determine oxygen saturation if not performed routinely.

At times when a newborn infant cries, a transient increase in right atrial pressure occurs and results in a small right-to-left shunt through the foramen ovale, causing the infant to appear dusky. This transient desaturation must be distinguished from infants with cyanotic heart disease who may also appear dusky initially only with crying or feeding. Although not apparently cyanotic at rest, infants with cyanotic congenital heart disease show some degree of oxygen desaturation by pulse oximetry at all times, whereas the normal newborn infant has normal oxygen saturation at rest.

The differential diagnosis of **decreased systemic perfusion** includes obstructive heart disease and myocardial dysfunction from sepsis, hematological abnormalities (anemia and polycythemia), or endocrine/metabolic disorders such as hypocalcemia, hypoglycemia, and metabolic acidosis. Neonatal sepsis is common, especially in the setting of prolonged rupture of the membranes. Hematological abnormalities are associated with placenta abruptio, twin-to-twin transfusion, placental insufficiency, post-term delivery, or small-for-gestational age infants. A positive family history is often present in newborns with endocrine/metabolic diseases. Newborns with obstructive heart disease rarely have a positive perinatal history. These infants typically are stable during the first hours of life, but eventually develop poor feeding, pallor, diaphoresis, and tachypnea with respiratory distress. This may occur as late as 3 to 4 weeks after birth, so it is extremely important for every infant to be carefully assessed at the time of discharge and at subsequent visits during the first month of life. Subtle findings of irritability, pallor, poor feeding, or diaphoresis may reflect inadequate systemic perfusion.

Tachypnea is often a subtle finding that develops over days or weeks, as pulmonary vascular resistance and hemoglobin concentration decline. Thus, tachypnea immediately after birth, in the absence of signs of cyanosis or decreased systemic perfusion, usually points to pulmonary disease rather than heart disease. Parents rarely appreciate that an infant is breathing more rapidly than normal. Poor feeding with associated failure to thrive and diaphoresis is common; murmurs may be absent. Thus, an infant with unexplained failure to thrive, particularly in association with tachypnea and diaphoresis, should be evaluated for possible congenital heart disease.

■ FAMILY HISTORY

A family history of congenital cardiovascular defects or cardiomyopathy is relevant to the outcome of the fetus as a positive family history increases the risk for subsequent children. Genetic abnormalities are increasingly recognized to contribute to congenital heart disease and are discussed in Chapter 15.

■ PHYSICAL EXAMINATION

Pulse Oximetry as a Screening Test

For the past several years there has been a controversy as to whether screening pulse oximetry should be performed in all newborns shortly after birth. Because this issue is essential to resolve before presenting the physical examination of the newborn, this section of the chapter will present a discussion of the issue at this juncture.

In the past, a number of studies have shown that physical examination by pediatric residents is unreliable for the detection of critical heart disease. However, more recent studies have demonstrated that even the expert cardiologist and neonatologist frequently miss such diseases. In a highly reputable neonatal unit in England, the timing of the diagnosis of critical heart disease was followed for 20 years, from 1985 through 2004. Of the over 600 patients diagnosed, 25% were diagnosed in living infants after discharge from hospital and 5% were diagnosed after death. There was no trend to a decrease in these percentages over the 20 years. In another large study from Sweden, by 2 days of age, 20% of newborns with critical heart disease were discharged without diagnosis, and the percentage actually increased over the 8 years of study, from 13% to 26%. Even more concerning was the finding that 75% of newborns with ductal dependent pulmonary circulation and 60% of newborns with ductal dependent systemic circulation were not diagnosed by 2 days of age, the time by which most term newborns in the United States have been discharged from the hospital. If one accepts our conservative estimate at the beginning of this chapter that 20% of infants with critical heart disease are discharged from the hospital without diagnosis in the United States, about 700 newborns are sent home without diagnosis. There is no doubt that the morbidity and mortality of these infants far exceeds that of newborns diagnosed as fetuses or after birth but prior to discharge.

The ability of a screening test such as pulse oximetry to detect critical heart disease (true positive), and the frequency and cost of false-positive findings are important to consider. A number of investigators have studied the course of oxygen saturation as determined by pulse oximetry after birth. Using newer oximeters with an error of less than 3%, Levesque and his colleagues measured pulse oximetry at birth, at 24 hours, and at discharge in nearly 1800 normal term newborns. The overall mean saturation over their course in hospital was 97.2%, and the saturation two standard deviations below the mean was 94%.

Importantly, the saturation increased on average only 0.17% over the course of hospitalization, indicating that oxygen saturation becomes normal very soon after birth. Also, there was no difference between newborns born vaginally and those born by cesarean section. Several other studies demonstrate similar findings, so that most investigators recommend an oxygen saturation of 95% or greater as normal. Of course, normal levels will vary among institutions depending on altitude, the pulse oximeter used, and the method of measurement.

The general practice in those institutions using pulse oximetry for screening is to record the oxygen saturation around 24 hours of age, with the newborn at rest, and on the foot, in order not to miss left heart obstruction. For example, the newborn with severe coarctation of the aorta often presents at birth with normal upper body saturations and mildly decreased lower body saturations. Because such infants usually have adequate lower body blood flow in the first few days of life because the ductus arteriosus remains patent (Chapter 8), this lesion constitutes the most common form of critical heart disease in which the patient is discharged without appropriate diagnosis. This is particularly concerning to the cardiologist because infants with coarctation are usually easily repaired surgically, yet many are left with severe morbidity, or die, because of late diagnosis. Some institutions also perform pulse oximetry on the right hand, in order to diagnose the rare patient with transposed great arteries and aortic coarctation, who might have normal saturations in the lower body.

Newborns with saturations under 90% are usually referred for cardiology evaluation, and those with saturations between 90% and 94% and without clinical findings undergo a second screen within 12 hours. Using this approach, the overall false-positive rate across a number of studies is less than 0.20%, and less than 0.05% if performed on the second day of life. This compares very favorably to a study from the Swedish group which found a false-positive rate of nearly 2% from clinical examination without pulse oximetry, and a false-positive rate of only 0.18% using pulse oximetry.

The low false-positive rate (assuming the addition of a second screen for borderline saturations) and the low cost of the test are (largely limited to the cost of the probe; even lower if the probe is reused) combined to minimize the overall financial impact of false-positive results. Considering the cost of the tests and of a cardiology evaluation for newborns who fail two tests, the cost of false-positive pulse oximetry screening is far less than that of false-positive results from newborn metabolic screening performed commonly in the United States. Conversely, the true-positive cost of pulse oximetry compares very favorably to newborn metabolic screening. From a meta-analysis of a large number of studies on pulse oximetry screening, Hoffman has estimated that the true-positive cost is about $9000 per critical heart disease patient diagnosed. When compared to the cost associated with the increased morbidity of late diagnosis, not to mention the devastation to the family of a neonatal death, this cost is acceptable. Lastly, the false-negative rates are quite low, and almost all of such patients had coarctation of the aorta. Careful evaluation of upper and lower body pulses in such patients can improve their timely diagnosis (Chapter 8).

Given the likely benefits and relatively low costs, it is time to incorporate routine pulse oximetry screening in the evaluation of all newborns.

The Cardiovascular Examination

The physical examination should be performed systematically. Each step determines if the infant falls into a specific mode of presentation (cyanosis, decreased systemic perfusion, or excessive pulmonary blood flow), and once defined, into a specific hemodynamic category. Ancillary tests assist in establishing specific diagnoses and defining the most appropriate therapy for each infant.

The general examination includes vital signs and observation of the unclothed and warm infant. The vital signs of temperature, heart rate, respiratory rate, and blood pressure are measured, in conjunction with respiratory status, perfusion, and color. As discussed above, we consider pulse oximetry to be a vital sign in the newborn and believe that it is essential to measure oxygen saturation in one foot at birth, and if less than normal (95% in most hospitals), it should be measured again no more than 12 hours later. Weight, length, and head circumference are measured and plotted on growth charts to aid in identifying growth impairment. Any postnatal decrease in weight percentiles compared to length and head circumference should raise the possibility of heart disease. This is of particular importance in lesions of excessive pulmonary blood flow—the other signs of cyanosis and hypoperfusion are not present, and there may be no murmurs or discernible respiratory distress.

The first sign to assess on general observation is **cyanosis**. Peripheral cyanosis (acrocyanosis) is common in newborn infants, and reflects the normally unstable peripheral vasomotor tone. Central cyanosis, which is indicative of arterial oxygen desaturation, is the important sign to recognize. Thus, vascular beds with little vasoconstrictor tone such as the tongue, gums, and the buccal mucosa should be evaluated (not the hands, feet, or perioral region). It is also important to evaluate the patient during conditions such as feeding or crying which are most likely to produce central cyanosis. Cyanosis is difficult to perceive until arterial oxygen saturation is less than about 85% and decreased hemoglobin concentration makes detecting cyanosis more difficult. Thus, oxygen saturation should be measured if there is any question of cyanosis. Measuring oxygen saturation simultaneously in the right hand and a lower extremity by use of two pulse oximeters is necessary to evaluate whether the upper and lower bodies are perfused, at least partially, by different ventricles. A difference in oxygen saturation of only 3% to 5% may be significant, but most oximeters are only accurate to within ±2% to 3%. For this reason, it may be helpful to reverse the probes to ensure that any difference (or absence of a difference) is real and not just related to inherent variations in the probes or oximeters. Less commonly, it may be necessary to measure the oxygen saturation in an ear lobe if aortic arch and arch vessel anomalies are suspected (Chapter 6).

Next, the **respiratory status** should be carefully evaluated. Infants who have isolated cyanosis are usually tachypneic but do not otherwise exhibit increased work of breathing. In contrast, the increased pulmonary venous pressures and pulmonary edema seen in patients with hypoperfusion cause respiratory distress in addition to tachypnea. In that case, variable intercostal and/or subcostal retractions, nasal flaring, and grunting may be observed.

Signs of **decreased systemic perfusion** including the temperature and color of the skin, blood pressure, peripheral pulses, and capillary refill in each extremity should be assessed next. Lower extremity pulses are more easily palpated in the feet rather than in the inguinal area. If the infant has a normal dorsalis pedis or posterior tibial pulse, then pulsatile blood flow to the lower extremity is not impaired. Blood pressure should be measured in the upper and lower extremities; normally the lower extremity blood pressure is slightly greater than that in the upper extremity. The left subclavian artery arises from the aortic isthmus and may be involved in a coarctation. Thus, the systolic pressures in the right arm and either leg should be measured simultaneously. If the pulses are decreased and no blood pressure differential is detected, the carotid arteries should be palpated. If they are increased, the infant may have a coarctation or interruption of the aorta and also have a right subclavian artery arising anomalously from the descending aorta.

The periphery, head, and neck should be examined for dysmorphic features of syndromes associated with heart disease, such as 22q11 deletion (DiGeorge) syndrome and trisomy 21 (Chapter 15).

At this point in the examination, it has been determined whether the infant has cyanosis, decreased systemic perfusion, or tachypnea. Examination of the abdomen, lungs, and heart then assists in defining the hemodynamic category. Heart murmurs are common in many normal infants and are absent in about 50% of infants with symptomatic cardiovascular disease. Thus, the mere presence of a murmur is of little value to the examination, as is its absence. However, specific murmurs are much more likely to be appreciated if the clinician has a differential diagnosis in mind at the time when auscultation is performed. Moreover, the presence of a nonspecific murmur is of much less concern in an infant who has an otherwise normal examination.

The abdomen should be palpated because hepatomegaly is often a sign of right atrial hypertension or increased circulating volume from excessive pulmonary blood flow. The location of the liver and stomach is reversed in situs inversus. The liver may be midline in situs ambiguous, either appearing to be two right lobes (right atrial isomerism, or asplenia syndrome) or two left lobes (left atrial isomerism, or polysplenia syndrome).

Examination of the lungs includes inspection of the pattern and work of breathing, the symmetry of chest movement, and auscultation. Because of the small size of the patient, normal breath sounds in one lung field may reflect ventilation of the other lung.

The cardiac examination begins with palpation of the precordium to assess right ventricular pressure and volume load. Unlike the older patient, the normal newborn infant has a parasternal and subxiphoid impulse, because the sternum is thin and the right ventricle is thick-walled. The parasternal and subxiphoid impulses are increased in most infants with cyanotic heart disease because the right ventricle is ejecting at or above systemic pressure into a transposed aorta or against right ventricular outflow obstruction. A decreased right ventricular impulse in a cyanotic patient is suggestive of inflow obstruction to the right ventricle, either tricuspid atresia or hypoplastic right heart syndrome. A parasternal thrill suggests the presence of a ventricular septal defect, but only a small minority of

infants with ventricular septal defects have thrills at birth. Therefore, the absence of a thrill is not useful in excluding the presence of a ventricular septal defect, but its presence is very helpful in a cyanotic newborn. The presence of a parasternal thrill in a cyanotic infant is diagnostic of tricuspid atresia with ventricular septal defect, because this is only form of cyanotic heart disease in which the ventricular shunt is directed anteriorly toward the sternum from the left ventricle to the right ventricle. The left ventricular apical impulse is not usually palpable in a normal newborn infant because the dominant right ventricle displaces the left ventricle posteriorly. A palpable left ventricular impulse usually indicates increased left ventricular volume load as the ventricular cavity dilates and extends anteriorly and laterally. In contrast, increased left ventricular pressure load often does not cause a palpable impulse. A suprasternal notch thrill is suggestive of turbulence from valvar, or supravalvar aortic stenosis.

Auscultation should be performed in a systematic manner. The first heart sound is rarely helpful, but may be louder than normal in the infant with a complete atrioventricular septal defect. The quality of the second heart sound provides important information. Although it is often difficult to appreciate splitting of the second heart sound in the newborn because of the rapid heart rate, the presence of a clearly split second heart sound is suggestive of markedly increased pulmonary blood flow. This may lead the clinician toward the diagnosis of total anomalous pulmonary venous connection or a large arteriovenous malformation. Most cyanotic infants have a single heart sound because the pulmonary valve is either diminutive or atretic, or because it is malposed, posterior to the aorta. The presence of a split second heart sound in a cyanotic infant strongly suggests total anomalous pulmonary venous connection.

After listening to the normal heart sounds, the presence of clicks and gallops should be evaluated. Clicks may be difficult to hear, but when present usually indicate a bicuspid aortic valve or persistent truncus arteriosus. A click is not present in patients with severe aortic or pulmonic stenosis because valve mobility is greatly decreased. In contrast, truncus arteriosus can frequently be diagnosed in the patient with tachypnea and modest desaturation based on the presence of an ejection click. Such clicks are commonly heard because the truncal valve is almost always dysplastic. The click is often closer to the apex rather than in the region of the semilunar valve. Mid-systolic clicks are rarely heard, but may be present in Ebstein anomaly or in newborns with severe mitral valve prolapse that occur in neonatal Marfan patients. Gallop rhythms may be present in newborn infants with severe left ventricular dysfunction.

Auscultation of heart murmurs may define specific diagnoses based upon unique features of the murmurs. A murmur is best localized by determining the location of its highest-frequency components because high-frequency sounds radiate very short distances as compared to lower frequency sounds. Loudness may be a poor indicator of the site of origin because most clinicians hear low-frequency components as being louder than high-frequency components. Thus, when the highest-frequency components of a murmur are heard in the left axilla, the source is likely extracardiac in origin, and the diagnosis of peripheral pulmonary artery stenosis in a normal newborn infant can be made. In addition to localization of the source of a murmur, focusing on its frequency allows the clinician to determine whether more than one murmur is present. While following the radiation of a murmur, if there is an increase in the frequency after a decrease, it is likely that a second systolic murmur is present.

The frequency of a murmur reflects the degree of turbulence, which correlates directly with the pressure gradient. A high-frequency murmur indicates a high-pressure gradient and a low-frequency murmur indicates a low gradient. Mid-diastolic murmurs are difficult to appreciate because they are of very low frequency, and are often noticed as the absence of silence in diastole. Conversely, early diastolic murmurs caused by semilunar valve insufficiency are usually easy to hear because the pressure gradient is greater and the murmur is thus in an easily audible frequency range. If a murmur of semilunar valve insufficiency is heard in a newborn without significant respiratory distress, the diagnosis is usually truncus arteriosus. Stenotic aortic and pulmonary valves are rarely insufficient at birth. If the newborn has severe respiratory distress in addition to the diastolic murmur of semilunar valve insufficiency, the diagnosis is usually absent pulmonary valve syndrome. In this lesion, the patient has very large pulmonary arteries which compress the bronchi, leading to severe respiratory distress. The cardiac disease is usually a mild form of tetralogy of Fallot, and the absence of pulmonary valve tissue leads to a characteristic to-and-fro murmur.

■ ANCILLARY TESTS

Arterial Blood Gases

As mentioned earlier, measurement of oxygen saturation by pulse oximetry should be performed in all newborns at some time in the first 1 to 2 days of life. It should be done at least in one foot, and many centers will also measure it in the right hand. In a newborn with any findings suggestive of heart disease, oxygen saturation should definitely be measured in the right hand and one foot, and any abnormality should lead to further investigation including the measurement of arterial blood gases. It is also important to measure arterial blood gases in any infant who has respiratory distress, even with normal pulse oximetry. Blood gases determine not only the oxygen content of arterial blood, but also the extent of the oxygen debt and an infant's ability to compensate for a metabolic acidosis by decreasing CO_2, which is particularly valuable in patients who might have decreased systemic perfusion.

Electrocardiogram

Unless an arrhythmia is present (Chapter 10), an electrocardiogram is of limited value in making a specific diagnosis at birth for many defects. The right ventricle is dominant in utero, and thus a pattern of right ventricular hypertrophy is present in the normal newborn: right axis deviation, prominent R waves and upright T waves in the right precordium, and septal Q waves positioned very laterally, between V_5 and V_7. The electrocardiogram recorded at birth is normal in patients with common symptomatic heart disease, such as d-transposition of the great arteries, coarctation of the aorta, and tetralogy of Fallot. It is not until 5 to 10 days after birth when the pattern of right ventricular hypertrophy regresses in the normal infant (the T waves become inverted in the right precordium) that the electrocardiogram in such patients is abnormal. However, as discussed in subsequent chapters, some defects are associated with abnormal and in some cases, pathognomonic, electrocardiograms, so that electrocardiography can be of value in assisting in the diagnosis of certain defects. It is important to emphasize that a normal electrocardiogram does not exclude heart disease in the newborn.

Chest Radiograph

The chest radiograph provides information about the heart size and contour, pulmonary blood flow, and the lung parenchyma. Absence of a thymic shadow may contribute to the diagnosis of 22q11 deletion (DiGeorge) syndrome. The absence of a rightward deviation of the trachea and a contour on the right side of the spine are suggestive of a right aortic arch, which is highly associated with this syndrome. The main pulmonary artery is often malposed (as in d-transposition of the great arteries) or diminutive (as in tetralogy of Fallot) and thus the normal convexity in the left upper mediastinum is absent. Other defects associated with abnormalities of the contour or size of the heart include l-transposition of the great arteries, truncus arteriosus, and Ebstein anomaly, among others.

Increased pulmonary blood flow is often difficult to assess by conventional chest radiography at birth because even when pulmonary blood flow is three to four times systemic flow, the pulmonary vessels may not appear large. Small proximal vessels can conduct large quantities of blood as long as the distal vasculature is well developed. It is not until many days or weeks later that the arteries enlarge in response to increased flow. Conversely, pulmonary venous congestion can be appreciated very soon after birth, as pulmonary blood flow increases dramatically. That increased flow rapidly increases pulmonary venous pressures when the left side of the heart is critically obstructed. Lesions such as total anomalous pulmonary venous connection with obstruction show increased venous markings and pulmonary edema within hours of birth.

Echocardiography

Echocardiography is the mainstay of the diagnosis of the newborn with symptomatic heart disease and has largely replaced cardiac catheterization. However, to understand the pathophysiology and to offer the best care, it is important to take a systematic approach at each point of the evaluation and to use each piece of information to build upon that understanding. Two-dimensional echocardiography clearly visualizes the anatomy of the heart and the central great vessels, even in the smallest premature infants. Demonstrating blood flow by use of color Doppler studies is essential for evaluating the atrial septum, the aortopulmonary septum, and the pulmonary veins because imaging alone may fail to identify these very thin structures.

Pulsed and continuous wave Doppler studies add information about the physiology of the heart and great vessels beyond two-dimensional imaging. For example, peak instantaneous pressure differences can be estimated from the Bernoulli equation

$$\Delta P = 4 \cdot v^2$$

where P is pressure difference in mm Hg and v is velocity measured by Doppler study in $m \cdot s^{-1}$. This equation is based on a discrete narrowing in a rigid tube. If the

obstruction is relatively long or the geometry of the structures is not linear, the gradient is often overestimated. Acquiring the velocity at angles greater than about 30° from parallel tends to underestimate velocity, and thus underestimate the pressure difference. Within these limitations, however, Doppler studies are invaluable for estimating the severity of defects and pressures in chambers and arteries not accessible by other noninvasive methods. Right ventricular systolic pressure can be estimated by the peak instantaneous Doppler velocity of the tricuspid insufficiency jet, which correlates with the peak systolic pressure difference between the right ventricle and right atrium. In addition, the velocity of the flow across a defect in the ventricular septum provides an estimate of the peak systolic pressure difference between the left and right ventricles. Pulmonary arterial mean pressure can be estimated by the velocity of a pulmonary insufficiency jet. Doppler studies are also helpful in evaluating patients with noncardiac disease. For example, right ventricular pressure and pulmonary arterial mean pressure can be estimated in patients with pulmonary hypertension of the newborn.

In some cases, magnetic resonance imaging and magnetic resonance angiography can be very helpful in defining the anatomy and physiology. These imaging techniques are especially useful in defining the extracardiac and great vessel anatomy. Magnetic resonance imaging may be an important component of the evaluation of infants with coarctation of the aorta, interrupted aortic arch, and anomalous pulmonary venous connections. It is expected that the application of these techniques will expand as the technology improves to provide accurate information regarding blood flow, ventricular volume and function, and pressure gradients in the small infant.

Genetics Evaluation

Every infant with congenital heart disease should be carefully evaluated for evidence of dysmorphic features. As more extensively described in Chapter 15, a number of relatively common syndromes such as DiGeorge syndrome, trisomy 21, trisomy 18, Williams syndrome, Turner syndrome, and Alagille syndrome have characteristic features that may be evident on physical examination. These conditions have a high incidence of significant congenital heart defects. It is often helpful to involve specialists in clinical genetics to assist in the diagnostic evaluation of the infant and the family. Even a relatively low index of suspicion should prompt a genetics evaluation. Chromosome analysis or other specialized genetic testing may be indicated and should be performed in a rational and targeted manner. This will become increasingly important in the near future, as more information becomes available regarding the molecular genetics of congenital heart disease.

■ INITIAL TREATMENT

Timely initiation of medical therapy in patients with congenital heart defects is necessary to prevent and/or reverse clinical deterioration. The general approach to a term or preterm infant with heart disease should follow the usual guidelines for management of a critically ill (or potentially critically ill) infant. It is beyond the scope of this text to review specific details of ventilator use, fluid and electrolyte management, monitoring, maintenance of a neutral thermal environment, and general supportive care of newborns. However, it is useful to review a few commonly applied guidelines that are particularly relevant to infants with heart disease. More detailed information regarding specific medical and surgical care is provided in the chapters that describe individual defects and postoperative care.

General Principles

Oxygen

Supplemental oxygen is often administered to infants with known or suspected heart disease without full consideration of the goals of therapy and of the possible adverse effects. As with any other therapy, rational use of oxygen must be founded on sound principles of pathophysiology and include setting endpoints of efficacy and toxicity. Depending on the specific pathophysiology, newborns with heart disease may be prone to inadequate systemic output with overcirculation in the pulmonary vascular bed. An example is an infant with single ventricle physiology and unrestricted pulmonary blood flow (either through a large patent ductus arteriosus or antegrade from the heart in the absence of pulmonary stenosis). In this setting, the balance of pulmonary to systemic blood flow is determined by the relative resistances of the pulmonary and systemic vascular beds. Pulmonary overcirculation with inadequate systemic output is manifest by deterioration in pulmonary mechanics, a fall in urine output and evidence of decreased systemic perfusion (metabolic acidosis, diminished cutaneous perfusion). A common response in this setting is to increase the fraction of inspired oxygen in an attempt to maintain "normal" oxygen saturation or arterial pO_2. However, this response will almost certainly result in further deterioration because it

will lead to further systemic vasoconstriction and pulmonary vasodilation, and thus even more pulmonary blood flow at the expense of systemic output. A vicious cycle is perpetuated unless proper steps are taken to reduce pulmonary and increase systemic blood flow. Simply reducing the fraction of inspired oxygen to 0.21 (room air) is the first step in reversing this pathophysiologic spiral. It is often better to accept lower oxygen saturations, in the 80s, to maintain effective systemic circulation and limit pulmonary blood flow. It must be remembered at all times that systemic blood flow and hemoglobin concentration are as important as arterial oxygen saturation in determining systemic oxygen delivery, and that increased pulmonary blood flow worsens pulmonary mechanics and thus increases oxygen consumption, which in turn decreases oxygen reserve.

In the patient with suspected heart disease, an oxygen challenge test is sometimes performed. This is only rarely of value in assisting in the diagnosis and may promote constriction of the ductus arteriosus, which can be severely deleterious to the newborn with an undiagnosed ductal-dependent cardiac defect. If performed, it should be done over a few minutes, oxygen saturation should be measured by pulse oximetry in both the upper and lower bodies, and if oximetry shows a saturation of 97% or higher, arterial blood should be drawn for measurement of arterial oxygen tension.

Mechanical Ventilation

Mechanical ventilation of the infant whose primary symptom is cyanosis is often not necessary. If arterial blood gases show adequate spontaneous ventilation, intubation and mechanical ventilation usually will not improve oxygenation significantly. In contrast, mechanical ventilation and sedation are often very beneficial to the infant with decreased systemic perfusion and inadequate systemic oxygen delivery, because decreasing (or removing) the work of breathing decreases oxygen consumption. Although it is generally desirable to maintain normal acid-base and electrolyte status to optimize cardiac function, in some settings it may be perfectly acceptable to allow the pCO_2 to rise (permissive hypercapnia). Again, this strategy may be particularly useful in manipulating the ratio of pulmonary to systemic blood flow by promoting pulmonary vasoconstriction. Infants often require intermittent sedation to achieve appropriate control of ventilation, and some even require muscle relaxants. Monitoring ventilatory status, blood gases, urine output, and the clinical examination are all important in caring for neonates with heart disease who are being mechanically ventilated.

Fluids

Careful attention to fluid status and urine output is essential when managing newborns with congenital heart disease. In general, on the first day or two of life, newborn infants with congenital heart disease manifest the same fluid, glucose, and electrolyte requirements as infants without congenital heart disease. Depending on the particular defect, however, fluid and electrolyte management may change dramatically. For example, an infant with a single ventricle or large unrestricted ventricular septal defect and no pulmonary stenosis will exhibit progressively greater left-to-right shunting as the pulmonary vascular resistance falls postnatally. Consequently, signs and symptoms of heart failure may develop, because of increased pulmonary blood flow, reduced systemic output, and compensatory sodium and water retention. Free water restriction and diuretic therapy are indicated to reduce total body sodium and water. It is not unusual for mild hyponatremia to occur, which should not prompt administration of additional sodium. Instead, this most likely represents dilution due to excess water retention and should be treated with further reduction of free water intake. In contrast to hyponatremia, hypokalemia and hypocalcemia should be treated with supplemental administration of potassium and calcium. Urine output, serum electrolytes, and body weight must be monitored and used to guide water and electrolyte administration. Requirements may change rapidly during the first few days and weeks after birth since circulatory patterns and hemodynamics may change considerably during this time period. Thus, it is important to constantly reassess and be willing to modify therapy as conditions change.

Just as with oxygen therapy, fluid resuscitation must be considered carefully and from a physiologic perspective in the treatment of the newborn with critical heart disease. Just as the reflex response of administering oxygen to a cyanotic infant may be deleterious, the reflex response of administering large volumes of fluid to the hypotensive infant may be similarly so. Unlike hypovolemic or septic shock, venous pressures in the infant with decreased systemic perfusion may be, and usually are, increased. As is discussed in Chapter 8, decreased systemic perfusion is caused by either impaired myocardial function or obstruction to the left heart. In both instances, pulmonary venous pressures increase. In the newborn, this leads to a marked increase in pulmonary arterial pressures, because the arteries are still highly muscularized. The subsequent elevation in right ventricular pressures, in concert with decreased oxygen delivery to the heart, results in secondary right ventricular failure and elevation of right atrial pressures. In the presence of elevated right and left atrial pressures, fluid resuscitation could be extremely harmful, increasing pulmonary interstitial fluid and further dilating an already dilated right ventricle, leading to further ventricular failure. In the newborn with signs of cardiovascular collapse which might be caused by critical heart disease, the clinician must evaluate filling pressures, by palpating the liver and looking for evidence of pulmonary edema. If venous filling pressures are found to be increased, excess fluid administration is contraindicated; only the other measures to improve oxygen delivery or decrease oxygen demand (mechanical ventilation, inotropic support, vasomodulating agents, PGE_1, bicarbonate, calcium, etc) should be considered.

Prostaglandin E_1 (PGE_1)

More than any other therapy, PGE_1 has been lifesaving for newborns with critical congenital heart disease. The ductus arteriosus normally begins to close immediately after birth, but many critical cardiovascular defects require patency of the ductus arteriosus to maintain either pulmonary or systemic blood flow. Although oxygen is the primary effector of ductal closure, the ductus arteriosus still constricts within the first day of life in most patients with systemic arterial desaturation. Thus, effective therapy to maintain ductal patency is necessary for the healthy survival of infants with ductal dependent heart defects. PGE_1 is that therapy in most instances. Its appropriate use is not only lifesaving but allows time for careful diagnosis, evaluation, and formulation of a rational treatment plan. The clinical pharmacology of PGE_1 is presented in Chapter 12.

The decision to initiate therapy with PGE_1 is usually not very difficult. The two general indications are either inadequate pulmonary blood flow due to pulmonary outflow obstruction (eg, critical pulmonary stenosis or pulmonary atresia) or inadequate systemic blood flow due to obstructed aortic flow (eg, critical aortic stenosis, coarctation or interrupted aortic arch, hypoplastic left heart syndrome). In addition, PGE_1 is commonly used in infants with d-transposition of the great arteries to increase pulmonary blood flow. In this setting, the increased volume return to the left atrium promotes atrial left-to-right shunting, which will increase systemic oxygenation.

If a newborn infant is suspected of having a structural defect for which either pulmonary or systemic blood flow depends upon flow through the ductus arteriosus, then an infusion of PGE_1 should be started immediately. With proper attention to the potential side effects of PGE_1, the risk of its administration, even in infants later found not to have heart disease, is slight, and the benefit to the infant found to have ductus-dependent heart disease is lifesaving. The main risks are hypotension, which can be treated with infusions of drugs such as dopamine with vasoconstrictor properties, and hypoventilation, which can be treated with intubation and mechanical ventilation. Both of these therapeutic modalities must be readily available upon institution of PGE_1.

Infants with ductus-dependent pulmonary blood flow generally present with severe hypoxemia. In contrast to infants with lung disease, they rarely have dramatic increase in their work of breathing, and the arterial pO_2 does not increase significantly in response to administration of 100% oxygen. An infusion of PGE_1 should be started in any infant younger than 2 weeks suspected of having cyanotic congenital heart disease. Infants with ductus-dependent systemic blood flow typically present between 3 and 14 days of age and with signs of cardiogenic shock. In these conditions dilation of the ductus arteriosus allows the right ventricle to perfuse the descending aorta. In general, any infant younger than 2 weeks presenting with shock, decreased pulses, cardiomegaly, and/or hepatomegaly should be considered a candidate for treatment with PGE_1. Confirmation of the diagnosis should not delay initiation of therapy. It is generally advisable to initiate PGE_1 therapy for an infant with suspected heart disease before transporting to a tertiary care center for more definitive diagnosis and treatment. If after further evaluation, the infant is found to not have structural heart disease, then the PGE_1 infusion can be discontinued.

Administration of PGE_1 will almost always maintain patency of the ductus arteriosus and will dilate a ductus that has recently constricted. Although PGE_1 has been shown to be able to open a ductus arteriosus in left-sided obstructive lesions up to 100 days after birth, it will not open a ductus that is anatomically closed and as such, often will not be effective in older infants. Certainly, infants younger than 2 weeks are candidates for treatment but infants older than 4 weeks are much less likely to benefit. It is reasonable to attempt to open the ductus arteriosus in infants between 2 and 4 weeks, but the success rate is much lower than that in newborn infants. If the ductus has not reopened within 1 to 2 hours at a maximal dose of PGE_1 (0.10 µg/kg/min), then it is very unlikely that the ductus will open. The infusion should be discontinued and the infant should be considered for urgent surgical or catheter-based intervention.

Hematological Considerations

Newborn infants with congenital heart disease rarely have intrinsic hematological problems. However, there are several aspects of the care of these infants that warrant consideration.

Because all newborns are at some risk of graft-versus-host disease, it is recommended that they receive irradiated blood if donated from a first- or second-degree relative, and all newborns should receive blood that is CMV-negative and less than 5 days old, if possible. Particular care should be given to infants with deletion 22q11 (DiGeorge) syndrome, who often have abnormal immune function because of the thymic defects. If transfusion therapy is required for an infant with known or suspected deletion 22q11 syndrome, blood products should be treated before administration to decrease the chances of a graft-versus-host reaction. This is especially important to consider in infants with significant structural defects who require urgent surgical intervention in the first few days of life. In these cases, the results of genetic and chromosomal analyses may not be completed before surgery so it is important to follow these recommendations even if the definitive diagnosis has not been confirmed. A high index of suspicion is necessary for infants with cardiac defects commonly associated with deletion 22q11 syndrome (eg, interrupted aortic arch, truncus arteriosus, anomalous origin of the pulmonary artery from the aorta, and tetralogy of Fallot, especially with pulmonary atresia or absent pulmonary valve). Cyanotic congenital heart disease may be associated with secondary hematological abnormalities (eg, thrombocytopenia), but these generally do not develop until later in life and are therefore beyond the scope of this textbook. However, it is important to note that infants with cyanosis are especially prone to iron deficiency. The hemoglobin and hematocrit alone may not be sufficient for making this diagnosis, since a cyanotic infant with "anemia" may actually have hemoglobin and hematocrit values within the ranges that are considered normal. It may be useful to measure the mean corpuscular volume (MCV) or serum ferritin levels. Infants with cyanotic heart disease are typically polycythemic and they should not be allowed to develop iron deficiency. Iron deficiency, even without anemia, predisposes patients to thrombosis and cerebral vascular accidents (for reasons that are not entirely clear). Lastly, because systemic oxygen delivery is at risk of being impaired in nearly all infants with uncorrected or palliated symptomatic heart disease, the infant should receive iron supplementation on discharge from the hospital unless there is a specific reason not to do so.

Recognition and Management of Hypercyanotic Spells

Infants with tetralogy of Fallot (and other types of congenital cardiovascular defects with similar pathophysiology) are at risk for hypercyanotic spells. These episodes are rare in the newborn period, but may have their onset in the first few months of life in infants waiting for more definitive intervention. Hypercyanotic spells are characterized by intense cyanosis with abnormal respirations and a change in the level of consciousness. The episode usually begins with irritability and crying. The degree of cyanosis increases and the respirations become rapid and occasionally labored. Untreated, the infant may develop lethargy and loss of consciousness. During a hypercyanotic spell, the systolic ejection murmur of pulmonary stenosis becomes very soft or disappears completely. As the infant recovers, the murmur returns. These findings are consistent with an acute reduction in pulmonary blood flow and an increase in the magnitude of the right-to-left shunt during a hypercyanotic episode.

Initial treatment of a hypercyanotic episode includes placing the infant in a knee-chest position (this helps increase systemic vascular resistance, which in turn forces more of the output toward the lungs), administration of oxygen and morphine sulfate (0.1 mg/kg subcutaneously or intravenously if a vascular catheter is already in place). These measures are generally sufficient to interrupt the spell. If the infant is unresponsive or deeply cyanotic, a crystalloid infusion should be started and a vasopressor (eg, phenylephrine) should be infused; these actions increase preload and thus ventricular output, and systemic vascular resistance, to decrease the relative right-to-left shunt. If these measures are not successful, then an infusion of esmolol (a short acting β-adrenergic receptor blocker) should be started. This acts by a variety of mechanisms to decrease the severity and duration of the episode. It decreases oxygen consumption, heart rate (which then increases preload for each beat), and the rate of pressure generation by the ventricles (and thus the extent of the obstruction during early ejection). If

despite all of these efforts, the spell cannot be interrupted, then the infant should be anesthetized and mechanically ventilated in anticipation of either emergency surgical intervention or extracorporeal oxygenation.

SUGGESTED READINGS

Physical Examination and Ancillary Tests

Allen HD, Phillips JR, Chan DP. History and physical examination. In: Allen HD, Driscoll DJ, Shaddy RE, Feltes TF, eds. *Moss and Adams' Heart Disease in Infants, Children, and Adolescents Including the Fetus and Young Adult*. 7th ed. Philadelphia, PA: Lippincott Williams & Wilkins; 2008: Chapter 3.

Brown KL, Ridout DA, Hoskote A, et al. Delayed diagnosis of congenital heart disease worsens preoperative condition and outcome of surgery in neonates. *Heart*. 2006; 92(9): 1298-1302.

Chang RK, Gurvitz M, Rodriguez S. Missed diagnosis of critical congenital heart disease. *Arch Pediatr Adolesc Med*. 2008;162(10):969-974.

Gaskin PR, Owens SE, Talner NS, et al. Clinical auscultation skills in pediatric residents. *Pediatrics*. 2000 Jun;105(6): 1184-1187.

Hoffman JI, Kaplan S. The incidence of congenital heart disease. *J Am Coll Cardiol*. 2002 Jun 19;39(12):1890-1900.

Hoffman JIE. *The Natural and Unnatural History of Congenital Heart Disease*. Oxford, United Kingdom: Wiley-Blackwell; 2009.

Kimball TR, Michelfelder EC. Echocardiography. In: Allen HD, Driscoll DJ, Shaddy RE, Feltes TF, eds. *Moss and Adams' Heart Disease in Infants, Children, and Adolescents Including the Fetus and Young Adult*. 7th ed. Philadelphia, PA: Lippincott Williams & Wilkins; 2008: Chapter 6.

Mellander M, Sunnegardh J. Failure to diagnose critical heart malformations in newborns before discharge—an increasing problem? *Acta Paediatr*. 2006 Apr;95(4): 407-413.

Moller JH, Hoffman JIE, eds. *Pediatric Cardiovascular Medicine*. Philadelphia, PA: Churchill Livingstone; 2000.

Park MK. *The Pediatric Cardiology Handbook*. 4th ed. Philadelphia, PA: Mosby Elsevier; 2010.

Phoon CKL. *A Guide to Pediatric Cardiovascular Physical Examination*. Philadelphia, PA: Lippincott-Raven Publishers; 1998.

Rudolph AM. *Congenital Diseases of the Heart: Clinical-Physiological Considerations*. Chichester, United Kingdom: Wiley-Blackwell; 2009: Chapter 4—Functional Assessment.

Wren C, Reinhardt Z, Khawaja K. Twenty-year trends in diagnosis of life-threatening neonatal cardiovascular malformations. *Arch Dis Child Fetal Neonatal Ed*. 2008 Jan;93(1):F33-F35.

Pulse Oximetry as a Screening Test

Aamir T, Kruse L, Ezeakudo O. Delayed diagnosis of critical congenital cardiovascular malformations (CCVM) and pulse oximetry screening of newborns. *Acta Paediatr*. 2007;96(8):1146-1149.

Ainsworth S, Wyllie JP, Wren C. Prevalence and clinical significance of cardiac murmurs in neonates. *Arch Dis Child Fetal Neonatal Ed*. 1999 Jan;80(1):F43-F45.

de-Wahl Granelli A, Wennergren M, Sandberg K, et al. Impact of pulse oximetry screening on the detection of duct dependent congenital heart disease: A Swedish prospective screening study in 39,821 newborns. *BMJ*. 2009;338:a3037.

Hoffman JIE. It is time for routine neonatal screening by pulse oximetry. *Neonatology*. 2010;99(1):1-9.

Levesque BM, Pollack P, Griffin BE, Nielsen HC. Pulse oximetry: what's normal in the newborn nursery? *Pediatr Pulmonol*. 2000 Nov;30(5):406-412.

Mahle WT, Newburger JW, Matherne GP, et al. Role of pulse oximetry in examining newborns for congenital heart disease: a scientific statement from the American Heart Association and American Academy of Pediatrics. *Circulation*. 2009 Aug 4;120(5):447-458.

Meberg A, Brugmann-Pieper S, Due R, Jr., et al. First day of life pulse oximetry screening to detect congenital heart defects. *J Pediatr*. 2008 Jun;152(6):761-765.

Thangaratinam S, Daniels J, Ewer AK, Zamora J, Khan KS. Accuracy of pulse oximetry in screening for congenital heart disease in asymptomatic newborns: a systematic review. *Arch Dis Child Fetal Neonatal Ed*. 2007 May;92(3):F176-F180.

Initial Treatment

Fetus and Newborn Committee, Canadian Paediatric Society. Red blood cell transfusions in newborn infants: revised guidelines. *Paediatr Child Health*. 2002;7(8):553-566.

Nichols DG, ed. *Rogers' Textbook of Pediatric Intensive Care*. 4th ed. Philadelphia, PA: Lippincott Williams & Wilkins; 2008.

Nichols DG, Cameron DE, eds. *Critical Heart Disease in Infants and Children*. 2nd ed. St. Louis, MO: Mosby-Year Book Inc; 2006.

Rudolph AM. Oxygen uptake and delivery. In: *Congenital Diseases of the Heart: Clinical-Physiological Considerations*. Chichester, United Kingdom: Wiley-Blackwell; 2009. Chapter 3.

Approach to the Cyanotic Infant

■ INTRODUCTION

Cyanosis is the most common manifestation of symptomatic heart disease in the newborn infant. Moreover, cyanosis in the absence of significant respiratory distress is almost always caused by structural cardiovascular disease because pulmonary disease severe enough to cause cyanosis is usually associated with severe respiratory distress. Congenital heart defects that cause primarily cyanosis in newborn infants are reviewed in this chapter. Infants who have decreased systemic perfusion as the primary symptom, even if cyanosis is also present, are discussed in Chapter 8.

■ PATHOPHYSIOLOGY OF CYANOSIS

Oxygen Delivery

Adequate oxygen delivery to meet metabolic needs is essential for healthy survival. The amount of oxygen delivered to the tissues is dependent on systemic blood flow, hemoglobin concentration, and hemoglobin oxygen saturation (Table 6-1). At birth, oxygen consumption increases nearly threefold to meet the energy costs of breathing and thermoregulation. Normally, systemic blood flow at least doubles and systemic arterial oxygen saturation and content increase by about 25% in the immediate newborn period (reviewed in Chapter 3). Thus, despite the increase

■ TABLE 6-1. Calculation of Oxygen Delivery and Blood Flows

$$SOD = Q_S \cdot C_{SA}$$

$$Q_S = \frac{VO_2}{(C_{SA} - C_{SV})}$$

$$Q_P = \frac{VO_2}{(C_{PV} - C_{PA})}$$

$$Q_{EP} = \frac{VO_2}{(C_{PV} - C_{SV})}$$

$$C = c \cdot Hb \cdot S$$

SOD, systemic oxygen delivery. Q_S, systemic blood flow. C_{SA}, oxygen content of systemic arterial blood. VO_2, oxygen consumption. C_{SV}, oxygen content of mixed systemic venous blood. Q_P, pulmonary blood flow. C_{PV}, oxygen content of pulmonary venous blood. C_{PA}, oxygen content of pulmonary arterial blood. Q_{EP}, effective pulmonary blood flow. C, oxygen content. c, constant describing the oxygen carrying capacity of a unit of hemoglobin (each gram of hemoglobin can carry 136 mL of oxygen per liter of blood). Hb, blood hemoglobin concentration. S, oxygen saturation of a given source of blood.

■ TABLE 6-2. Congenital Cardiovascular Defects Presenting With Cyanosis Caused by Decreased Pulmonary Blood Flow

Anatomic level	Structural defect
Tricuspid valve	Tricuspid valve regurgitation
	Tricuspid valve stenosis or atresia
	Ebstein anomaly
Right ventricle	Hypoplastic right ventricle
	Tetralogy of Fallot (subpulmonic stenosis with ventricular septal defect)
Pulmonary valve	Pulmonary valve stenosis or atresia with intact ventricular septum
	Pulmonary valve stenosis or atresia with ventricular septal defect (± single ventricle, malposed aorta, or aortopulmonary collateral vessels)
	Absent pulmonary valve syndrome
Pulmonary artery	Supravalvar pulmonary artery stenosis
	Branch pulmonary artery stenosis

in oxygen consumption, oxygen delivery increases similarly and the reserve to extract oxygen remains large in normal infants. In contrast, newborn infants with cyanotic congenital heart disease cannot increase systemic arterial oxygen saturation and, in fact, oxygen saturation often falls precipitously soon after birth. These infants are therefore at risk for inadequate systemic oxygen delivery, which, if untreated, may result in anaerobic metabolism, metabolic acidosis, and death.

Hemodynamic Categories of Cyanotic Heart Disease

Decreased pulmonary blood flow (Table 6-2) and *malposition of the aorta over the systemic venous ventricle (transposition complexes)* are the two main pathophysiological mechanisms responsible for severely decreased systemic arterial saturation in newborn infants with cyanotic heart disease. In the normal circulation, all of the poorly saturated systemic venous blood is directed through the right heart structures to the pulmonary arteries; the oxygen saturations of the blood in the systemic veins and pulmonary arteries are therefore equal. This blood becomes nearly fully saturated as it gains oxygen in the pulmonary capillary bed and returns to the heart via the pulmonary veins. Pulmonary venous blood then passes through the left heart structures to the aorta. Thus, the oxygen saturations in the pulmonary veins and systemic arteries are the same

and pulmonary blood flow is equal to systemic blood flow (Table 6-1).

In conditions of *decreased pulmonary blood flow* (Table 6-2), systemic venous blood returns to the right atrium, but some of this desaturated blood does not reach the pulmonary arteries for oxygen uptake. Rather, a portion passes to the left heart structures and aorta where it mixes with pulmonary venous blood, resulting in decreased systemic arterial saturation. In addition, a portion of pulmonary venous blood often returns to the lungs (eg, via a ductus arteriosus) and does not contribute to oxygen uptake. "Effective pulmonary blood flow" denotes the volume of systemic venous blood delivered to the pulmonary arteries for oxygen uptake and is directly proportional to the oxygen saturation in the aorta (Table 6-1).

In conditions of *malposition of the aorta over the systemic venous ventricle (transposition complexes)* cyanosis also occurs despite the fact that pulmonary blood flow is normal or even increased. For example, when the aorta is malposed over the ventricle that receives the systemic venous return (typically the right ventricle), most of the systemic venous blood is ejected into the aorta. Depending on the position of the pulmonary artery and the presence or absence of a ventricular septal defect, varying amounts of pulmonary venous blood are ejected into the aorta and pulmonary artery. In the most common defect in this category, d-transposition of the great arteries with intact ventricular septum (Figure 6-1A), all of the pulmonary venous blood flows back to the pulmonary arteries when there is no communication between the two sides of the heart. Thus, although pulmonary blood flow is normal (or even increased if the ductus arteriosus is patent), the newborn infant is severely hypoxemic because the systemic arterial saturation is similar to that in the systemic veins (instead of that in the pulmonary veins). The situation in which the systemic and pulmonary circulations are entirely in parallel rather than in series is not compatible with life. Survival is dependent upon at least some volume

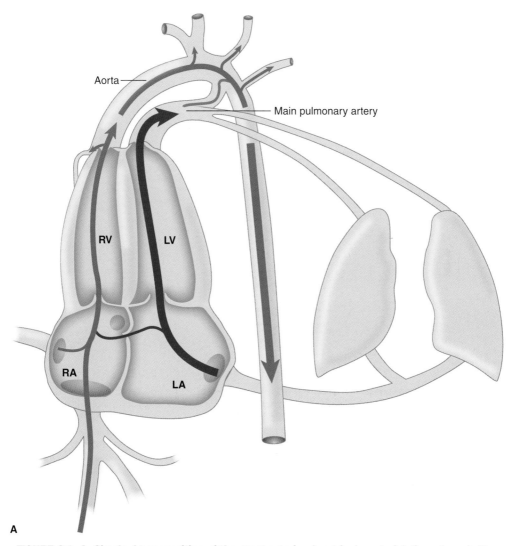

A

FIGURE 6-1. A. Simple d-transposition of the great arteries (ventricular-arterial discordance). The immediate postnatal circulation shows pulmonary venous blood returning to the pulmonary artery and systemic venous blood returning to the aorta, causing severe cyanosis. The shunt through the foramen ovale, if present, passes in a left-to-right direction. The shunt through the ductus arteriosus is mixed, with a small right-to-left in early systole, and a much larger left-to-right shunt in diastole. Red arrows indicate oxygenated blood and blue arrows indicate desaturated blood. Abbreviations: LA, left atrium; LV, anatomic left ventricle; RA, right atrium; RV, anatomic right ventricle.

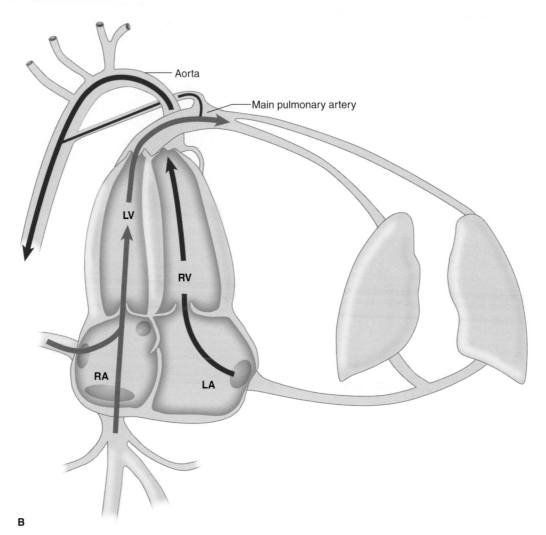

B

FIGURE 6-1. B. l-transposition of the great arteries (atrial-ventricular and ventricular-arterial discordance). The immediate postnatal circulation shows systemic venous blood returning normally to the right atrium, and then flowing to the anatomic left ventricle and pulmonary artery. Pulmonary venous blood returns to the left atrium and then flows to the anatomic right ventricle and aorta. Aortic saturation is normal and there is a small left-to-right ductal shunt. The aorta arises anteriorly and to the left (l-loop) and ascends to the right. Red arrows indicate oxygenated blood and blue arrows indicate desaturated blood. The abbreviations are the same as for Figure 6-1A.

of pulmonary venous blood entering the aorta. Because the ventricular septum is intact, this must occur either at the atrial level (eg, from the left atrium across the foramen ovale into the right atrium, right ventricle, and then the aorta) or at the arterial level (the ductus arteriosus), or both. Patency of the ductus arteriosus is often essential to maintain adequate oxygen delivery via the aorta. Flow

through the ductus arteriosus increases pulmonary blood flow so that left atrial volume and pressure increase, which in turn causes a large left-to-right atrial shunt.

Transposition of the great arteries is called ventricular-arterial discordance because the ventricles connect to the wrong arteries. In simple d-transposition of the great arteries, there is atrial-ventricular concordance because the right atrium connects normally to the anatomic right ventricle through a tricuspid valve and the left atrium connects normally to the anatomic left ventricle through a mitral valve. However, atrial-ventricular discordance can also occur. In that case the right atrium connects via the mitral valve to the left ventricle, and the left atrium connects via the tricuspid valve to the right ventricle (Figure 6-1B). If both atrial-ventricular discordance and ventricular-arterial discordance are present together, blood flow patterns are normal. Thus, this condition is often called "corrected" transposition of the great arteries. l-transposition of the great arteries is a more appropriate term because the embryologic abnormality is failure of the primitive heart tube to rotate to a rightward (d-looped) position. Instead, rotation is to the left (l-looping). Associated cardiovascular defects are commonly present in infants with l-transposition of the great arteries (see following text).

Clinical Presentation of Cyanotic Heart Disease

Cyanosis is a critically important clinical finding to detect in the newborn infant. It is the primary presentation of heart disease which manifests symptomatically in the newborn infant. If cyanosis due to congenital heart disease is not recognized, the neonate may experience rapid and severe cardiovascular decompensation. Evaluation of cyanosis is discussed in Chapter 5, but the critical features of cyanotic congenital heart disease are

- Systemic arterial hypoxemia is manifested clinically by central rather than peripheral cyanosis.

- Cyanosis is often not present immediately after birth, particularly in infants who have defects that cause decreased pulmonary blood flow, because the ductus arteriosus is still widely patent.

- Cyanosis is not evident until a significant amount of reduced hemoglobin is present. If an infant has a systemic arterial oxygen saturation above 85%, cyanosis may be quite difficult to detect by visual inspection. Oxygen saturation should be measured by pulse oximetry if there is any suggestion that central cyanosis may be present.

- Oxygen saturation may differ between the upper and lower body. The ascending and descending aorta may be perfused by different ventricles if the ductus arteriosus is patent. Pulse oximetry should be performed on the right hand, which receives blood from the ascending aorta in the normal aortic arch, and on either foot, which receives blood from the descending aorta. Certain conditions are associated with different relationships in oxygen saturation between the upper and lower body; defining the relationship may be very helpful to identify the specific defect causing cyanosis (Table 6-3). It should also be remembered that, rarely, the right subclavian artery arises from the descending aorta and does not reflect ascending aorta saturation (Chapter 5).

- Infants with cyanotic heart disease are hypoxemic and thus breathe rapidly. However, they rarely have respiratory distress (ie, no retractions or nasal flaring) and arterial CO_2 levels are usually decreased because of hyperventilation. Thus, these defects are rarely confused with primary lung disease.

■ **TABLE 6-3.** Possible Diagnoses by Defect Groups in Newborn Infants With Upper Body Oxygen Desaturation and With Variable Lower Body Desaturation

Lower body oxygen saturation (relative to upper)	Defect groups possible	Defect groups excluded
Same	Decreased pulmonary blood flow Transposition complexes Pulmonary hypertension	None
Higher	Transposition complexes	Decreased pulmonary blood flow Pulmonary hypertension
Lower	Pulmonary hypertension	Decreased pulmonary blood flow Transposition complexes

■ DEFECTS WITH DECREASED PULMONARY BLOOD FLOW

Obstruction to blood flow within the right heart or pulmonary arteries, or severe regurgitation of the tricuspid or pulmonary valve causes decreased pulmonary blood flow (Table 6-2). Obstructive defects are far more common than defects in which valvar regurgitation is the dominant problem. In all of these situations, a portion of the systemic venous blood is shunted from the right atrium through the foramen ovale to the left atrium where it mixes with pulmonary venous blood, resulting in systemic arterial desaturation. In certain defects, a right-to-left shunt across a ventricular septal defect is also present. Because obstruction or regurgitation almost always occurs

proximal to the ductus arteriosus, upper and lower body saturations are always similar in this group of defects, even if the ductus arteriosus is patent. This is a very important finding that differentiates this group of newborns from those with transposition complexes or persistent pulmonary hypertension of the newborn (Table 6-3).

Fetal Physiology

During fetal life, inflow or outflow obstruction to the right ventricle without a ventricular septal defect causes a large portion of blood, which would otherwise enter the right ventricle, to cross the foramen ovale into the left atrium. In the extreme case of either tricuspid atresia or pulmonary atresia with intact ventricular septum (Figure 6-2), all

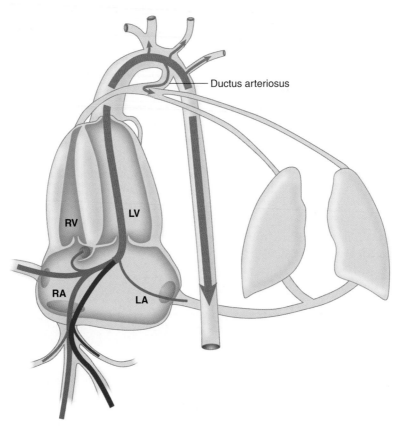

FIGURE 6-2. Hypoplastic right heart syndrome. Fetal flow patterns show systemic and umbilical venous return passing through the foramen ovale, causing it to be a large communication. The ascending aorta receives all of the ventricular output so that the aortic arch and isthmus are large and the ductus arteriosus, in which flow is reversed, is vertically oriented and small. Red lines indicate oxygenated blood and blue lines indicate desaturated blood. The intermediate purple arrows illustrate mixing of the venous return so that systemic blood has decreased oxygen saturation. Abbreviations: LA, left atrium; LV, left ventricle; RA, right atrium; RV, right ventricle.

systemic venous return passes through the foramen ovale. Thus, the foramen ovale is extremely large in utero. Postnatally, a secundum atrial septal defect is present. This defect is essentially a stretched foramen ovale in which the flap does not fully close the foramen after birth. Thus, the atrial septal defect is almost always nonrestrictive after birth and systemic venous return to the left heart is unobstructed. However, in rare cases, the opening in the atrial septum is too small and an emergency atrial septostomy is necessary to maintain systemic output.

In these conditions, the left ventricle receives much more of the combined venous return because of the increased blood flow into the left atrium across the foramen ovale. The coronary and upper body circulations receive a normal amount of combined ventricular output, so that the excess output passes through the aortic arch and isthmus to the descending aorta. This enlarges the aortic isthmus so that coarctation of the aorta does not occur in association with these defects. This is another important finding which differentiates these defects from the transposition complexes, in which coarctation of the aorta can occur.

Flow across the foramen ovale is *not* increased in a second group of infants with obstruction to pulmonary blood flow because of the coexistence of a ventricular septal defect. For example, in patients with tetralogy of Fallot, venous return passes normally to the right ventricle but, rather than passing entirely into the main pulmonary artery, some of the right ventricular output is diverted into the ascending aorta through a subaortic ventricular septal defect (Figure 6-3). Thus, blood flow through the ascending aorta and aortic arch is increased and again, coarctation of the aorta is not present. To summarize, the ascending aorta and aortic arch are enlarged and coarctation of the aorta is never present in infants with defects that cause decreased pulmonary blood flow.

Decreased Pulmonary Blood Flow With Inflow Obstruction

An extremely useful clinical finding in infants with cyanosis is the quality of the right ventricular impulse. Normally, the right ventricle is easily palpated along the lower sternum or in the subxiphoid area. This is because the right ventricle is the dominant ventricle during fetal life and is anteriorly positioned, and because the sternum is relatively pliable. The right ventricular impulse is either normal or increased in patients with right ventricular outflow tract obstruction, transposition complexes, or persistent hypertension of the newborn. However, the right

ventricle does not fill normally and thus cannot contract to a normal extent if inflow obstruction is present. The right ventricular impulse is therefore decreased in these patients. Thus the presence of a deceased right ventricular impulse in a newborn infant with cyanosis quickly limits the differential diagnosis to the few defects in which right ventricular inflow obstruction is present (Table 6-2), the two most common of which are presented next.

Tricuspid Atresia

Anatomic and physiologic considerations. In tricuspid atresia, the tricuspid valve fails to form normally, resulting in an atretic valve with total obstruction of inflow to the right ventricle from the right atrium. Consequently, all of the systemic venous blood crosses the foramen ovale to the left atrium and ventricle. The degree of right ventricular hypoplasia is variable. In the large majority of these infants, a ventricular septal defect is present, promoting the development of a small right ventricle as blood flows from the left ventricle through ventricular septal defect to right ventricle and pulmonary arteries in utero. The great arteries are usually normally related, but d-transposition of the great arteries is present in a small percentage of infants. When the great arteries are transposed, pulmonary blood flow is elevated because the pulmonary valve arises directly from the left ventricle, whereas systemic blood flow depends on the size of the ventricular septal defect, so that coarctation of the aorta may occur.

Clinical presentation. On physical examination the infant is cyanotic and the oxygen saturations are similar in all extremities. Tachypnea may be present but respiratory distress is absent. The peripheral pulses and perfusion are normal, and the remainder of the noncardiac examination is usually noncontributory. The right ventricular impulse is decreased, an important finding directing the clinician to consider this diagnosis. Even more specific is a thrill, which may be present when blood flows anteriorly from the left ventricle to the right via a restrictive ventricular septal defect. This is pathognomonic of tricuspid atresia in a cyanotic newborn infant; in all other cyanotic defects with a ventricular septal defect, blood flows from the right ventricle posteriorly to the left, so that a thrill is not present. The first heart sound is normal. No extra sounds or clicks are heard. The second heart sound depends on associated defects. It is usually single, but will be split if the flow across the ventricular septal defect and pulmonary valve is large. However, at the normal rapid heart rates present at birth, a split second heart sound is difficult to

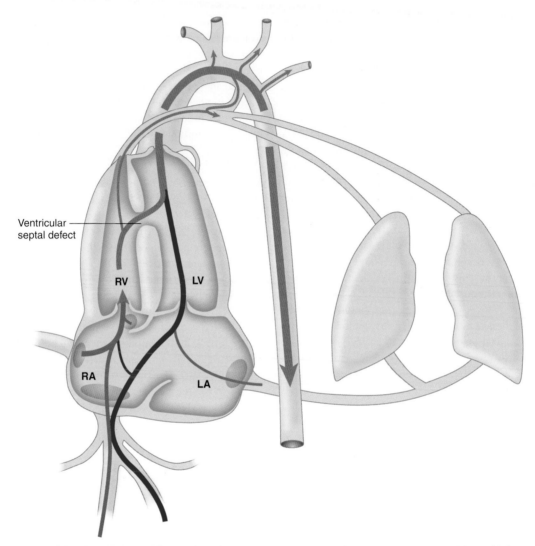

FIGURE 6-3. Tetralogy of Fallot. Fetal flow patterns show normal venous return to the right and left ventricles, but some right ventricular output is directed to the ascending aorta, enlarging the aortic arch and causing the ductus arteriosus to shunt left to right. Red lines indicate oxygenated blood and blue lines indicate desaturated blood. The intermediate purple arrows illustrate mixing of the venous return so that systemic blood has decreased oxygen saturation. Abbreviations: LA, left atrium; LV, left ventricle; RA, right atrium; RV, right ventricle.

appreciate. If the great arteries are transposed, the aortic component of the second heart sound may be loud. A murmur may be heard as a result of flow through a ventricular septal defect or right ventricular outflow tract obstruction.

Ancillary tests. Based upon clinical findings alone, it is usually possible to limit the differential diagnosis in these infants to cyanosis caused by defects that result in right ventricular inflow obstruction (Table 6-2). Simple ancillary tests usually can then differentiate tricuspid atresia from pulmonary atresia with intact ventricular septum, and determine whether there is associated d-transposition of the great arteries. The electrocardiogram usually shows right atrial enlargement and decreased right ventricular forces in all of these defects, but the axis is inferior with a normal clockwise loop in pulmonary atresia with intact septum, whereas it is superior ($0°$ to $-60°$) with a counterclockwise loop in tricuspid atresia. Infants with tricuspid atresia and d-transposition of the great arteries usually have a similar axis to those with pulmonary atresia ($0°$ to $+90°$). The chest radiograph shows a narrow mediastinum when the arteries are transposed and a normal mediastinum when they are normally related.

Echocardiography is definitive and shows no tricuspid valve tissue in the atrioventricular groove which between the right atrium from the right ventricle. Obligatory flow across the foramen ovale (or secundum atrial septal defect) into the left atrium is present and is often directed by a large eustachian valve in the right atrium. The size of the atrial communication, the presence of a ventricular septal defect, the size of the right ventricle and right ventricular outflow tract, the relationship of the great arteries, and the patency of the ductus arteriosus should all be evaluated.

Therapeutic considerations. These infants are considered to have a functional single ventricle because the right ventricle will never function as an adequate pumping chamber in the absence of an adequate inlet. Most infants require a systemic-to-pulmonary artery shunt shortly after birth because of severe cyanosis. Some centers are providing pulmonary blood flow by transcatheter placement of a stent in the ductus arteriosus rather than via a surgical aortopulmonary shunt. Subsequently a bidirectional Glenn shunt (superior cavopulmonary connection) and then a modified Fontan operation are performed (see following text). Infants who have a relatively well-developed right ventricle and pulmonary valve because of the presence of a ventricular septal defect are only minimally cyanotic and may not need a systemic-to-pulmonary artery shunt. Instead, they may undergo a Glenn shunt as the first stage, usually by 4 to 6 months of age. Infants with transposed great arteries often develop functional subaortic obstruction (restrictive bulboventricular foramen) and may need a Damus-Kaye-Stansel operation (see following text) to be performed at the time of either the bidirectional Glenn shunt or modified Fontan operation.

Pulmonary Atresia With Intact Ventricular Septum and Diminutive Right Ventricle (Sometimes Called Hypoplastic Right Heart Syndrome)

Anatomic and physiologic considerations. A second category of right ventricular inflow obstructive defects

occurs when the tricuspid valve is present but is severely hypoplastic. This is associated with hypoplasia of the right ventricle and atresia of the pulmonary valve. After birth, pulmonary blood flow is entirely dependent upon patency of the ductus arteriosus. The systolic pressure in the right ventricle is often greater than the systemic systolic pressure because of the right ventricular outflow tract obstruction. As a result of the very high pressure within the right ventricular cavity, embryonic connections of the right ventricular cavity with coronary arteries may persist as coronary sinusoids (Figure 6-4). These connections may perfuse the myocardium with poorly saturated blood and may not communicate with the proximal coronary system, or they may connect to the coronary arteries but with severely stenotic openings. In these situations, part of the coronary arterial circulation is dependent on perfusion from the right ventricle ("right ventricle-dependent coronary circulation") which increases the risk of death because of myocardial ischemia.

Clinical presentation. On physical examination the infant is cyanotic and has similar oxygen saturations in all extremities. The peripheral pulses and perfusion are normal. Important noncardiac findings are rarely present. Although the right ventricle is usually generating systolic pressures that greatly exceed systemic pressure, the right

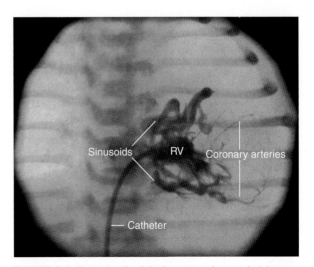

FIGURE 6-4. Hypoplastic right heart syndrome. A right ventricular angiogram demonstrating a very hypertrophied diminutive ventricle with extensive filling of the both coronary arterial systems by sinusoidal communications with the hypertensive ventricle. Abbreviation: RV, right ventricle.

ventricular impulse is often decreased because the right ventricle receives and ejects only a very small amount of blood. The first heart sound is normal. No extra sounds or clicks are heard. The second heart sound is single and of normal intensity. Murmurs are only occasionally present, and reflect either a narrow ductus arteriosus or tricuspid valve regurgitation.

Ancillary tests. The chest radiograph shows a small cardiac silhouette and normal mediastinum, similar to that seen in tricuspid atresia with normally related great arteries. The electrocardiogram shows decreased, normal or increased right ventricular forces depending on the mass of the right ventricular wall. In contrast to patients with tricuspid atresia, the axis is in the left inferior quadrant (+60° to 90°); this is an important differentiating point. The echocardiogram shows a small tricuspid valve annulus and a markedly hypertrophied right ventricle with little contraction and often evidence of endocardial fibrosis. The size of the tricuspid valve and right ventricle should be defined. There usually is no apparent right ventricular outflow tract and there is a unidirectional right-to-left atrial shunt. Color Doppler echocardiography may demonstrate flow in the coronary arterial sinusoids within the myocardial wall. Evaluation of whether or not the coronary arterial circulation is dependent on the right ventricle is mandatory and cardiac catheterization may be necessary to resolve this issue.

Therapeutic considerations. Treatment of these patients must be individualized and is often difficult and complicated. The major question is whether the tricuspid valve and right ventricle will grow enough to support the pulmonary circulation if right ventricular outflow obstruction is relieved or whether the patient must be treated as a functional single ventricle. Reconstruction of the right ventricular outflow tract establishes continuity between the right ventricle and pulmonary arteries and often results in remarkable growth of the tricuspid valve and right ventricle. In patients with a moderately hypoplastic right ventricle, placement of a systemic-to-pulmonary artery shunt may be necessary in addition to right ventricular outflow tract reconstruction to ensure adequate pulmonary blood flow. Patients with an extremely hypoplastic right ventricle, right ventricle–dependent coronary circulation, or a right ventricle that fails to grow adequately after relief of right ventricular outflow tract obstruction are treated as functional single ventricles. They require a systemic-to-pulmonary artery shunt and later are candidates for a bidirectional Glenn shunt and modified Fontan operation (see following text).

Decreased Pulmonary Blood Flow With Outflow Obstruction

Pulmonary Atresia With Intact Ventricular Septum and a Normal-Sized Right Ventricle

Anatomic and physiologic considerations. Pulmonary atresia with an intact ventricular septum is not necessarily associated with a hypoplastic right ventricle. When the right ventricular cavity is well-formed, the tricuspid valve is usually of nearly normal size, but may be severely insufficient. Coronary arterial sinusoids do not develop, likely in part because the right ventricle cannot generate high pressures because of the tricuspid regurgitation. Additionally, by the time the outflow obstruction develops during fetal life, the embryonic sinusoids may have already regressed. Interestingly, the pulmonary arteries are usually normally developed despite the fact that they only receive a small amount of the fetal combined ventricular output through the ductus arteriosus.

Clinical presentation. On physical examination the infant is cyanotic with similar oxygen saturations in all extremities. Mild tachypnea is present but respiratory distress is absent. The peripheral pulses and perfusion are normal, and the noncardiac examination is unremarkable. The large volume of blood passing into the right ventricle causes a normal to increased right ventricular impulse. The first heart sound is normal or may be obscured by the tricuspid regurgitation murmur. No extra heart sounds are present. The second heart sound is single. An early systolic murmur heard best at the left lower sternal border and radiating toward the right anterior chest is caused by the tricuspid valve regurgitation.

Ancillary tests. The chest radiograph usually shows an enlarged right atrium, and the central blood vessels are of normal size. The electrocardiogram is similar to that seen in pulmonary atresia with a hypoplastic tricuspid valve, except that right ventricular hypertrophy is more common and right atrial enlargement may be especially pronounced. The echocardiogram differs from that seen with a hypoplastic tricuspid valve and right ventricle in that the tricuspid valve annulus is nearly normal in size. The z-score, a measure of the number of standard deviations from the normal mean diameter, is usually greater than −2. Severe tricuspid regurgitation with an enlarged right atrium is often present. The right ventricle, which is well-formed (inflow, body, and outflow components are all present), contracts normally and endocardial fibroelastosis is not seen. The pulmonary arteries and pulmonary valve are normal in size and the pulmonary circulation is exclusively from blood passing through the ductus arteriosus.

Therapeutic considerations. These infants require administration of prostaglandin E_1 to maintain adequate pulmonary blood flow through the ductus arteriosus. Pulmonary valvuloplasty performed in the cardiac catheterization laboratory is the procedure of choice. Access to the pulmonary artery from the right ventricle usually is achieved by radiofrequency perforation of the atretic valve and then the balloon valvuloplasty is performed. Many infants do very well after this procedure but it also may be necessary to maintain the infant on prostaglandin E_1 after the procedure or to perform a systemic-to-pulmonary artery shunt, even after a successful valvuloplasty. This occurs when the ventricle is so hypertrophied and non-compliant that it cannot accept an adequate amount of systemic venous return despite relief of the obstruction. The ventricle, though, often rapidly remodels, and the prostaglandin E_1 infusion or the shunt may only be necessary for a short period of time.

Critical Pulmonary Valve Stenosis

Anatomic and physiologic considerations. Critical pulmonary valve stenosis is very similar to pulmonary atresia with a normal-sized right ventricle and is likely caused by similar events during cardiovascular development. Instead of an imperforate pulmonary valve, forward flow of blood is present. The distinction between critical and severe stenosis is based upon a systemic arterial desaturation below some arbitrary level, usually about 90% to 92%, in the absence of a patent ductus arteriosus. Both critical and severe stenosis of the pulmonary valve cause right ventricular systolic pressures to be at or most often, higher than systemic levels. If the degree of stenosis is critical, the ventricle cannot eject the entire systemic venous return across the pulmonary valve. In that case, some of the systemic venous return crosses the foramen ovale to the left atrium, causing systemic arterial desaturation.

Clinical presentation. The clinical presentation of infants with critical pulmonary valve stenosis is similar to that of infants with pulmonary atresia. The right ventricular impulse may be increased if there is a large amount of tricuspid regurgitation. The second heart sound is single. Although there is forward flow across the pulmonary valve, it is so minimal that it cannot be heard and the limited valve opening is not associated with an ejection click. A murmur of tricuspid regurgitation is usually present.

Ancillary tests. The electrocardiogram and chest radiograph are similar to those seen in pulmonary atresia. Coronary sinusoids are rarely present. Echocardiography is also similar to that seen in pulmonary atresia, except for the flow across the pulmonary valve. Forward flow may be so limited that it cannot be distinguished from the turbulence in the main pulmonary artery caused by ductal flow striking the atretic valve. Thus, definitive evidence of valve patency is often a small jet of pulmonary regurgitation visualized by color Doppler in the right ventricular outflow tract.

Therapeutic considerations. Although infants with severe pulmonary valve stenosis may be stable, those with critical obstruction of the pulmonary valve require administration of prostaglandin E_1 to maintain adequate pulmonary blood flow through the ductus arteriosus. Many infants do very well after a pulmonary valvuloplasty performed in the catheterization laboratory. Similar to patients with pulmonary atresia, it may be necessary to establish a second source of pulmonary blood flow, at least temporarily, via a systemic-to-pulmonary artery shunt even after a successful valvuloplasty.

Dextroposition Syndromes (Including Tetralogy of Fallot)

Anatomic and physiologic considerations. An entirely separate group of defects with right ventricular outflow obstruction are those associated with anterior malalignment of the outlet ventricular septum relative to the trabecular septum, resulting in right ventricular outflow tract obstruction. Tetralogy of Fallot is the most common of these defects and is characterized by anterior displacement of the infundibular or outlet septum, a large and anteriorly malaligned outlet ventricular septal defect, and narrowing of the right ventricular outflow tract (Figure 6-3). The aortic root is dextroposed and the amount of aortic valve overriding is variable (15%-90%). However, the aorta is still committed to the left ventricle, because the aortic valve remains in fibrous continuity with the mitral valve. The type of pulmonary stenosis is also highly variable and may occur at subvalvar, valvar, and /or supravalvar levels.

In the extreme situation, pulmonary atresia is present. If so, the pulmonary arteries may arise from a variety of sources. To understand the possible sources of pulmonary blood flow, one must be aware of the embryology of the pulmonary vascular bed. The central pulmonary arteries and ductus arteriosus arise from tissues derived from the sixth aortic arch. The peripheral pulmonary arteries are derived from an entirely different embryologic source, the capillary plexus of the embryonic lung. In the normal situation, the central pulmonary arteries invade the parenchyma of the lung along with intersegmental vessels of the descending aorta, such as the bronchial arteries. Normal central pulmonary arteries present in any lung segment are thought to send inhibitory signals that prevent connections with the intersegmental arteries. When pulmonary valve atresia occurs in the absence of a ventricular septal defect, the aortic arch tissues develop normally and normal central pulmonary arteries develop because they receive blood flow through the ductus arteriosus. However, the dextroposition syndromes develop in part because of abnormalities in the embryological development of the aortic arches, and thus the central pulmonary arteries are often very hypoplastic and may not connect to every lung segment.

In the absence of a connection between the central pulmonary artery and the distal vascular bed in a given lung segment, the inhibitory signals are absent, and other connections are made. Most commonly, intersegmental vessels from the descending aorta, called direct major aortopulmonary collateral vessels, connect to the lung segment (Figure 6-5A). Occasionally, these vessels do not develop and indirect collateral vessels derived from the head and neck vessels supply that segment (Figure 6-5B). In either situation, small central pulmonary arteries may fill with blood in a retrograde fashion from diminutive connections peripherally but central connections are not present (Figure 6-5C).

Clinical presentation. The initial presentation of the infant with any of these "dextroposition" defects depends entirely on the amount of pulmonary blood flow. Pulmonary blood flow increases greatly as pulmonary vascular resistance falls after birth in those infants with severe obstruction and a patent ductus arteriosus. These infants may be cyanotic very transiently, if noted at all, and soon do not appear cyanotic at rest. Typically, during the first hours of life these infants are cyanotic only when crying or feeding. Over the first few hours and days, the ductus arteriosus begins to close and cyanosis becomes more apparent.

On physical examination a variable degree of cyanosis is present and although the infant may be tachypneic, respiratory distress is not evident. Because pulmonary arterial resistance is less than systemic arterial resistance, any shunt across the ductus arteriosus must be from the aorta to the pulmonary artery so that upper and lower body arterial oxygen saturations are the same, a finding which can help to differentiate these infants with dextroposition defects from those with d-transposition of the great arteries (Table 6-3). The pulses are normal or increased if there is a large ductus arteriosus or aortopulmonary collateral flow. The cardiac examination shows a normal to increased precordial impulse and a single second heart sound. A systolic or continuous murmur reflecting flow through the collateral vessels is heard best over the lung fields and is often prominent in the back.

The remainder of the physical examination is normal except when the cardiac defect occurs in the presence of a specific syndrome. Unlike infants with other forms of cyanotic heart disease, associated noncardiac findings are quite common, particularly when the aortic arch is right sided (Chapter 15). A relatively large proportion of patients are syndromic or have chromosomal anomalies. The group of syndromes with a microdeletion on the short arm of chromosome 22 (deletion 22q11 syndrome) include DiGeorge syndrome, CATCH-22, velocardiofacial syndrome, conotruncal face anomaly, and Shprintzen syndrome, all of which have overlapping clinical findings. These findings, which include hypertelorism, low set ears, micrognathia, and palatal anomalies are commonly present in affected infants. These infants should undergo testing to assess for genetic defects.

Ancillary tests. The electrocardiogram is normal during the first few days of life, showing the normal right ventricular dominance pattern of upright T waves and dominant R waves in the right precordium. However, unlike the electrocardiogram from a normal infant in which the T waves become inverted during the first week of life, the upright T waves persist because the systolic pressure in the right ventricle remains at systemic levels. The chest radiograph shows a dominant right ventricular contour with absence

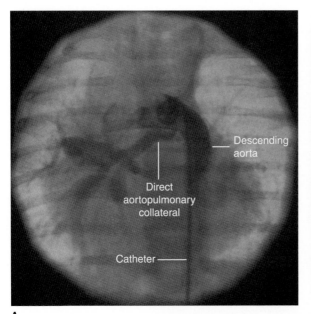

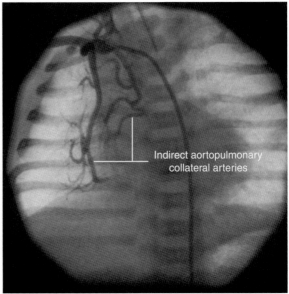

A

B

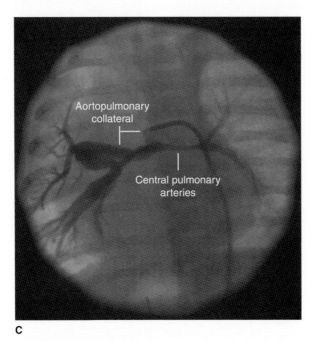

C

FIGURE 6-5. Aortic or selective angiograms performed in a patient with pulmonary atresia, ventricular septal defect, and aortopulmonary collateral vessels. A. Descending aortic angiogram shows large direct aortopulmonary collateral vessels arising from the mid-thoracic aorta. **B.** An angiogram performed in the right innominate artery demonstrates indirect collateral vessels arising from the right subclavian artery and perfusing the right lung. **C.** A selective angiogram in a direct aortopulmonary collateral vessel demonstrates distal filling of diminutive bilateral true pulmonary arterial circulation.

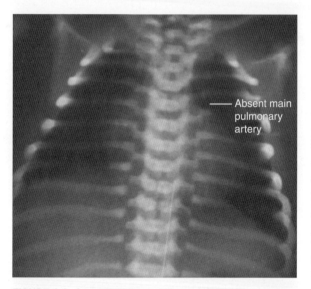

— Absent main
pulmonary
artery

FIGURE 6-6. A chest radiograph in an infant with tetralogy of Fallot demonstrates a narrow mediastinum by absence of the normal pulmonary arterial contour in the upper left heart border, and the dominant right ventricular contour making the left border take on a horizontal, or boot-shaped appearance. An umbilical artery catheter is present.

overriding the ventricular septum to a variable degree. The anatomy of the right ventricular outflow tract and pulmonary valve, the central pulmonary arterial anatomy, associated muscular ventricular septal defects, the coronary arterial anatomy, the side of the aortic arch, and the anatomy of the ductus arteriosus should be defined. In the presence of a patent ductus arteriosus and a patent pulmonary valve, it may not be possible to determine whether blood flow through the ductus arteriosus is necessary for healthy survival until the ductus arteriosus closes. However, the size of the outflow tract and pulmonary valve usually reflect the degree of right ventricular outflow tract obstruction. In pulmonary atresia, it is particularly important to clearly define the anatomy of the ductus arteriosus. Differentiating the ductus arteriosus from an aortopulmonary collateral vessel is sometimes difficult. If the ductus arteriosus is present, it may also connect to only one lung. If the pulmonary valve is atretic, a ductus arteriosus may or may not be present. Thus, newborns with pulmonary atresia and ventricular septal defect usually undergo cardiac catheterization and/or magnetic resonance imaging to ensure precise definition of anatomy.

Therapeutic considerations. Infants with reasonably well-developed pulmonary arteries undergo complete repair of their defects, usually within the first few months of life. Infants who require intervention but are either too premature or are at excessive risk from cardiopulmonary bypass because of secondary organ dysfunction may undergo a palliative procedure first. The palliation may be via a catheter approach, consisting of a balloon pulmonary valvuloplasty or stenting of the ductus arteriosus, or may be a surgical systemic-to-pulmonary artery shunt.

Therapy is much more complex in patients with hypoplastic central pulmonary arteries because the sources of pulmonary blood flow are complicated and different in every patient. Those infants in whom the blood supply to one or both lungs arises from the ductus arteriosus require surgery in the newborn period to preclude loss of these lung segments when the ductus closes. In contrast, surgery may be delayed for weeks or months in those infants whose pulmonary blood flow is supplied by aortopulmonary collateral vessels. The goal of therapy for these infants is reconstruction of the pulmonary arteries such that closure of the ventricular septal defect is possible, but this often involves a series of procedures in the catheterization laboratory and operating room.

of the main pulmonary artery contour and shows the classic "boot-shaped" heart (Figure 6-6). Evaluation of the central pulmonary vessels is important. Decreased central vascularity is often present, but this does not necessarily reflect decreased pulmonary blood flow. Pulmonary blood flow is not dependent upon the size of the central vessels, but rather upon the conductance of the peripheral vascular bed. A large quantity of blood may be passing through a ductus arteriosus or through aortopulmonary collateral vessels to the lungs without enlarging the central arteries. The oxygen saturation may be in the low to mid 90s in many infants with small central pulmonary arteries; this indicates pulmonary blood flow that is about three times the normal systemic blood flow. The presence of a right aortic arch is an important finding, which is commonly present in dextroposition defects and increases the likelihood of a chromosome 22 microdeletion. The absence of a rightward deflection of the trachea or of a left-sided aortic knob, and the presence of a descending aorta to the right of the spine are all suggestive of the presence of a right aortic arch on the chest radiograph.

The echocardiogram shows the internal cardiac anatomy of an outlet ventricular septal defect and an aorta

Heterotaxy Syndromes (Right and Left Atrial Isomerism)

Anatomic and physiologic considerations. Heterotaxy syndromes represent constellations of cardiac and noncardiac findings in which the situs of the neonate is uncertain (Chapter 1), and thus these are also called situs ambiguous. They may be divided into apparent bilateral right sidedness, also known as asplenia syndrome, and bilateral left sidedness or polysplenia syndrome. This is based upon the fact that the spleen is a left-sided structure, but unfortunately, the presence or absence of functioning splenic tissue does not fully track with the finding of right or left sidedness. Of all the findings that occur in one or the other syndrome, the most reproducible is the anatomy of the atrial appendages. The right and left appendages are very different. The right atrial appendage is blunt, has a wide opening to the atrium, and has pectinate muscles that extend to the anterior wall of the atrium. In contrast, the left atrium is long and fingerlike, has a narrow opening to the atrium and limited pectinate muscles that do not extend anteriorly. Because of these reproducible differences in the atrial appendages, the heterotaxy syndromes have been termed "right atrial isomerism" or "left atrial isomerism" (although the term refers to the appendages rather than to the body of the atrium).

In right atrial isomerism, obstruction of the pulmonary outflow is extremely common and atresia of the pulmonary valve is frequently present. The heart may be in either side of the thorax. Associated cardiac and noncardiac findings are numerous. Additional cardiovascular findings include bilateral superior vena cavae, bilateral sinus nodes, absence of the coronary sinus, a complete atrioventricular septal defect or atresia of one of the atrioventricular valves (rarely are two separate atrioventricular valves present), dextroposition of the aorta, and an almost pathognomonic finding of juxtaposition of the inferior vena cava and descending aorta. The pulmonary arterial anatomy usually mirrors that of the bronchi, exhibiting bilateral right-sided morphology. The pulmonary veins usually connect anomalously, often to one or both superior vena cavae. If they connect directly to the atria, they do so symmetrically into both atria. The hepatic veins also frequently connect abnormally, directly to the atria and separate from the inferior vena cava. Noncardiac findings include a midline liver, bilateral right bronchial and lung morphology, absence of a functioning spleen, and malrotation of the intestine.

Clinical presentation. The clinical presentation of the newborn with right atrial isomerism is similar to that of any infant with ductal-dependent pulmonary blood flow. Initially the saturations are high enough that cyanosis may only be appreciated when the infant is crying or feeding, but eventually cyanosis increases as the ductus arteriosus closes. Rarely, pulmonary venous obstruction is severe enough to cause significant pulmonary edema, which is associated with both severe respiratory distress and cyanosis. Specific clinical findings include a midline liver. Frequently, the heart is located in the right side of the thorax so the cardiac impulse and heart sounds are in the right chest. The second heart sound is single and murmurs are often absent, but if present, are usually heard best over the lung fields.

Ancillary tests. The electrocardiogram is highly variable because of the variability in the position of the heart and the intracardiac findings. There are usually prominent anterior forces since the ventricular chamber ejects into the anterior aorta, but those forces may be in the right or left chest, and there is usually no evidence of a septal Q wave in the precordial leads on either side of the chest. The chest radiograph often shows a right-sided heart and/or stomach, a midline liver, decreased central pulmonary vascularity, and occasionally bilateral minor fissures, indicative of two lungs of right-sided morphology. The mediastinum is often difficult to interpret because the aorta usually arises abnormally and bilateral vena cavae are present. The echocardiogram demonstrates most of the findings in right atrial isomerism if performed in a careful and thorough manner.

Therapeutic considerations. These patients all have a functional single ventricle. Almost all will need a systemic-to-pulmonary artery shunt in the newborn period. Subsequently, a bidirectional Glenn shunt (usually bilateral bidirectional because there are two superior vena cavae) and modified Fontan operation may be performed (see following text).

Left atrial isomerism presents with a wide constellation of findings as well, but usually is not associated with significant obstruction to pulmonary blood flow. Occasionally, however, there may be significant obstruction with associated cyanosis, so that this syndrome should be considered in the infant presenting with cyanosis and uncertain situs. The constellation of findings seen in left atrial isomerism is discussed in Chapter 7.

l-malposition of the Aorta With Pulmonary Stenosis/Atresia

Anatomic and physiologic considerations. l-malposition of the aorta is often associated with a ventricular septal defect and subvalvar and valvar pulmonic stenosis. In this condition, abnormal l-looping of the heart and rotation of the outflow tracts are present. As described earlier, there is both atrial-ventricular and ventricular-arterial discordance (Figure 6-1B). The tricuspid valve (which is the left, or pulmonary venous, atrioventricular valve), connects to the systemic right ventricle, and often has an Ebstein malformation (inferior displacement of the septal leaflet, see following text). However, tricuspid regurgitation is rarely severe in this defect. Occasionally, there is dextrorotation of the heart and more rarely, true situs inversus, which often lead to the erroneous diagnosis of a heterotaxy syndrome. In the presence of pulmonary outflow tract obstruction, a ventricular septal defect is almost always present, so that some of the desaturated blood that enters the left ventricle from the right atrium passes through the ventricular septal defect into the ascending aorta. Sometimes both atrioventricular valves empty into the left ventricle, a condition known as double-inlet left ventricle. If this occurs, the right ventricle is usually only a rudimentary outflow chamber and the physiology is that of a functional single ventricle. Mixed pulmonary and systemic venous blood passes through the ventricular septal defect and small right ventricle and then into the aorta. The size of the ventricular septal defect must be evaluated to ensure that it is large enough that all of the systemic output can pass through it without obstruction. Alternatively, instead of double-inlet left ventricle, the tricuspid valve may override the ventricular septum (tricuspid valve straddling).

Clinical presentation. The physical findings are dependent upon the specific defect present. The precordial impulse is usually normal or mildly increased in the absence of situs inversus, since the left ventricle is located adjacent to the normal right ventricle. The quality of second heart sound often provides a clue to the diagnosis. Because the aorta lies anteriorly and leftward (or rightward in situs inversus), the second heart sound is single, very loud, and heard more laterally than usual. A harsh midfrequency systolic murmur is heard in the mid-parasternal area and reflects flow through the ventricular septal defect. This murmur is difficult to separate from the pulmonary outflow murmur, which may be of somewhat higher frequency and which radiates into both lung fields.

Ancillary tests. The electrocardiogram is variable, depending on the location of the heart in the chest, but it frequently shows Q waves in the anterior precordial leads and evidence of biventricular hypertrophy, with prominent R and S waves. Atrioventricular block occurs occasionally but it is much more frequent in left atrial isomerism. If Ebstein anomaly of the tricuspid valve is present, preexcitation may be seen, and supraventricular tachycardia may occur. The chest radiograph shows mesocardia and an unusual left heart contour as a result of the l-transposed aorta, especially in older infants. The left-sided aorta is seen at the left upper mediastinal border (Figure 6-7). The echocardiogram shows the findings discussed in the preceding discussion. It is important to clearly determine the atrial-ventricular connections to exclude double-inlet left ventricle or straddling of the tricuspid valve, both of which affect the ultimate surgical approach to the patient. The morphology and function of the tricuspid valve, the ventricular septum, the subpulmonary region, and the pulmonary valve should also be defined.

Therapeutic considerations. The approach to therapy in an individual patient depends on the associated defects. Infants without associated intracardiac abnormalities do

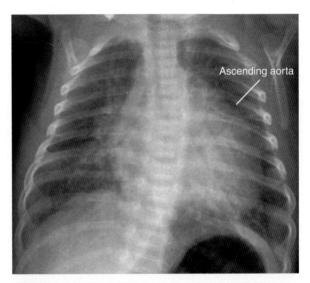

FIGURE 6-7. A chest radiograph in an infant with l-transposition of the great arteries shows a prominent shadow in the left upper mediastinum that is caused by the leftward ascending aorta. This gives the left heart border a straight appearance that is characteristic of this defect.

Ascending aorta

not require specific therapy. However, even in the absence of other defects, long-term follow-up studies indicate a high incidence of acquired systemic ventricular dysfunction, heart failure, systemic atrioventricular valve (tricuspid) regurgitation, arrhythmias, and sudden death. A ventricular septal defect is the most commonly associated defect and will often require surgical closure. Because of the abnormal course of the conduction system, complete atrioventricular block is common after closure of a ventricular septal defect and many patients will need permanent pacemaker placement. In addition, there is an incidence of acquired atrioventricular block in later life, even in the absence of surgical intervention.

Decreased Pulmonary Blood Flow With Valvar Regurgitation

Valvar regurgitation is a rare cause of decreased pulmonary blood flow, but regurgitation of the tricuspid valve is much more common than that of the pulmonary valve. Regurgitation of the tricuspid valve causes regurgitation of blood into the right atrium and thus increases right atrial pressures. This causes a right-to-left atrial shunt and cyanosis. Pulmonary valve regurgitation is extremely rare and occurs almost exclusively as part of a syndrome called tetralogy of Fallot with absent pulmonary valve (see following text). Pulmonary valve regurgitation does not increase right atrial pressures.

The course of cyanosis in the neonate with valvar regurgitation is often quite different from that of an infant with obstruction of pulmonary blood flow. Although both may have progressive cyanosis in the first few hours to days of life as the ductus arteriosus closes, the neonate with outflow obstruction requires intervention, whereas the neonate with valvar regurgitation may show a spontaneous increase in arterial oxygen saturation after a few days of very low saturations. This is because pulmonary vascular resistance affects the amount of valvar regurgitation but not the amount of proximal obstruction. Over the first weeks of life, pulmonary vascular resistance decreases, beginning at the same time but over a longer time course than the closure of the ductus arteriosus. The neonate with valvar regurgitation may be dependent on blood flow through the ductus arteriosus while the pulmonary vascular resistance is high. However, as pulmonary vascular resistance decreases during the first weeks of life, the degree of valvar regurgitation decreases and allows more blood to enter the pulmonary vasculature.

Ebstein Anomaly

Anatomic and physiologic considerations. Ebstein anomaly is characterized by varying degrees of inferior displacement of the septal and posterior (mural) leaflets of the tricuspid valve. This is the most common cause of cyanosis resulting from valvar regurgitation. Displacement of the leaflets into the right ventricle prevents proper coaptation of the leaflets and thus produces severe tricuspid regurgitation. Because the leaflet is displaced below the atrioventricular groove, the regurgitation is not only into the right atrium, but also into a component of the right ventricle. This is called the atrialized right ventricle, which may dilate greatly along with the right atrium.

In the fetus, the severe regurgitation and displacement of the septal leaflet of the tricuspid valve in Ebstein anomaly drastically reduces blood flow across the right ventricular outflow tract and increases flow across the foramen ovale. Thus, there may be a secondary abnormality in the development of the right ventricular outflow, the most severe abnormality being pulmonary valve atresia. Also, the large increase in flow across the foramen ovale is usually associated with a large secundum atrial septal defect. The increased right atrial pressures in the fetus also may be associated with hydrops fetalis, which may lead to fetal demise.

Clinical presentation. The neonate with Ebstein anomaly, even of only moderate severity, usually presents with profound cyanosis when the ductus arteriosus begins to close. Peripheral pulses and perfusion are usually normal. The liver is usually normal, although it occasionally is large and pulsatile. The precordium is hyperactive because a large volume of blood is passing back and forth between the right atrium and ventricle. Heart sounds are often complex and difficult to interpret, because multiple systolic clicks may be present. It is worthwhile remembering that a cyanotic infant with too many heart sounds is likely to have Ebstein anomaly. A loud, harsh systolic murmur at the lower left sternal border reflecting tricuspid regurgitation is heard and radiates to the right.

Ancillary tests. The electrocardiogram usually shows marked right atrial enlargement (peaked P wave in leads II, III, and V_1) and variable right ventricular forces. A short PR interval and a delta wave of preexcitation are sometimes present and supraventricular tachycardia may occur in these infants. The chest radiograph is often dramatically abnormal. The heart appears globular and markedly dilated, filling much of the chest, and the pulmonary vascular markings are decreased. Ebstein anomaly is one of the very few conditions that presents with marked cardiomegaly at birth. The echocardiogram is diagnostic, except in the rare infant in whom inferior displacement of the tricuspid valve is uncertain and other causes of tricuspid regurgitation must be considered. Usually, a large degree of separation between the hinge point of the leaflet and the atrioventricular groove is present, and the mural leaflet is small and dysplastic. Another pathognomonic finding is the location of the orifice of the valve, indicated by the origin of the regurgitation jet. Whereas color Doppler demonstrates regurgitation beginning near the atrioventricular groove in other causes of tricuspid regurgitation, in Ebstein anomaly the jet begins well down toward the apex of the ventricle. It is important to carefully evaluate the size of the true right ventricle, outflow tract, and pulmonary valve, because this often determines whether the cyanosis will regress spontaneously or whether neonatal surgery will be necessary. The absence of forward flow of blood across the pulmonary valve is not diagnostic of pulmonary valve atresia. Pulmonary arterial pressures may be maintained at systemic levels by flow through a patent ductus arteriosus. If the pulmonary arterial pressure exceeds the pressure that the right ventricle can generate because of the presence of tricuspid regurgitation, the pulmonary valve will not open. In the absence of forward flow, color Doppler evidence of pulmonary regurgitation verifies the patency of the valve. This is very important because neonatal surgery still carries significant mortality and may be unnecessary. The pulmonary arteries are well developed even if the pulmonary valve is atretic, and the left-sided structures are normal.

Therapeutic considerations. The fact that tricuspid regurgitation often improves as the pulmonary vascular resistance decreases over the first few weeks of life should be considered when planning therapy for these patients. As discussed earlier, cyanosis may gradually decrease and it is advisable to continue an infusion of prostaglandin E_1 for several weeks rather than to perform a potentially unnecessary systemic-to-pulmonary artery shunt or complex tricuspid valve surgery. Newer corrective surgical techniques are being developed, and the cone reconstruction has shown very good early results. The atrial septal defect is large and is often sufficient to maintain adequate systemic output and thus an atrial septostomy is not necessary at birth. Later in life it is often necessary to close the

atrial septal defect, even in patients with mild Ebstein anomaly.

Other Causes of Tricuspid Regurgitation

Other causes of tricuspid regurgitation are much less common than Ebstein anomaly. The tricuspid valve may be dysplastic but without displacement of the septal leaflet, causing severe regurgitation. The clinical presentation, results of ancillary tests, and therapy depend on the amount of regurgitation and are similar to that described above for Ebstein anomaly. Ischemic damage to the papillary muscles of the tricuspid valve related to perinatal asphyxia is discussed in Chapter 9.

Absent Pulmonary Valve Syndrome

Anatomic and physiologic considerations. Pulmonary regurgitation is extremely rare and occurs almost exclusively as tetralogy of Fallot with absent pulmonary valve syndrome. The pulmonary valve annulus is mildly hypoplastic but has only vestigial valve remnants. The central branch pulmonary arteries are massively dilated, sometimes asymmetrically. A ductus arteriosus rarely exists, and its absence has been implicated in the dramatic pulmonary arterial enlargement. This enlargement may also be caused by a primary defect in the wall of the pulmonary arteries, and histology shows disruption of the elastic layer. Although the unrestricted pulmonary regurgitation in association with the infundibular narrowing and the ventricular septal defect causes right-to-left ventricular shunting and cyanosis, compression of the central bronchi by the dilated pulmonary arteries often contributes to the severe cyanosis.

Clinical presentation. On physical examination, the infant is cyanotic but, unlike in infants with other causes of cyanotic heart disease, is in severe respiratory distress. The distress is both inspiratory and expiratory and may improve dramatically when the infant is placed in a prone position, an important finding that should be considered in evaluating and treating the infant. However, many infants are in such distress that they require endotracheal intubation and mechanical ventilation. The pulses are normal and the noncardiac examination is usually noncontributory. The precordial impulse is usually markedly increased. The heart sounds often are difficult to appreciate because of the loud murmur. It is best described as a sawing murmur, loudest at the left upper sternal border but radiating to the entire chest. Few murmurs will be confused with this dramatic sound, except perhaps that of truncal valve stenosis and regurgitation in a neonate with persistent truncus arteriosus (although infants with truncus arteriosus rarely have the same degree of respiratory distress).

Ancillary tests. The electrocardiogram is similar to that of the neonate with tetralogy of Fallot. It is usually normal, but may show right ventricular hypertrophy, particularly after several days when the right precordial T waves have not inverted normally. The chest radiograph is often dramatically abnormal, showing a massively dilated right or left pulmonary artery, or both. The cardiac silhouette is often large. The pulmonary vascular markings may appear increased despite reduced pulmonary blood flow because of the marked pulsatility caused by the pulmonary valve regurgitation. The echocardiogram shows a mild form of tetralogy of Fallot but with massively dilated proximal pulmonary arteries. Little obvious valve tissue is present in the pulmonary annulus and severe pulmonary regurgitation is present.

Therapeutic considerations. The pulmonary complications of this syndrome are the principal determinants of successful therapy. The ventricular septal defect is closed and conduits are used to reconstruct the right ventricular outflow tract. Despite reparative surgery, tracheobronchial obstruction secondary to the markedly dilated pulmonary arteries often results in chronic respiratory insufficiency.

■ d-TRANSPOSITION COMPLEXES

The other main hemodynamic category of defects that cause cyanosis is the d-transposition complexes. The aorta is "transposed" to the opposite side of the ventricular septum and thus arises from the morphologic right ventricle in patients with d-transposition. In the most common form, simple d-transposition of the great arteries (Figure 6-1A), the heart is normally or d-looped. The right atrium is connected normally to the right ventricle (atrial-ventricular concordance) which, in turn, is connected to the aorta (ventricular-arterial discordance). The left atrium is connected normally to the left ventricle and the pulmonary artery is also transposed over the ventricular septum and thus arises from the left ventricle. Desaturated systemic venous blood returns to the right atrium and flows across the tricuspid valve into the right ventricle and out the aorta, resulting in profound cyanosis. The pulmonary artery may arise from the left ventricle or may arise with the aorta from the right ventricle. This is associated with a subpulmonary ventricular septal defect and is called double-outlet right ventricle of the Taussig-Bing type. Other cardiovascular abnormalities are frequently present in patients with the d-transposition complexes and include an atrial septal defect, a ventricular septal defect, subvalvar pulmonary stenosis, subvalvar aortic stenosis (in the presence of Taussig-Bing anomaly), and coarctation of the aorta.

Fetal Physiology

Blood flow patterns are abnormal in the fetus with d-transposition of the aorta, but these patterns are not as dramatically altered as in the fetus with obstruction of blood flow within the right heart. Because the left and right ventricles eject blood under similar pressures in both the normal fetus and in those with transposition, their relative ability to receive blood (passive compliance) is similar. Thus, venous return enters the ventricles and crosses the foramen ovale in a normal pattern.

The right ventricle ejects blood containing somewhat less oxygen and glucose to the upper body. The brain and heart accommodate the decreased oxygen and glucose delivery by use of local vasodilatory mechanisms that increase blood flow, although there is recent evidence suggesting that metabolic adaptations are incomplete and that neurodevelopmental problems may begin in utero (Chapter 14). The left ventricle, which receives a larger portion of the placental return, ejects blood with relatively high oxygen saturation and glucose concentration to the lower body and placenta. This may cause the pancreas to produce more insulin. Hyperinsulinemia may explain the apparent association, at birth, of d-transposition of the great arteries with macrosomia and hypoglycemia.

Blood flow around the aortic arch is normal or somewhat increased in the fetus with simple d-transposition. Thus, these infants rarely have coarctation of the aorta. More commonly, coarctation occurs when there is a subpulmonic ventricular septal defect, which directs some of the right ventricular output to the pulmonary artery and through the ductus arteriosus to the lower body thus decreasing blood flow around the aortic arch. A subpulmonary ventricular septal defect may occur if the pulmonary artery is committed to the left ventricle (d-transposition with ventricular septal defect), but it is much more frequent when the pulmonary artery is committed to the right ventricle (double-outlet right ventricle of the Taussig-Bing type). In this defect, the great vessels are often side by side, which compromises the aortic out-flow tract, causing subaortic stenosis in addition to the aortic coarctation.

Simple d-Transposition of the Great Arteries

Anatomic and physiologic considerations. Pulmonary blood flow increases dramatically after birth, which raises left atrial pressure and causes the flap of the foramen ovale to close. The likelihood that this flap is insufficient, as occurs in a secundum atrial septal defect, is no higher in infants with d-transposition than in a normal new-born infant. If the flap of the foramen closes, pul-monary venous return does not enter the right atrium and right ventricle, and the pulmonary and systemic circulations are thus completely separated. In the pres-ence of d-transposition of the great arteries, this prevents the ascending aorta from receiving highly saturated pul-monary venous return and results in severe cyanosis, requiring urgent intervention.

The frequent presence of higher oxygen saturations in the lower extremities in d-transposition of the great arteries is explained by understanding the abnormal blood flow patterns (Table 6-3). Although this is more common and severe when coarctation of the aorta is present, mildly increased lower extremity saturations still occur commonly in simple d-transposition without coarctation (especially before a balloon atrial septostomy is performed). This is because the normal postnatal left-to-right ductal shunt raises left atrial pressure if the foramen ovale is restrictive. The continued left-to-right shunting and increased left atrial pressure cause reflex pulmonary arterial vasoconstric-tion. This increases pulmonary vascular resistance to a level that right-to-left shunting occurs through the ductus arte-riosus so that highly saturated blood from the pulmonary artery flows to the descending aorta.

Clinical presentation. Simple d-transposition of the great arteries is the most common form of cyanotic heart dis-ease and one of the most common forms of symptomatic heart disease in the newborn. Unlike the infant with decreased pulmonary blood flow who generally does not have severe cyanosis at birth, the infant with d-transposi-tion of the great arteries is often profoundly cyanotic within minutes or hours after birth. Thus the newborn infant who presents early with profound cyanosis but without respira-tory distress most frequently has d-transposition of the great arteries.

On physical examination the infant is cyanotic in all extremities, although, as discussed earlier, pulse oximetry may show a higher oxygen saturation in the lower extrem-ities. The infant is tachypneic but not in respiratory distress. The pulses and perfusion are normal. The noncardiac examination is noncontributory. The precordium is active, but not increased compared to that of a normal newborn infant. The first heart sound is normal and the second sound is single and loud but not displaced. Murmurs are rarely present.

Ancillary tests. The electrocardiogram is normal at birth, although evidence of right ventricular hypertrophy is pres-ent by several days of age. The newborn chest radiograph classically shows an "egg-on-a-string" (Figure 6-8), in which the heart is of normal size but the mediastinum is narrow because of posterior and rightward malposition of the pulmonary artery. However, the thymus is frequently present and the narrow mediastinum may not be appreci-ated. Over the next few days, if the infant is untreated, the heart enlarges and pulmonary vascularity increases. d-transposition is rapidly diagnosed by two-dimensional echocardiography. Upon diagnosis, it is important to quickly define the patency of the ductus arteriosus and of

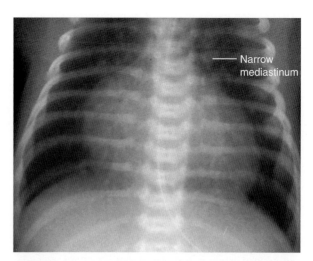

FIGURE 6-8. A chest radiograph in an infant with d-transposition of the great arteries shows a narrow medi-astinum caused by posterior and medial displacement of the pulmonary artery. The left ventricular contour is dominant making the apex of the heart point downward, like an "egg-on-a-string." A nasogastric tube is present.

the foramen ovale. Doppler echocardiography should be used to estimate the flow and the pressure difference across the foramen ovale. If a significant pressure difference between the right and left atria is found, the foramen ovale is said to be "restrictive." Associated abnormalities such as a ventricular septal defect, coarctation of the aorta, or subvalvar pulmonic stenosis should be defined. It is also important to describe the anatomy of the pulmonary and aortic valves, the alignment of their commissures and of the coronary arteries.

Therapeutic considerations. To maintain patency of the ductus arteriosus, prostaglandin E_1 (Chapter 12) should be administered to all newborn infants with d-transposition of the great arteries. Although shunting through the ductus arteriosus is typically bidirectional (right-to-left in early systole and left-to-right throughout diastole), only left-to-right shunting through the foramen ovale allows highly saturated blood to reach the ascending aorta. If the patient is profoundly cyanotic and the foramen ovale is small and restrictive, an emergency balloon atrial septostomy should be performed. This can usually be done under echocardiographic guidance at the infant's bedside as soon as the problem is recognized. After the septostomy, the increased pulmonary blood flow caused by the ductal shunt raises left atrial pressure, which may dramatically increase the left-to-right shunt across the foramen ovale, which in turn increases aortic oxygen saturation.

Definitive surgical repair of simple d-transposition of the great arteries is accomplished by performing the arterial switch procedure (usually in the first week or two of life). The aorta and pulmonary artery are transected just above their respective valves and then sewn to the appropriate ventricle. To maintain coronary perfusion with normal pressure and oxygen saturation, the coronary arteries must be transferred from the aorta to the pulmonary artery (which now becomes the neo-aorta). The anatomy of the coronary arteries is frequently abnormal in these patients, but in almost all instances, the coronary arteries can be successfully transplanted into the neo-aorta at the time of surgery.

d-Transposition of the Great Arteries With Ventricular Septal Defect

Anatomic and physiologic considerations. The cardiac defect most commonly associated with d-transposition of the great arteries is a ventricular septal defect. The defect usually lies in the perimembranous region, but may be muscular in location. When the ventricular septal defect is subpulmonic, it may be associated with redirection of some of the right ventricular output to the pulmonary artery, so that coarctation of the aorta is more likely to occur.

Clinical presentation. The clinical presentation of the infant with d-transposition of the great arteries who also has a ventricular septal defect may be the same or quite different than that of the infant with an intact ventricular septum. Blood tends to flow through the ventricular septal defect to the pulmonary arteries (left-to-right shunting) because the resistance in the pulmonary vascular bed is lower than that in the systemic bed. If the atrial septum is intact, the infant is profoundly cyanotic and an emergency balloon atrial septostomy is indicated despite the presence of a ventricular septal defect. The only distinguishing features from simple d-transposition may be a short systolic murmur and, occasionally, respiratory distress from the increased left atrial pressures and subsequent pulmonary edema. If, however, a relatively nonrestrictive foramen ovale is present, the left-to-right ventricular shunt increases left atrial filling and causes a large left-to-right atrial shunt which does not decrease with closure of the ductus arteriosus. Thus, these infants may have quite high arterial oxygen saturations, and, indeed, occasionally they are not diagnosed until several weeks of age when they present with evidence of excessive pulmonary blood flow. The implementation of pulse oximetry screening in the newborn should greatly decrease such delayed diagnoses.

Ancillary tests. The electrocardiogram is similar to that seen in simple d-transposition of the great arteries. The chest radiograph shows an enlarged heart and increased vascularity at an earlier time. The echocardiogram shows the location and shunting of the ventricular septal defect. The flow and pressure difference across the patent foramen ovale must be assessed. Possible associated defects such as pulmonary stenosis and coarctation of the aorta should be defined.

Therapeutic considerations. Definitive surgical repair is accomplished by the arterial switch procedure and closure of the ventricular septal defect. If a subaortic ventricular septal defect is present, the presence of fixed subvalvar and valvar pulmonary stenosis prevents this approach.

Instead, a Rastelli procedure is performed, but this is usually delayed for several months or years. In this operation, the ventricular septal defect is closed in such a fashion that the left ventricle ejects into the aorta (an interventricular baffle). Connection of the right ventricle to the pulmonary artery often requires an external conduit but occasionally, the right ventricular outflow tract also can be internally baffled, to connect to the pulmonary valve without significant obstruction.

Taussig-Bing Anomaly

Anatomic and physiologic considerations. Double-outlet right ventricle of the d-transposition type is commonly referred to as Taussig-Bing anomaly. There is disagreement about what constitutes double-outlet right ventricle as compared to d-transposition with ventricular septal defect. Perhaps the best way to differentiate the two defects is that a subpulmonic conus or infundibulum is present in double-outlet right ventricle but not in d-transposition with a ventricular septal defect. The conus is a structure that is part of the embryologic outflow tract, which is incorporated into the future right ventricle. Thus, the presence of a conus below the pulmonary valve suggests that it is committed to the right ventricle rather than to the left ventricle. This is more than a semantic consideration. The presence of a subpulmonic conus indicates that the pulmonary valve is located more anteriorly and leftward than occurs in simple d-transposition. This position is more likely to encroach upon the subaortic outflow tract, and the right ventricle is likely to eject more of its output across the pulmonary valve. Thus, subaortic stenosis and coarctation of the aorta are far more likely to occur in Taussig-Bing anomaly, and complete interruption of the aorta is common.

Clinical presentation. On physical examination, the infant is cyanotic but usually not as severely as the newborn with simple d-transposition. There commonly is a significant discrepancy between upper and lower body oxygen saturations, and the lower body pulses may be decreased if coarctation of the aorta is present. If so, respiratory distress and decreased systemic perfusion may be present. The precordium is active, the second heart sound is single, and a short systolic murmur is present.

Ancillary tests. The electrocardiogram and chest radiograph are not different than those seen in d-transposition of the great arteries with ventricular septal defect. The echocardiogram demonstrates the abnormal relationships of the great arteries and shows both the subpulmonic conus and a separate subaortic conus. The subpulmonic ventricular septal defect is readily demonstrated. The anatomy of the subaortic region, the aortic arch, and the coronary arteries should be defined. The relative size of the great arteries should also be evaluated because major size discrepancies may complicate the arterial switch operation.

Therapeutic considerations. Definitive surgical repair is accomplished in early infancy by the arterial switch procedure and closure of the ventricular septal defect, although marked discrepancy in semilunar valve size, coronary artery abnormalities, and the obstruction of the left ventricular outflow tract after closure of the ventricular septal defect all adversely affect the long-term outcome. Associated defects such as coarctation of the aorta are repaired at the same time.

■ PALLIATIVE PROCEDURES

Systemic-to-Pulmonary Artery Shunts

A shunt may be placed between the aorta or branch of the aorta and pulmonary artery in two groups of infants who do not have enough pulmonary blood flow because of severe pulmonary stenosis or pulmonary atresia: those who are too small to undergo open-heart repair of all defects and those in whom open-heart repair is not feasible. The shunt must be large enough to provide adequate pulmonary blood flow as the patient grows but not so large that the patient develops ventricular dysfunction because of volume overload. In addition, placement of the shunt should avoid distortion of the pulmonary artery.

The Blalock-Taussig shunt was one of the first surgeries performed in children with congenital heart disease. As originally described, the subclavian artery was divided and the proximal end was anastomosed to the main branch pulmonary artery on the same side (Figure 6-9). More commonly, a modified Blalock-Taussig shunt is performed by placing a Gore-Tex tube graft between the subclavian artery and the branch pulmonary artery on the same side. The size of the shunt is determined by the size of the Gore-Tex tube graft. A central shunt is performed by placing a Gore-Tex tube graft between the ascending aorta and main

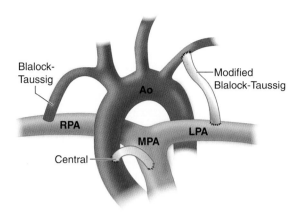

FIGURE 6-9. Diagram of most commonly performed systemic-to-pulmonary artery shunts. Abbreviations: LPA, left pulmonary artery; MPA, main pulmonary artery; RPA, right pulmonary artery.

pulmonary artery (Figure 6-9). This shunt has a very low likelihood of causing distortion of the pulmonary artery. In patients with very hypoplastic or otherwise distorted pulmonary arteries, atypical shunts are most often constructed with a piece of Gore-Tex tubing connecting the aorta or subclavian artery to a branch pulmonary artery. Alternatively, some avoid surgery and use transcatheter placement of a stent in the ductus arteriosus to maintain pulmonary blood flow.

After surgical or catheter-based placement of a systemic-to-pulmonary artery shunt, the magnitude of pulmonary blood flow is largely determined by shunt size and the relation of the systemic-to-pulmonary vascular resistances. The goal is usually to keep the oxygen saturations 75% to 85%, which usually provides adequate systemic oxygen delivery and does not create excessive volume overload for the ventricle(s) (see following discussion).

Patients who have had a shunt procedure are at risk of infectious endocarditis, paradoxical embolism, brain abscess, and shunt thrombosis. Low-dose aspirin is often administered daily to decrease the risk of shunt thrombosis and clopidogrel has been added in some high-risk patients although studies as to its efficacy and safety are ongoing. Shunt thrombosis should always be considered if a patient becomes acutely hypoxemic and the shunt murmur becomes very soft or absent.

Approach to the Patient With a Functional Single Ventricle

Anatomy

Unfortunately many complex cardiac defects result in a functional single ventricle. The possible anatomic variations are numerous; the most common defects are discussed in Chapters 6 to 8 and complete lists may be found in standard textbooks.

Physiology

Mixing of the systemic and pulmonary circulations occurs in infants with a functional single ventricle. The output from the single ventricle is divided between the two circulations; the proportion going to the systemic and pulmonary vascular beds is determined by the relative resistance to flow within the respective circulation. Resistance to pulmonary blood flow is determined by the amount of subvalvar and valvar pulmonary obstruction, the size of the ductus arteriosus (or surgically placed shunt) if present, and the pulmonary vascular resistance. The resistance to systemic blood flow is determined by the degree of subvalvar and valvar aortic obstruction, aortic arch hypoplasia or coarctation, the size of the ductus arteriosus, and the systemic vascular resistance.

Initial Treatment

Patients with a functional single ventricle usually have too much or too little pulmonary blood flow. Those without enough pulmonary blood flow usually have pulmonary atresia or severe pulmonary stenosis. At birth they are cyanotic and are dependent on flow of blood through the ductus arteriosus to maintain pulmonary blood flow. Once the ductus arteriosus begins to close, cyanosis increases. These infants require prostaglandin E$_1$ administration (Chapters 5 and 12) and then placement of a systemic-to-pulmonary artery shunt (see earlier discussion).

Some patients have a mild amount of pulmonary stenosis shortly after birth that limits pulmonary blood flow and prevents severe congestive heart failure. The degree of pulmonary stenosis tends to increase with time and so these patients become progressively more cyanotic. A systemic-to-pulmonary artery shunt may be necessary at 2 to 3 months of age but some patients may be able to wait until they are candidates for a bidirectional Glenn shunt (see following text).

Other patients have excessive pulmonary blood flow as they have little or no obstruction between the heart and pulmonary artery (Chapter 7). The high pulmonary vascular resistance present at birth usually prevents symptomatic pulmonary overcirculation in the neonatal period. However, as the resistance decreases over the first few weeks of life, pulmonary blood flow increases and the patient develops tachypnea, diaphoresis, and poor feeding associated with congestive heart failure. These infants may not appear cyanotic as the large pulmonary blood flow may result in saturations > 85%. Seldom however, will the oxygen saturation be > 95% and a pO_2 in 100% oxygen almost always will be < 100 mm Hg. Placement of a pulmonary artery band may be indicated (Chapter 7). Alternatively some surgeons prefer to ligate the pulmonary artery and place a shunt with a goal of more precise control of pulmonary blood flow.

The overall goal of therapy for patients with a functional single ventricle is to divide the output of the single ventricle between the systemic and pulmonary vascular beds such that systemic oxygen delivery is adequate and the volume load to the functional single ventricle is minimized. Assuming a normal systemic output and normal pulmonary venous saturation, a systemic arterial saturation of 75% to 85% reflects a pulmonary to systemic flow ratio of 1.0 to 2.0. The hematocrit should be at least 40% to 45% to assist in maintaining adequate systemic oxygen delivery in the presence of moderate hypoxemia.

As discussed earlier, patients may be born with excessive pulmonary blood flow (eg, hypoplastic left heart syndrome) or have pulmonary blood flow supplied via the ductus arteriosus or systemic-to-pulmonary artery shunts (eg, tricuspid atresia). In either case, if the pulmonary vascular resistance is too low, pulmonary blood flow may increase at the expense of systemic blood flow. If this occurs, the oxygen saturation will be > 90% and the peripheral pulses and perfusion will be decreased. Metabolic acidosis may be present because even though the oxygen saturation is fairly high, systemic oxygen delivery is decreased as a result of the low systemic blood flow. Management of this problem involves taking advantage of the fact that hypoxia is a potent pulmonary vasoconstrictor. Supplemental oxygen should be avoided and the infant should be breathing room air. If the oxygen saturation remains > 90%, supplemental inspired nitrogen (or sometimes carbon dioxide) will increase pulmonary vascular resistance by inducing alveolar hypoxia. If necessary, endotracheal intubation,

neuromuscular blockade, and mechanical ventilation may be used such that the pCO_2 is maintained at 40 to 50 mm Hg. In contrast, if the patient has oxygen saturations < 70%, modest hyperventilation (pCO_2 25-35 mm Hg) will often decrease pulmonary vascular resistance and improve pulmonary blood flow. Constant vigilance at the bedside is necessary to monitor and to adjust the variables that modulate distribution of ventricular output to the pulmonary and systemic vascular beds. These temporizing measures are necessary to maintain adequate systemic perfusion and prepare the infant for surgical intervention.

Rationale for Modified Fontan Operation

Before the 1970s, patients who either received a shunt or a pulmonary artery band as a neonate, often developed ventricular failure in part because the functional single ventricle pumped blood to both the systemic and pulmonary circulations. In addition, they were at risk for cerebrovascular accidents and brain abscesses because of right-to-left shunting. The average lifespan for these patients was 15 to 25 years of age.

The principle of the modified Fontan operation is that systemic venous return (superior and inferior vena caval blood) flows passively to the pulmonary arteries through surgically constructed anastomoses. The pulmonary venous return flows into the functional single ventricle and then is pumped to the aorta. Thus the pulmonary and systemic circulations are completely separate and flow in series. The patient is acyanotic and theoretically not at risk of paradoxical emboli. In addition the functional single ventricle is pumping to one, not to two, circulations and is thus considered "volume unloaded."

Characteristics of a Good Candidate for a Modified Fontan Operation

Careful patient preparation and selection are critically important to attain a good long-term result after this procedure. From the time of initial diagnosis in the newborn period, it is incumbent upon cardiologists and surgeons to be aware of the following considerations when planning treatment of patients with functional single ventricles.

- For blood to flow passively to the pulmonary arteries, the pulmonary arteries must be well developed and the pulmonary artery pressures and resistances must be within normal limits. Distortion of the pulmonary arteries at the time of surgery must be avoided and congenital stenoses should be relieved to allow proper growth and development of the pulmonary arterial vasculature.

- The function of the single ventricle must be within normal limits. If the end-diastolic pressure of the ventricle is increased (which is transmitted to the pulmonary vascular bed), passive pulmonary blood flow will be limited which will result in cyanosis and poor cardiac output. Thus prolonged volume loading and outflow obstruction must be avoided.

- There should be no or only mild atrioventricular valve regurgitation. Moderate or more severe degrees of regurgitation will increase left atrial pressure which in turn increases pulmonary pressures, therefore limiting pulmonary blood flow. Minimizing the volume load to the ventricle decreases the risk of atrioventricular valve regurgitation.

- Aortopulmonary collaterals vessels increase the volume load to the functional single ventricle and should be ligated, coiled, or unifocalized with the true pulmonary arteries.

Superior Cavopulmonary Anastomosis

The modified Fontan operation was originally performed all at one operation, that is, the venous return through *both* the superior and inferior vena cavae was directed to the pulmonary arteries. This procedure was often associated with considerable morbidity. Additionally, patients seem to have a better long-term outcome when their single ventricle is volume unloaded at a relatively early age. It is not usually practical to perform the Fontan operation on patients < 12 to 18 months of age. For these reasons the modified Fontan operation is usually separated into two stages.

The first stage is a superior cavopulmonary anastomosis, which can be performed in a patient as young as 4 to 6 months of age. This current approach is a modification of the original Glenn shunt (end-to-end anastomosis of the superior vena cava to the right pulmonary artery) and is sometimes referred to as a bidirectional Glenn shunt. However, most centers have further modified the procedure so the term superior cavopulmonary anastomosis is more accurate. Typically, the superior vena cava is divided and the cephalic end is connected end-to-side to the ipsilateral pulmonary artery (Figure 6-10). If a patient has bilateral superior vena cavae, then bilateral superior cavopulmonary anastomoses are performed. A variation in surgical technique, called a hemi-Fontan, is preferred by

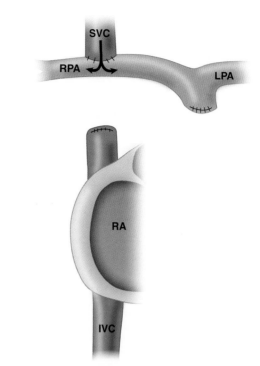

FIGURE 6-10. Superior cavopulmonary anastomosis. The superior vena cava is anastomosed to the right pulmonary artery. Abbreviations: IVC, inferior vena cava; LPA, left pulmonary artery; RA, right atrium; RPA, right pulmonary artery; SVC, superior vena cava.

some surgeons. The hemi-Fontan does not divide the superior vena cava but excludes inferior vena caval blood from the pulmonary arteries by means of a temporary intra-atrial patch.

Modified Fontan Operation

Most patients will have had a superior cavopulmonary anastomosis (or hemi-Fontan) as a first stage. The modified Fontan operation is performed anywhere from 1 to 3 years later. The goal of this procedure is to direct flow from the inferior vena cava to the pulmonary arteries. The exact method by which the modified Fontan operation is performed depends on the patient's anatomy and preference of the physicians. This may involve a right atrial to pulmonary arterial anastomosis, a lateral tunnel in which a baffle is created within the atrium to direct the inferior vena caval blood flow to the pulmonary artery, or an extracardiac conduit (Figure 6-11). Some believe that creation of a fenestration within the Fontan circuit (the fenestration functions physiologically like an atrial septal

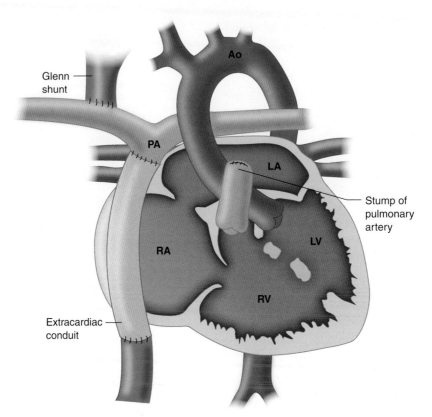

FIGURE 6-11. Diagram of a modified Fontan operation showing a bidirectional Glenn shunt and an extracardiac conduit. MPA indicates main pulmonary artery.

defect) decreases the morbidity associated with the procedure. Some fenestrations close spontaneously; whether the fenestrations that remain open should be closed is unknown.

Long-term outcome studies have shown that patients who have undergone successful modified Fontan operations live longer than those who were treated with shunts and/or pulmonary arterial banding. Most surviving patients are in New York Heart Association Class I-II. Their exercise capacity is about 60% of normal. However, the modified Fontan operation is a less than perfect solution to the complex problem of functional single ventricle. Some of these patients are reasonably asymptomatic but many eventually develop atrial arrhythmias, intracardiac thromboses, protein-losing enteropathy, and/or significant ventricular dysfunction. Some eventually require cardiac transplantation.

Damus-Kaye-Stansel Operation

This procedure is performed primarily for patients with functional single ventricle in whom the aorta arises from a hypoplastic ventricular chamber that has a small communication (bulboventricular foramen) with a functional single ventricle. These patients thus have the equivalent of subaortic stenosis. Resection of the ventricular septum is associated with high morbidity and mortality. For this reason, as shown in Figure 6-12, a connection is placed between the main pulmonary artery and ascending aorta. The pulmonary valve and proximal main pulmonary artery becomes the main outlet to the systemic circulation. Depending on the exact anatomy, the connection can be a tube graft as shown or a patch which creates a side-to-side anastomosis when the aorta and pulmonary artery are close to each other. Flow to the pulmonary arteries is supplied by a shunt.

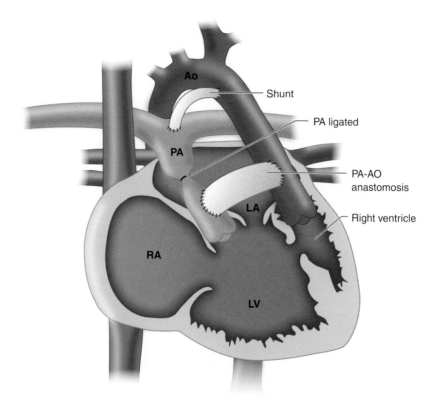

FIGURE 6-12. Damus-Kaye-Stansel procedure. A small communication between the left and right ventricles creates physiologic subaortic stenosis. In this example a tube graft has been placed between the main pulmonary artery and ascending aorta to provide unobstructed blood flow to the systemic circulation (PA-AO anatomosis). The pulmonary artery is ligated distally and pulmonary blood flow is supplied by a systemic-to-pulmonary artery shunt. Abbreviations: Ao, aorta; LA, left atrium; LV, left ventricle; PA, pulmonary artery; RA, right atrium.

SUGGESTED READINGS

General

Allen HD, Driscoll DJ, Shaddy RE, Feltes TF, eds. *Moss and Adams' Heart Disease in Infants, Children, and Adolescents Including the Fetus and Young Adult.* 7th ed. Philadelphia, PA: Lippincott Williams & Wilkins; 2008.

Hoffman JIE. *The Natural and Unnatural History of Congenital Heart Disease.* Oxford, United Kingdom: Wiley-Blackwell; 2009.

Moller JH, Hoffman JIE, eds. *Pediatric Cardiovascular Medicine.* Philadelphia, PA: Churchill Livingstone; 2000.

Rudolph AM. *Congenital Diseases of the Heart: Clinical-Physiological Considerations.* Chichester, United Kingdom: Wiley-Blackwell; 2009.

Defects With Decreased Pulmonary Blood Flow

Cohen MS, Anderson RH, Cohen MI, et al. Controversies, genetics, diagnostic assessment, and outcomes relating to the heterotaxy syndrome. *Cardiol Young.* 2007;17. (suppl 2): 29-43.

da Silva JP, Baumgratz JF, da Fonseca L, et al. The cone reconstruction of the tricuspid valve in Ebstein's anomaly. The operation: early and midterm results. *J Thorac Cardiovasc Surg.* 2007;133:215-223.

Daubeney PE, Delany DJ, Anderson RH, et al. Pulmonary atresia with intact ventricular septum: range of morphology in a population-based study. *J Am Coll Cardiol.* 2002; 39:1670-1679.

Jacobs JP, Franklin RC, Wilkinson JL, et al. The nomenclature, definition and classification of discordant atrioventricular connections. *Cardiol Young.* 2006;16 (suppl 3):72-84.

Rosenthal E, Qureshi SA, Chan KC, et al. Radiofrequency-assisted balloon dilatation in patients with pulmonary valve atresia and an intact ventricular septum. *Br Heart J.* 1993;69:347-351.

Schmidt KG, Cloez JL, Silverman NH. Changes of right ventricular size and function in neonates after valvotomy for pulmonary atresia or critical pulmonary stenosis and intact ventricular septum. *J Am Coll Cardiol.* 1992;19:1032-1037.

Shinkawa T, Polimenakos AC, Gomez-Fifer CA, et al. Management and long-term outcome of neonatal Ebstein anomaly. *J Thorac Cardiovasc Surg.* 2010;139:354-358.

d-Transposition Complexes

Griselli M, McGuirk SP, Ko CS, et al. Arterial switch operation in patients with Taussig-Bing anomaly—influence of staged repair and coronary anatomy on outcome. *Eur J Cardiothorac Surg.* 2007;31:229-235.

Jouannic JM, Gavard L, Fermont L, et al. Sensitivity and specificity of prenatal features of physiological shunts to predict neonatal clinical status in transposition of the great arteries. *Circulation.* 2004;110:1743-1746.

Konstantinov IE. Taussig-Bing anomaly: from original description to the current era. *Tex Heart Inst J.* 2009;36:580-585.

Leobon B, Belli E, Ly M, et al. Left ventricular outflow tract obstruction after arterial switch operation. *Eur J Cardiothorac Surg.* 2008;34:1046-1050.

Pasquali SK, Hasselblad V, Li JS, et al. Coronary artery pattern and outcome of arterial switch operation for transposition of the great arteries: a meta-analysis. *Circulation.* 2002;106:2575-2580.

Palliative Procedures

Alwi M, Choo KK, Latiff HA, et al. Initial results and medium-term follow-up of stent implantation of patent ductus arteriosus in duct-dependent pulmonary circulation. *J Am Coll Cardiol.* 2004;44:438-445.

Anderson, PAW, Sleeper, LA, Mahony, L, et al. Contemporary outcomes after the Fontan procedure: a pediatric heart network multicenter study. *J Am Coll Cardiol.* 2008;52:85-98.

Blaufox AD, Sleeper LA, Bradley DJ, et al. Functional status, heart rate, and rhythm abnormalities in 521 Fontan patients 6 to 18 years of age. *J Thorac Cardiovasc Surg.* 2008;136:100-107.

Cowgill LD. The Fontan procedure: a historical review. *Ann Thorac Surg.* 1991;51:1026-1030.

Giardini A, Hager A, Pace Napoleone C, et al. Natural history of exercise capacity after the Fontan operation: a longitudinal study. *Ann Thorac Surg.* 2008;85:818-821.

Khairy P, Poirier N, Mercier LA. Univentricular heart. *Circulation.* 2007;13:800-812.

Murphy AM, Cameron DE. The Blalock-Taussig-Thomas collaboration: a model for medical progress. *JAMA.* 2008;300:328-330.

Approach to the Infant With Excessive Pulmonary Blood Flow

■ INTRODUCTION

Respiratory distress in the setting of normal peripheral perfusion and without overt cyanosis is the least common manifestation of symptomatic heart disease in the newborn. Particularly in the absence of a murmur, the diagnosis of heart disease is often delayed or missed entirely because respiratory distress alone in an acyanotic infant with normal perfusion is most often caused by lung disease rather than intrinsic cardiac disease. Furthermore, symptoms usually develop gradually over the first few days or weeks of life and are often rather subtle. It may take several weeks or more to recognize that the infant is growing poorly and that heart disease may be the cause. This chapter reviews structural cardiovascular defects that can cause respiratory distress; cardiomyopathies and arrhythmias are discussed in Chapters 9 and 10, respectively and heart failure is discussed in Chapter 11.

■ PATHOPHYSIOLOGY OF INCREASED PULMONARY BLOOD FLOW

Clinical Presentation

A diverse group of congenital structural cardiovascular defects share the common feature of increased pulmonary blood flow as the main pathophysiologic process. It is this common characteristic that is the basis for the majority of symptoms caused by this group of defects. The arterial oxygen saturation, although sometimes mildly decreased, is not so low that either cyanosis is appreciated or systemic oxygen delivery is compromised. The primary symptom in these infants is **tachypnea**, often accompanied by mildly increased work of breathing.

In addition to tachypnea, many of these infants exhibit other signs and symptoms of the heart failure syndrome (Chapter 11). These infants have heart failure with high cardiac output ("high output failure"), which is very different than the low output failure that occurs in adults with acquired heart disease and in neonates with decreased systemic perfusion (Chapters 8 and 11). In addition to increased pulmonary blood flow, systemic blood flow is often increased in response to the increased metabolic demands resulting from the greater respiratory effort. The increased cardiac output leads to greater circulating blood volume to maintain normal filling pressures. The heart is hypercontractile and venous filling pressures are usually normal on both sides of the heart. Peripheral edema does not occur because venous pressures are not increased. However, **hepatomegaly** is a fairly constant finding because the liver and hepatic veins are very compliant and enlarge to accommodate the increased circulating blood volume.

Oxygen consumption or metabolic demand is increased for a variety of reasons. The major contributor is the increased work of breathing. In a normal infant, breathing is a large component of basal oxygen consumption (20%), which is similar to the metabolic requirements for growth. As the work of breathing increases, it may comprise 30% to 40% of oxygen consumption. An increase in adrenergic drive is necessary to maintain the increased combined ventricular output and this too increases oxygen consumption, particularly by its effect on brown fat metabolism. This increased adrenergic drive is mediated by both neural and hormonal mechanisms and causes two other common signs of high-output heart failure, **tachycardia** and **diaphoresis**. In infants, diaphoresis is observed on the forehead and scalp, especially during feeding.

Lastly, **failure to thrive** is an important and frequent component of the clinical presentation. It is caused by the increased caloric requirements associated with increased oxygen consumption and by decreased caloric intake. These infants feed poorly because of their increased respiratory effort, and vomit frequently because of gastroesophageal reflux in the presence of increased intra-abdominal pressure, which in turn is caused by increased respiratory effort. The caloric intake required for growth in a normal infant is about 100 to 120 kcal/kg/d. Failure to thrive occurs because the infant in high-output failure may take in only a fraction of this amount. These infants may actually require 160 to 180 kcal/kg/d to maintain a normal growth rate because of increased metabolic demands.

Pathophysiology of Tachypnea

The mechanism for the tachypnea seen in infants with increased pulmonary blood flow is not known. Left atrial pressures are generally normal. Ventilation and oxygenation are also not impaired, which suggests that significant alveolar edema is not present. The increased amount of fluid in the thorax caused by increased pulmonary blood flow, particularly distributed in the pulmonary veins, may make it more difficult for the infant to breathe by increasing the weight of the lungs, but this has never been shown to be an independent factor in respiratory work. More likely, the increased production of interstitial fluid with the attendant increase in lymphatic flow is the primary cause of tachypnea in these infants.

As blood flows normally through the lungs, interstitial fluid is produced. This fluid is drained from the interstitial spaces by the lymphatic vessels. As blood flow increases, lymphatic flow increases similarly. Defects with high pulmonary arterial pressures increase precapillary pressures which further increase lymphatic flow. As interstitial fluid production increases, the ability of the lymphatics to drain the fluid may be exceeded, causing accumulation of interstitial fluid. The fluid is predominantly peribronchial, which may impair bronchial function. Airway size may decrease and airway resistance may increase, further increasing the work of breathing. In addition, the infant may be more likely to develop wheezing, as only a small further decrease in airway lumen would impair air exchange. This scenario explains not only the tachypnea universally seen in infants with a symptomatic increase in pulmonary blood flow, but also the radiographic findings of increased vascular markings, the presence of peribronchial edema, and other manifestations of interstitial, but not of alveolar, fluid.

Infants with normal lung size and function and no abnormalities other than heart disease do not develop tachypnea and failure to thrive until pulmonary blood flow is very high, usually exceeding two and one-half times the normal flow. The onset of symptoms tends to track with the time course over which pulmonary blood flow increases after birth. In the normal infant, systemic blood flow peaks at around 6 to 10 weeks of age, at the time of the nadir of hemoglobin concentration. Pulmonary vascular resistance also decreases during this time period. Thus, pulmonary blood flow increases greatly during this time in the infant with a heart defect associated with increased pulmonary blood flow because of the increase in systemic blood flow associated with physiologic anemia and an increase in the relative proportion of blood flow to the lungs (an increased pulmonary-to-systemic blood flow ratio) related to the decreased pulmonary vascular resistance.

In contrast, infants with intrinsic pulmonary disease who also have excessive pulmonary blood flow may develop tachypnea and heart failure at a level of pulmonary blood flow only modestly higher than normal. A common situation is an infant born prematurely who develops bronchopulmonary dysplasia. The presence of even a minor cardiac structural defect (such as an atrial septal defect) that would not cause symptoms in a normal-term infant may result in significant symptoms in this setting. The onset of symptoms and the requirement for medical and/or surgical intervention are often accelerated in this subset of infants.

Classification of Defects That Result in Increased Pulmonary Blood Flow

Many congenital cardiovascular defects cause an increase in pulmonary blood flow as the dominant pathophysiological process, yet some are categorized according to other manifestations that are of less importance with regard to the clinical presentation. Truncus arteriosus and total anomalous pulmonary venous connection without obstruction are good examples. Because some degree of systemic arterial desaturation occurs in both of these conditions, they are often classified as "cyanotic heart disease." However, in contrast to classical cyanotic defects (such as d-transposition of the great arteries and tetralogy of Fallot), truncus arteriosus and total anomalous pulmonary venous connection without obstruction are associated with only modest systemic arterial desaturation. Furthermore, the predominant symptoms are tachypnea and failure to thrive, which are secondary to excessive pulmonary blood flow, not cyanosis. These defects should therefore be categorized among those that cause excessive pulmonary blood flow rather than cyanosis.

Defects that cause excessive pulmonary blood flow can be divided into two distinct subgroups. In both subgroups, excessive pulmonary blood flow occurs because a large volume of fully saturated pulmonary venous blood is diverted back into the pulmonary arteries via an abnormal communication (ie, a large left-to-right shunt is present).

In the first subgroup, only a left-to-right shunt is present. No desaturated systemic venous blood is diverted into the systemic arterial bed. Thus, systemic arterial saturation is normal and equals that in the pulmonary veins (Figure 7-1). The second subgroup of defects also has a large left-to-right shunt but this subgroup is distinguished by the additional presence of a right-to-left shunt, that is, systemic venous blood is diverted back into the systemic arterial circulation before passing through the pulmonary arterial system (Figure 7-2). Thus, some degree of systemic arterial desaturation is present in these infants. However, the dominant (or net) shunt is still left-to-right. Pulmonary blood flow is markedly increased and systemic blood flow is normal or mildly increased. Consequently, the extent of systemic arterial desaturation is only modest and the clinical effects of that desaturation are negligible.

These principles are illustrated by considering an infant with truncus arteriosus with the following scenarios: (1) all systemic and pulmonary venous blood mixes completely in the combined outflow tract so that aortic and pulmonary arterial blood oxygen saturations are the same; (2) pulmonary blood flow has increased to four times the systemic normal blood flow after 1 week of life; (3) pulmonary venous blood is nearly fully saturated at 98%; and (4) systemic venous blood is less saturated than normal at 50% because of the increased respiratory work and decreased systemic arterial saturation. Therefore, four volumes of pulmonary venous blood mix with one volume of systemic venous blood in the ventricular outflow and that blood is ejected out the aorta and pulmonary arteries. When these five volumes of blood mix, the oxygen saturation of the fully mixed blood is:

$$\frac{[(4 \times 0.98) + (1 \times 0.50)]}{5} \times 100 = 88.4$$

Thus, this infant has a systemic arterial saturation of about 88%. The infant may not appear cyanotic because the threshold for observing cyanosis is about 85% with a normal hemoglobin concentration and even lower at a few weeks of age because of the normal physiologic anemia. In addition, oxygen delivery to the tissues is not impaired because normally only about 25% of the oxygen delivered is consumed. Tachypnea would be a prominent manifestation because of high pulmonary blood flow, and failure to thrive would be likely for the reasons described earlier. Thus, categorizing such an infant as having "cyanotic heart disease" is not consistent with either the physical examination or the pathophysiology of the defect.

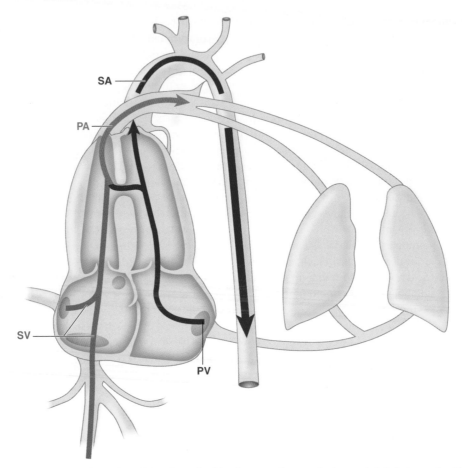

FIGURE 7-1. Exclusive left-to-right shunt. In this diagram of a ventricular septal defect, much of the fully saturated pulmonary venous blood (PV) passes through the ventricular septal defect to join the poorly saturated systemic venous blood (SV). This left-to-right shunt increases the saturation of pulmonary arterial blood (PA) above systemic venous saturation. However, none of the systemic venous blood crosses the ventricular septal defect to enter the aorta. Thus the oxygen saturation of systemic arterial blood (SA) is normal and equal to that in the pulmonary veins.

Instead, categorizing truncus arteriosus as a defect with "excessive pulmonary blood flow" is more appropriate on both accounts.

Infants with excessive pulmonary blood flow can therefore be categorized as having an exclusive left-to-right shunt or as having bidirectional shunting but with a dominant left-to-right shunt. Within each category, the defects can be considered according to the anatomic level, beginning arbitrarily with left-to-right shunts which empty into the right atrium and progressing through the right ventricle, pulmonary arteries, and the systemic veins (Tables 7-1 and 7-2).

■ LEFT-TO-RIGHT SHUNTS

This section will only consider congenital cardiovascular defects with exclusive left-to-right shunts that present symptomatically in the otherwise normal infant. Several defects associated with left-to-right shunting will not be considered because they do not cause symptoms. For example, left-to-right shunting across an **atrial septal defect** occurs when the stiffness of the left ventricle is greater than that of the right ventricle. Newborn infants have a right ventricle that is of equal or greater thickness and stiffness as the left ventricle so that the left-to-right

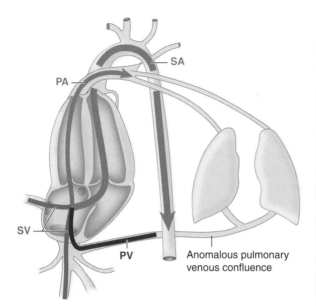

PA

SA

SV

PV   Anomalous pulmonary
venous confluence

FIGURE 7-2. Predominant left-to-right shunt with an associated right-to-left shunt. In this idealized diagram of total anomalous pulmonary venous connection, the large volume of fully saturated pulmonary venous blood (PV) fully mixes in the right atrium with the smaller volume of systemic venous blood (SV). The majority of this fully mixed blood passes into the right ventricle to enter the pulmonary artery, and a lesser amount crosses the foramen ovale to the left side of the heart and into aorta. Thus, pulmonary arterial (PA) and systemic arterial blood (SA) have the same oxygen saturation, which is determined by the relative volumes of pulmonary venous and systemic venous blood flows.

■ **TABLE 7-1.** Congenital Cardiovascular Malformations That Result in an Exclusive Left-to-Right Shunt. Defects in **Bold** Letters Commonly Cause Symptoms During the Neonatal Period.

Anatomic level	Structural defect
Atrial septum	Secundum atrial septal defect
	Primum atrial septal defect
	Sinus venosus atrial septal defect
Atrioventricular septum	**Complete atrioventricular septal defect**
	Partial atrioventricular septal defect
Ventricular septum	**Inlet ventricular septal defect**
	Perimembranous ventricular septal defect
	Muscular ventricular septal defect (may cause symptoms if a large mid-muscular defect is present)
	Outlet ventricular septal defect
Truncal/ aortopulmonary septum	**Aortopulmonary window**
	Anomalous origin of the right pulmonary artery from the ascending aorta
Arterial communication	**Patent ductus arteriosus**
	Arteriovenous malformation
Venous communication	Partial anomalous pulmonary venous connection

■ **TABLE 7-2.** Congenital Cardiovascular Malformations With Bidirectional Shunts and Excessive Pulmonary Blood Flow

Anatomic level	Structural defect
Atrial septum	Common atrium (usually left atrial isomerism)
Atrioventricular septum	Complete atrioventricular septal defect with common ventricle (usually left atrial isomerism)
Ventricular septum	Single ventricle physiology:
	1. Double-inlet left ventricle (usually l-malposed aorta) and unobstructed outflow tracts
	2. AV valve atresia/stenosis (mitral or tricuspid) with large ventricular septal defect and unobstructed outflow tracts
Truncal/ aortopulmonary septum	Truncus arteriosus
Venous communication	Total anomalous pulmonary venous connection without obstruction

shunt at birth is small or nonexistent (Chapter 3). Although pulmonary vascular resistance begins to fall immediately at birth, it takes months for the right ventricle to remodel and accept a significantly greater amount of blood than the left ventricle. In addition, pulmonary arterial pressures are normal so that less interstitial fluid is produced for the same level of pulmonary blood flow. Thus, unless the infant has lung disease, even a large atrial septal defect does not cause symptoms in newborns and young infants.

At the atrioventricular and ventricular levels (eg, a ventricular septal defect), the magnitude of the left-to-right shunt increases much more rapidly after birth. These shunts depend on the relative resistances of the pulmonary and systemic vascular beds. The shunt occurs almost exclusively in systole when the distal vascular bed (the resistance vasculature) is filled with blood from the previous contraction, which limits the extent of the shunt.

Although pulmonary vascular resistance falls precipitously immediately after birth, it does not fall so low that a systolic shunt will be large enough to cause symptoms. The further steady decline in pulmonary vascular resistance over the next several weeks of life occurs simultaneously with the normal decline in hemoglobin and hematocrit (physiologic "anemia" of infancy). Together, these processes promote a progressive increase in left-to-right shunting and pulmonary blood flow to levels high enough to cause symptoms. Typically, symptoms are manifest between 4 and 8 weeks of age. An exception is a small number of infants with an atrioventricular septal defect who have a direct communication between the left ventricle and the right atrium or severe mitral insufficiency. Both of these conditions lead to a large atrial left-to-right shunt; the shunt is **obligatory**, in that atrial pressure is always much lower than left ventricular pressure during ventricular systole. In the neonate, a very large left-to-right shunt may develop within the first days after birth, causing early symptoms of heart failure.

At the arterial level (eg, a patent ductus arteriosus), the shunt occurs during both systole and diastole. Diastolic shunts are always much larger than the corresponding systolic shunt because blood continues to flow from the resistance vessels of the lungs during diastole, affording much more vascular space to be filled. Thus, shunts at the arterial level are likely to cause high-output heart failure at an earlier age than shunts that occur at the ventricular level. These infants are frequently tachypneic when they leave the hospital after birth, but it may not be appreciated until they return for postnatal follow-up and are found to be failing to thrive.

Shunts that occur **at an arteriovenous level** (eg, a congenital arteriovenous malformation) are also obligatory shunts because, even in the fetus, arteriolar pressure far exceeds venous pressure. Thus the magnitude of the shunt is directly related to the size of the malformation, and the transition from fetus to newborn or newborn to older infant does not alter the magnitude of the shunt. The difference in compliance of the two vascular beds is so great that any increase in ventricular output merely passes into the systemic veins.

Lastly, exclusive left-to-right shunts **at a pulmonary venous level** (eg, partial anomalous pulmonary venous connection) drain into the right atrium or systemic veins. Partial anomalous pulmonary venous return presents similarly to an atrial septal defect, and it may take several months for a clinically significant shunt to develop, if ever.

Atrioventricular Septal Defect

Anatomic and Physiologic Considerations

Atrioventricular septal defects are often termed endocardial cushion defects or atrioventricular canal defects, but these terms assume an understanding of the embryologic origin, which has yet to be completely defined. The spectrum of defects which comprise atrioventricular septal defects, from the primum atrial septal defect and the cleft mitral valve to the complete atrioventricular septal defect, have one common finding—absence of the atrioventricular septum. Thus the term atrioventricular septal defect seems most appropriate. The septal leaflet of the tricuspid valve inserts inferiorly to the septal attachments of the mitral valve and it is the atrioventricular septum that separates the right atrium from the left ventricle. This portion of the septum is very small and is recognized on echocardiography by the more inferior hinge point of the septal leaflet of the tricuspid valve compared to the anterior leaflet of the mitral valve (Figure 7-3). In all forms of atrioventricular septal defect, this discrepancy is absent and the two valves lie in the same plane. Because of the absence of the atrioventricular septum, it is possible for blood to shunt directly from the left ventricle to the right atrium. As stated in the preceding discussion, this type of shunt is obligatory and can be quite large. However, the atrioventricular valve tissue usually prevents such a direct connection and in most cases of atrioventricular septal defects, a left ventricular-right atrial shunt is not present.

Clinical Presentation

A complete atrioventricular septal defect does not usually cause symptoms in the fetal or early neonatal periods. Newborn infants may not have a cardiac murmur because pulmonary vascular resistance is still relatively high. This is an especially important consideration in a newborn with trisomy 21, in whom the likelihood of an atrioventricular septal defect is high. The absence of a murmur is common in these infants because they frequently have lung hypoplasia, which contributes to the maintenance of high pulmonary vascular resistance. Thus, a pediatric cardiologist should evaluate every infant with trisomy 21, even in the absence of a murmur or other signs and symptoms. Most infants with a complete atrioventricular septal defect present within the first few weeks of life with tachypnea, diaphoresis, poor feeding, and failure to thrive.

On physical examination, the weight percentile is usually at least one or two standard deviations below the length percentile. If the infant has trisomy 21, it is important to

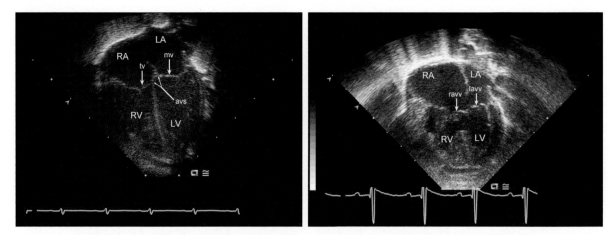

FIGURE 7-3. A. Apical four-chamber echocardiogram in a normal newborn infant. The atrioventricular septum (avs) lies between the medial hinge point of the mitral valve (mv) and the more inferiorly placed septal hinge point of the tricuspid valve (tv). **B. Apical four-chamber echocardiogram in a newborn infant with a complete atrioventricular canal defect.** Note that the right-sided component of the atrioventricular valve (ravv) hinges at the same level as the left-sided component (lavv) so that there is no atrioventricular septum. The absence of an atrioventricular septum occurs even in the presence of a partial atrioventricular canal defect (eg, a primum atrial septal defect) in which there is no ventricular septal defect. Abbreviations: LA, left atrium; LV, left ventricle; RA, right atrium; RV, right ventricle.

use growth charts specific to the syndrome, which show quite a different normal growth pattern than that of the normal population. There is often moderate resting tachycardia, in the 130 to 150 beats/min range. Tachypnea with intercostal and substernal retractions is common. The extremities are warm and well perfused and the peripheral pulses are strong, indicating that systemic blood flow is well maintained by peripheral vasodilation. Systemic oxygen saturation measured by pulse oximetry may be normal at rest but may be in the low 90s, especially during crying because of right-to-left intracardiac shunting. The liver is moderately enlarged with a sharp margin, and splenomegaly can often be appreciated. The precordium is diffusely hyperactive to palpation. The first heart sound is often normal but occasionally may be louder than normal. If the atrial or ventricular-atrial shunt is large and there is a right bundle branch block, the second heart sound may be widely split with little variation. More often, however, the rapid heart rate and high pulmonary arterial diastolic pressures make it difficult to appreciate splitting of the second heart sound. However, the second heart sound is almost always louder than normal because of high diastolic pulmonary arterial pressure. Extra heart sounds are not common, but occasionally an S_3 can be heard at the

apex. There is often a harsh mid-frequency systolic murmur along the mid-sternal border that may be holosystolic and which radiates throughout the chest. A separate systolic murmur of higher frequency may be appreciated at the apex if there is significant left-sided atrioventricular (mitral) valve insufficiency. This situation should be suspected if the pulses are decreased and the peripheral extremities are cool. A diastolic inflow rumble is often present at the apex or the lower left sternal border, though rapid heart rates may make it difficult to appreciate. More often, the absence of silence in diastole suggests that a diastolic murmur is present. The diastolic murmur is caused by excessive blood flow across the mitral valve and usually indicates that pulmonary blood flow is at least twice the normal.

Ancillary Tests

The electrocardiogram shows left axis deviation (QRS axis between 0° and −120°) with a counterclockwise loop. Right ventricular hypertrophy is demonstrated by persistence of upright T waves with prominent R waves in the right precordial leads (Figure 7-4). If a large ventricular shunt is present, the ECG shows biventricular hypertrophy, indicated by the presence of normal left-sided forces despite

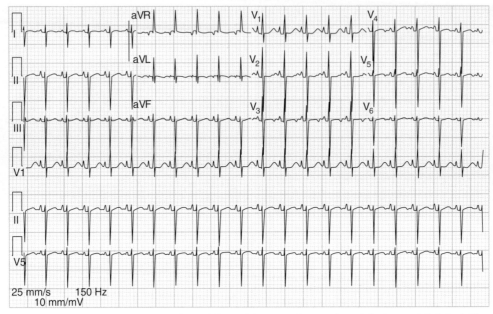

FIGURE 7-4. An electrocardiogram in an infant with a complete atrioventricular septal defect. The ECG shows left axis deviation (approximately –120°) and right ventricular hypertrophy (a dominant R wave with upright T waves in V_1 and deep S waves in V_6).

right ventricular hypertrophy. These left-sided forces are demonstrated by prominent S waves in the right precordial leads as well as left-sided forces (R waves) in V_6 and in the inferior limb leads. The chest radiograph shows generalized cardiomegaly with a globular heart, often including a prominent right contour indicative of right atrial enlargement and increased pulmonary vascularity.

The echocardiogram clearly demonstrates the common atrioventricular valve with atrial and ventricular septal defects. The attachments of the valve, the relative size of the two ventricles, and the degree of atrioventricular valve insufficiency are critical elements of the echocardiographic examination. Associated defects commonly occur, particularly secundum atrial septal defects and patent ductus arteriosus. The most important commonly associated defects are subaortic stenosis and coarctation of the aorta because of their deleterious effects on systemic perfusion.

Therapeutic Considerations

Treatment of heart failure and failure to thrive are important elements of the medical management of infants with atrioventricular septal defects. However, because of the large left-to-right shunt and propensity for the early development of

pulmonary vascular disease, it is important to plan for early surgical repair. Infants with complete atrioventricular septal defects generally undergo surgical repair in the second or third month of life, even in the absence of severe heart failure and failure to thrive. Repair in the first few months of life is associated with a more benign postoperative course and fewer problems related to residual pulmonary hypertension. Although several surgical techniques are utilized, the general approach involves closure of the atrial and ventricular septal defects and repair of the atrioventricular valve. Postoperatively, these infants may have residual atrioventricular valve insufficiency (or occasionally, atrioventricular valve stenosis). However, the prognosis is favorable and most infants and children are symptom-free after surgical repair.

Ventricular Septal Defect

Anatomic and Physiologic Considerations

The most common congenital cardiac structural malformation is a ventricular septal defect. Ventricular septal defects are categorized according to their position within the septum (Figure 7-5). The most common ventricular septal defects occur in the membranous septum, the very

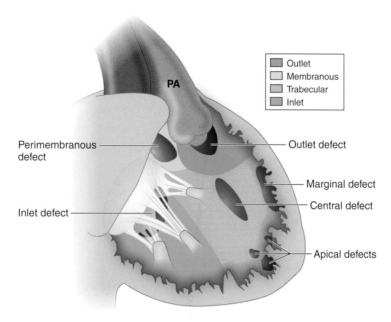

FIGURE 7-5. Schematic diagram of the ventricular septum. The sites of common ventricular septal defects are shown.

small component of the ventricular septum where the aortic, mitral and tricuspid valves attach and where there is no muscle in the septal wall. These defects extend from the membranous region in any direction, and are thus commonly termed perimembranous ventricular septal defects. Most commonly, they extend toward the outlet of the ventricles. In this situation, the outlet septum may be normally aligned with the inlet septum, allowing for unobstructed flow of blood from each ventricle to its respective great vessel. Less commonly, the outlet septum may be malaligned with respect to the inlet septum. If there is anterior deviation of the outlet septum, the defect is then subaortic and it is associated with subpulmonic and pulmonic valve stenosis (tetralogy of Fallot, Chapter 6). If there is posterior deviation of the outlet septum, the defect is subpulmonic and there is often associated subaortic stenosis and coarctation of the aorta (Figure 7-6).

Defects of the ventricular septum may also be isolated to the inlet portion, where the ventricular component of atrioventricular septal defects occurs (Figure 7-4). A defect may occur in the muscular septum, where they are often multiple. Tiny defects located in the apex of the muscular septum are common at birth and almost always close spontaneously. The most superior defects lie above the crista supraventricularis and directly under both the aortic and pulmonary valves and are termed "supracristal" or "doubly committed subarterial" ventricular septal defects. In this type of defect, the deficiency in the subvalvar region causes the noncoronary cusp of the aortic valve to not be properly suspended. This often results in prolapse of the noncoronary cusp into the defect, causing aortic insufficiency.

Clinical Presentation

An infant with an isolated ventricular septal defect is rarely symptomatic in the first weeks of life. Rather, if symptoms are to develop, they do so after a few weeks as the pulmonary vascular resistance falls and the hematocrit approaches its postnatal nadir.

The symptomatic infant with a ventricular septal defect presents similarly to the infant with an atrioventricular septal defect. The infant is tachycardic and tachypneic, often with retractions. Pulses and perfusion are normal or sometimes increased because of the increased sympathetic drive. Oxygen saturation measured by pulse oximetry is normal. Hepatomegaly occurs in association with the increased biventricular output. The lungs are generally clear to auscultation. The precordium is hyperactive. Right

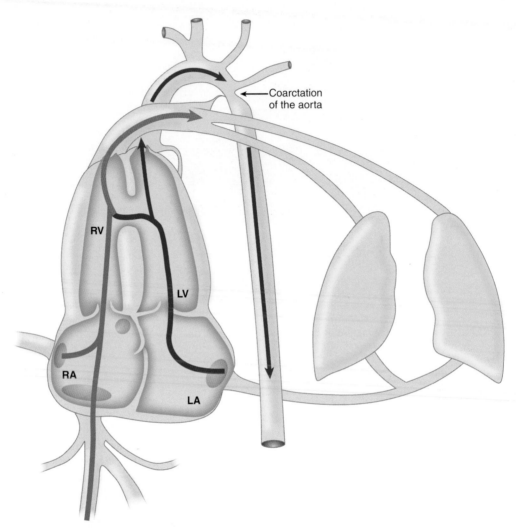

FIGURE 7-6. Posterior maligned ventricular septal defect. With posterior malignment of the outlet septum, the ventricular septal defect is subpulmonic and the aortic outflow tract is narrowed. This decreases flow in the ascending aorta in the fetus, leading to coarctation of the aorta. Abbreviations: LA, left atrium; LV, left ventricle; RA, right atrium; RV, right ventricle.

ventricular pressure is not necessarily increased because a pressure-restrictive defect (see following text) may still allow a large enough shunt to cause symptoms. A parasternal thrill is occasionally present if there is a pressure-restrictive defect with a high velocity jet across the septum that is directed anteriorly toward the sternum. The first heart sound is normal and the second heart sound depends on pulmonary arterial pressures. Splitting of the second heart sound is normal or may be decreased, and there is an increased pulmonic component if the defect is not pressure-restrictive. However, it is often difficult to appreciate the splitting and quality of the second heart sound because the murmur is usually loud and holosystolic. The frequency of the murmur is should be evaluated carefully—higher frequency components are associated with a more pressure-restrictive is the defect. A mid-diastolic inflow murmur is usually present in the symptomatic infant because of the increased flow across the mitral valve, as discussed earlier. This can be used to assess the general magnitude of the left-to-right shunt.

Ancillary Tests

The electrocardiogram usually shows a normal axis unless there is pulmonary hypertension, which may cause right axis deviation. Left ventricular hypertrophy is often present, and the presence or absence of right ventricular hypertrophy depends on the amount of pressure restriction across the defect. Left atrial enlargement is frequently evident as a wide (greater than 3 mm) and often bifid P wave in lead II. The chest radiograph shows cardiomegaly but, unlike the infant with an atrioventricular septal defect who also has an atrial level shunt, chamber enlargement is confined to the left side of the heart. Increased vascular markings are also present.

The echocardiogram is used to define the location, size, and number of ventricular septal defects, the alignment of the outlet septum, and the presence of associated defects as discussed earlier. Doppler echocardiography can be used to estimate right ventricular and pulmonary arterial pressures and the magnitude of the left-to-right shunt.

Therapeutic Considerations

The requirement for medical and surgical intervention in early infancy depends on the magnitude of the left-to-right shunt and severity of symptoms. Many infants with a small defect and minimal left-to-right shunt are asymptomatic and do not require any intervention. Small defects often resolve spontaneously during the first year or two of life (especially isolated defects located in the muscular septum). In contrast, infants with a large left-to-right shunt and failure to thrive despite adequate medical management require early surgical repair. The risks of surgical repair are low and there is no advantage to delaying surgical correction in most infants with symptoms due to a large ventricular septal defect. However, it should be recognized that the normal postnatal decline in hemoglobin and hematocrit may temporarily aggravate symptoms of heart failure. Thus, it may be reasonable to continue medical management until the normal physiologic anemia of infancy has resolved in those infants with mild or moderate symptoms.

Beyond early infancy, the decision to close a ventricular septal defect depends not on the size of the shunt and associated failure to thrive but on the size of the defect and/or associated defects. When the ventricular septal defect approaches the size of the aortic root, the defect is no longer pressure-restrictive. That is, right ventricular systolic pressure equals that in the left ventricle. The increased pressure is transmitted to the pulmonary arteries. In turn, pulmonary arterial hypertension creates excessive shear forces in the distal pulmonary vasculature. Initially this delays the normal postnatal regression of muscle in the walls of the arterioles. Over time, intimal hyperplasia, fibrosis, and ultimately vascular occlusion occur. The progression from reactive pulmonary hypertension to irreversible pulmonary vaso-occlusive disease in a patient with ventricular septal defect usually takes at least 18 months. A decision regarding closure of a nonrestrictive ventricular septal defect is usually made within 4 to 6 months so that the risk for vaso-occlusive disease is minimized.

Associated defects which lead the cardiologist to recommend surgical closure may develop over time but these rarely occur during infancy. They include membranous subaortic stenosis, double-chamber right ventricle (in which anomalous muscle bundles develop and obstruct blood flow into the right ventricular outflow tract), aortic insufficiency (caused by prolapse of an aortic valve leaflet into the defect, most commonly seen in supracristal defects), and recurrent bacterial endocarditis.

Occasionally a ventricular septal defect is closed surgically or by a transcatheter approach when the shunt remains large enough to cause left ventricular dilation but is not associated with pulmonary hypertension or other defects. Because of the propensity for ventricular septal defects to decrease in size over time, such defects are usually not closed before 5 years of age.

Aortopulmonary Window/Anomalous Origin of the Right Pulmonary Artery From the Ascending Aorta

Anatomic and Physiologic Considerations

These two structural defects are rare, but because they are related embryologically and present similarly, they are discussed together. In both defects, a direct communication between the ascending aorta and at least one pulmonary artery is present. However, because there are two semilunar valves, the shunt is exclusively left-to-right (unlike that of truncus arteriosus, described in the following discussion). Aortopulmonary window results from a deficiency in septation of the aortopulmonary septum, which thereby allows for a varying-sized communication between the ascending aorta and main pulmonary artery. It usually occurs midway between the semilunar valves and the bifurcation of the main pulmonary artery. This defect is thought to be embryologically distinct from persistent truncus arteriosus based upon observations that aortopulmonary window is not associated with chromosome

22 microdeletion syndromes (such as DiGeorge syndrome), nor is ablation of the cardiac neural crest tissue in experimental models associated with an aortopulmonary window. In utero, an aortopulmonary window often causes no abnormalities in blood flow patterns, but, if the left ventricle ejects a large portion of its output across the window and through the main pulmonary artery to the ductus arteriosus, interruption of the aortic arch may occur. Interestingly, aortopulmonary window is associated with type A interruption of the aortic arch (distal to the subclavian artery), rather than type B (between the carotid and subclavian artery), which is the most common site of interruption seen in infants with chromosome 22 microdeletion syndrome.

Anomalous origin of the right pulmonary artery from the aorta occurs more frequently than that of the left, but both are quite rare. Anomalous origin of the right pulmonary artery occurs in association with aortopulmonary window and with type A interruption of the aortic arch. Although it has been called "hemitruncus" this is a poor term because, as mentioned earlier, these defects are not embryologically related to persistent truncus arteriosus and two separate semilunar valves are present, a finding that excludes an abnormality of truncal septation. Anomalous origin of the left pulmonary artery is sometimes associated with tetralogy of Fallot, and thus does not present similarly to aortopulmonary window.

Clinical Presentation

The infant with aortopulmonary window or with anomalous origin of the right pulmonary artery from the ascending aorta is tachypneic very soon after birth, though it may not be recognized immediately. This is particularly true when no murmurs are present, which may happen when there is no stenosis of the communication, thus allowing for laminar flow through defect and central vessels. Inevitably, the infant exhibits poor growth and respiratory distress. On physical examination, the infant is generally warm with normal perfusion of the extremities. A hallmark finding is that of bounding pulses. The lungs are clear to auscultation. The liver is moderately enlarged. The precordium is hyperdynamic, indicative of a hypertensive right ventricle. Infants with anomalous origin of the right pulmonary artery often have left pulmonary arterial pressures that exceed systemic pressures; right ventricular systolic pressure is suprasystemic. The first heart sound is normal, and the second heart sound is narrowly split or single and is louder than normal. A harsh systolic murmur is may be present at the upper sternal border and radiates to one or both lung fields. Occasionally, the murmur is continuous and resembles that heard in an infant with a patent ductus arteriosus. A mid-diastolic murmur at the apex reflects the increased blood flow across the mitral valve resulting from the increased pulmonary blood flow.

Ancillary Tests

The electrocardiographic findings are variable, showing persistent right precordial upright T waves and prominent anterior forces beyond the first week of life, indicative of right ventricular hypertrophy. Often there is evidence of biventricular hypertrophy. Left atrial enlargement may be present. The chest radiograph shows generalized cardiomegaly with a prominent main pulmonary artery and increased vascularity. Pulmonary edema may be present, particularly when there is an associated interruption of the aorta arch (Figure 7-7). The echocardiogram shows an enlarged left atrium and left ventricle. It is often difficult to appreciate that there is a communication of the ascending aorta with one or both pulmonary arteries unless this is considered in the differential diagnosis. Right ventricular hypertension is usually present. The aortic arch should be carefully evaluated for the presence of obstruction.

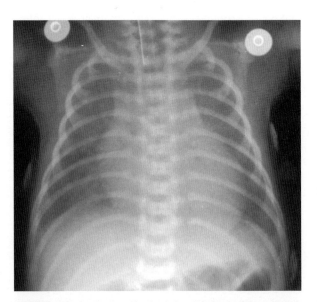

FIGURE 7-7. A chest radiograph in an infant with aortopulmonary window and interrupted aortic arch. The important findings include generalized cardiomegaly with a left ventricle-forming apex, a large main pulmonary artery, and passive congestion of the lungs. An endotracheal tube is present and ECG monitoring leads are evident on the shoulders.

Therapeutic Considerations

Both of these defects require surgical repair. It is important to intervene early to prevent pulmonary vascular disease. Repair of an aortopulmonary window is generally accomplished from a transaortic approach. It is important to correct any associated defects if present. There have been a few reports of catheter-based intervention to close an aortopulmonary window without the need for surgery. Surgical correction of an anomalous right pulmonary artery arising from the ascending aorta requires division of the right pulmonary at its origin and reimplantation into the main pulmonary artery. This may be accomplished directly or may require augmentation with prosthetic, autologous, or heterologous material.

Patent Ductus Arteriosus

Anatomic and Physiologic Considerations

A patent ductus arteriosus is a common problem in prematurely born infants but is relatively uncommon in term newborn infants. Moreover, unless it is quite large, a patent ductus arteriosus rarely causes symptoms in a term infant. In the term infant, normal postnatal closure of the ductus arteriosus occurs in two stages. Immediately after birth, contraction of the medial smooth muscle causes functional closure, usually within 12 to 24 hours. Thereafter, infolding of the endothelium causes disruption of the internal elastic lamina and proliferation of the subintimal layers. Necrosis of these layers occurs and, as the mounds continue to enlarge, there is progressive replacement of muscle fibers with connective tissue, resulting in permanent closure and converting the ductus to a ligamentum arteriosus. This process usually takes about 2 to 3 weeks. In the preterm infant, the initial functional closure frequently does not occur, and the decrease in pulmonary vascular resistance over the first few days of life causes an increasing left-to-right shunt through the ductus.

The initial closure of the ductus arteriosus and its failure to close in premature infants has been the subject of many investigations. Patency of the ductus arteriosus is mediated by the perfusing oxygen concentration and the levels of prostaglandin E_2 and I_2, although other vasoactive substances such as bradykinin and circulating catecholamines may contribute. The immature ductus is very sensitive to the dilating effects of prostaglandins and much less sensitive to the vasoconstricting effects of oxygen. As the ductus matures in the later stages of gestation, it becomes much more sensitive to oxygen and much less so to prostaglandins. Thus, the large increase in oxygen concentration likely induces complete closure of the ductus arteriosus in the term infant, but this is not the case in the preterm infant. Moreover, prostaglandin levels decrease to a greater extent in the term infant, further promoting ductal closure. Circulating prostaglandin levels are very high in the fetus. Because the pulmonary vascular musculature is less well developed in preterm infants, pulmonary vascular resistance is particularly low and shunts of a large magnitude can develop rapidly. In addition, pulmonary capillary permeability may be greater, allowing for the production of more interstitial edema in response to a moderate increase in pulmonary blood flow. Furthermore, the immature alveoli may be more sensitive to the presence of increased fluid. Because of these factors, a moderate left-to-right shunt through a ductus arteriosus has a far greater effect on the lung function in a preterm infant than in a term infant.

The effects of a patent ductus arteriosus on the systemic circulation are also much more prominent and deleterious in the preterm infant. In a term infant with a patent ductus arteriosus, the left ventricle is capable of greatly increasing output in response to the increases in preload and sympathetic nervous system activity. Despite a very large shunt, systemic blood flow usually is maintained and organ ischemia does not occur. In contrast, the left ventricle of the preterm infant is less capable of increasing its output. The ventricle is less compliant because of higher water content and less organized myocyte architecture. Therefore, end-diastolic volume cannot increase as much in response to an increase in pulmonary venous return, limiting the increase in stroke volume. End-diastolic pressure increases to a greater extent, contributing to alveolar edema. Additionally, resting heart rate is greater and near the level at which a further increase causes a decrease in stroke volume. For all of these reasons, systemic blood flow frequently falls in the premature infant with a large patent ductus arteriosus. This decrease in systemic blood flow may lead to serious consequences, including renal insufficiency, necrotizing enterocolitis, and intraventricular hemorrhage. Even the myocardium is susceptible to ischemia. Although coronary blood flow can increase greatly in response to stress, the very low diastolic pressures in the aorta of the preterm infant with a ductus arteriosus may not provide sufficient perfusion pressure to prevent subendocardial ischemia.

Clinical Presentation

A large ductus arteriosus in a preterm infant usually presents after a few days of age as the infant is recovering from respiratory distress syndrome. The earliest signs are often an increased need for respiratory support and increased arterial carbon dioxide levels due to alveolar edema. The widespread use of surfactant therapy has decreased the severity of respiratory distress syndrome but symptoms of a patent ductus arteriosus tend to occur earlier. Surfactant promotes alveolar patency and therefore improves oxygenation but pulmonary vascular resistance falls more rapidly. Pulses become more prominent and the pulse pressure widens, often with diastolic pressures falling into the mid to low twenties. The liver is enlarged. The precordial impulse is very prominent. The heart sounds are normal, and an S_3 gallop is occasionally heard. The murmur is not the usual continuous murmur in the left infraclavicular area that is classically described in older infants. Rather, the murmur in preterm infants is usually heard along the left sternal border and is predominantly systolic with limited diastolic spillover. There may be an associated mid-diastolic rumble at the apex, although the rapid heart rates make this difficult to appreciate.

Ancillary Tests

The electrocardiogram in the preterm infant with a large ductus arteriosus is usually normal because the presentation is rapid and there is little time for ventricular hypertrophy to develop. However, if the ductus is not appreciated immediately, left atrial enlargement, as manifested by a wide P wave in lead II, and left ventricular hypertrophy, with prominent inferior and lateral R waves and flattening of the ST-T waves, may be seen. Marked biventricular hypertrophy may be seen in older infants with a large patent ductus arteriosus. The chest radiograph shows an enlarged left ventricle and left atrium and interstitial and alveolar edema.

Echocardiography is essential for confirmation of the diagnosis and assessment of severity. The left atrium and ventricle are enlarged and there is often an associated left-to-right shunt across the foramen ovale. Pulsed and color Doppler echocardiography demonstrate the left-to-right shunt, which occurs primarily in diastole. Although the width of the color jet roughly estimates the diameter of the ductus arteriosus and the size of the left-sided chambers roughly estimate the size of the shunt, the magnitude and importance of the ductal shunt is best determined by evaluating flow in the systemic arteries. The presence and extent of retrograde flow in the descending aorta correlates with severity, as it reflects the amount of blood that is being directed away from the gastrointestinal tract and

kidneys. These organ systems are primarily perfused in diastole and are most susceptible to ischemic damage.

Therapeutic Considerations

Treatment of preterm infants with indomethacin has dramatically altered the management of patent ductus arteriosus. Indomethacin is administered either prophylactically or very early after recognition of the presence of a patent ductus arteriosus. A number of different dosing regimens have been proposed and local institutional practices vary. The key features are early administration and repeat dosing over a 24-hour period. It is important to repeat the echocardiogram if there is any suspicion of failure of the ductus to close or if reopening is suspected after initial closure. Repeat courses of indomethacin can be administered, but if ductal patency persists and the infant remains symptomatic, most authorities recommend an aggressive approach to surgical ligation of the ductus. In many institutions, this is accomplished in the neonatal intensive care unit, thereby avoiding potential problems associated with transporting a sick premature infant to and from the operating room. Recent studies have suggested that other prostaglandin synthesis inhibitors, such as ibuprofen, may be equally effective as indomethacin and may have fewer side effects. However, additional studies are necessary before ibuprofen is recommended as primary therapy.

A patent ductus arteriosus in a full-term infant rarely causes significant symptoms. However, closure is recommended if the ductus remains patent past infancy. Outside the neonatal period, the ductus arteriosus is not responsive to indomethacin and either a surgical or catheter-based approach to closure is necessary. Occlusion of the ductus in the catheterization laboratory has become commonplace and is generally recommended as the treatment of choice. At present, this approach is not technically feasible for small premature infants.

Arteriovenous Malformation

Anatomic and Physiologic Considerations

A systemic arteriovenous malformation has the same pathophysiological effects on pulmonary blood flow as an intracardiac defect such as ventricular septal defect. The excess portion of flow that enters the venous system through the abnormal arteriovenous malformation is directed through the right atrium, right ventricle, and pulmonary arteries. The magnitude of the increase in systemic venous flow can be sufficiently large to cause interstitial edema and all of the symptoms of excessive pulmonary blood flow.

Before birth, a very large arteriovenous malformation may cause heart failure by reducing systemic perfusion and elevating venous pressures, causing hydrops fetalis. An arteriovenous malformation commonly associated with hydrops occurs in the placental circulation and may not be appreciated after birth. The placenta should be carefully evaluated in all infants with hydrops of unknown etiology.

The most common site for arteriovenous malformations that present symptomatically is deep within the brain. These most commonly drain into a large vein of Galen and are associated with abnormal brain development. In addition, an unusually high incidence of sinus venous atrial septal defects is present in infants with vein of Galen malformations. The next most common site of arteriovenous malformation is in the liver. These are often associated with hepatic hemangioendotheliomas.

Clinical Presentation

After birth, the excessive venous flow is directed into the lungs as the foramen ovale and ductus arteriosus close. Unlike other causes of exclusive left-to-right shunts, the amount of shunting is not dependent on the slower, second phase of the decrease in pulmonary vascular resistance that occurs during the first few weeks of life. Furthermore, the shunt magnitude is only minimally affected by the postnatal decline in hemoglobin and hematocrit. In the presence of a large arteriovenous malformation, very high levels of pulmonary blood flow occur almost immediately after birth, and tachypnea can be apparent within hours. Occasionally, if the malformation is extremely large, systemic blood flow is compromised and decreased systemic perfusion may be the dominant finding. In this instance, the erroneous diagnosis of hypoplastic left heart syndrome or some other left-sided obstructive defect is often considered initially. If desaturation is prominent, persistent pulmonary hypertension is also a common misdiagnosis.

The physical examination of an infant with a symptomatic arteriovenous malformation is striking. The infant is tachycardic and tachypneic. Oxygen saturation may be normal but it also may be mildly decreased in the upper extremities because of a right-to-left atrial shunt, and further decreased in the lower extremities because of a right-to-left ductal shunt, mimicking pulmonary hypertension of the newborn. If systemic blood flow is not compromised, the extremities are warm and well-perfused and the

pulses are bounding. Even when perfusion is poor and the extremities are cool, the pulses are unusually strong. If appreciated clinically, this is a pathognomonic finding of arteriovenous malformations. The liver is moderately enlarged. The precordium is strikingly hyperactive. The dramatic increase in precordial activity is indicative of the greatly increased blood flow into the right ventricle and secondary pulmonary arterial hypertension. The first heart sound is normal, the second heart sound is usually single and loud, and there may be a nonspecific systolic ejection murmur. Bruits can always be heard over the location of the malformation. Auscultation of head and liver is extremely important in any infant with respiratory distress or decreased systemic perfusion at birth, especially if the pulses and precordial impulse are prominent.

Ancillary Tests

The electrocardiogram shows right ventricular hypertrophy, and often biventricular hypertrophy even at birth. Enlargement of one or both atria may also be apparent. The chest radiograph shows generalized cardiomegaly, including enlargement of the superior vena caval shadow in patients with a vein of Galen malformation. The echocardiogram shows generalized chamber enlargement. The right atrium and right ventricle are particularly large and the right ventricle appears to be hypercontractile. Dilation of the superior vena cava or inferior vena cava should be apparent, depending on the location of the malformation. The intracardiac anatomy should be defined and the specific presence of a sinus venosus atrial septal defect should be sought in infants with a vein of Galen malformation.

A thorough Doppler evaluation is extremely important, as this can indirectly locate the site of the arteriovenous malformation. The ascending aortic flow signal shows exaggeration of the forward flow in all instances, but retrograde diastolic flow in the aorta will occur distal to the origin of the vessels feeding the malformation. Thus, the entire aorta and head and neck vessels should be interrogated. Rapid and accurate diagnosis is essential, because these infants are often quite ill and require prompt intervention.

Therapeutic Considerations

Infants with a large arteriovenous malformation generally require stabilization with positive pressure ventilation and supportive measures to maintain effective systemic circulation. Once the infant has been stabilized, interventional catheterization should be performed promptly. The arteriovenous malformation can often be occluded either partially or completed using coils or other devices and materials. Even partial occlusion may be very helpful in reducing the magnitude of the shunt, thereby minimizing symptoms and allowing the infant to grow normally. Unfortunately, many infants with vein of Galen aneurysm malformations have severe neurologic injury before birth or may occur as a result of the intervention, which usually requires large numbers of coils and other methods to fully occlude the abnormal vasculature and may impair blood flow to normal brain tissue, as well. Complete neurologic evaluation with magnetic resonance imaging is performed before intervention and, in the presence of severe injury, palliative care is often recommended.

■ DEFECTS WITH BIDIRECTIONAL SHUNTS AND EXCESSIVE PULMONARY BLOOD FLOW

This category includes congenital cardiovascular malformations in which the dominant pathophysiologic process is excessive pulmonary blood flow, although the presence of an associated right-to-left shunt causes varying degrees of systemic arterial desaturation. Some of these defects cause symptoms of decreased systemic perfusion (total anomalous pulmonary venous connection with obstruction) or cyanosis (double-inlet left ventricle with subvalvar pulmonary stenosis), but only those conditions in which excessive pulmonary blood flow is the dominant pathophysiological process are considered in this chapter.

Total Anomalous Pulmonary Venous Connection Without Obstruction

Anatomic and Physiologic Considerations
The most proximal extracardiac connection that allows for mixing of systemic and pulmonary venous blood is the abnormal connection of the pulmonary veins either to the systemic veins, the coronary sinus or the right atrium directly. During normal development, the pulmonary veins from the five lobes of the lung approach the midline and coalesce, forming a single pulmonary venous confluence. This confluence then merges into the posterior left side of the primitive atrium, forming a large communication. The mature left atrium is composed of the pulmonary venous confluence and the left half of the primitive atrium.

When the pulmonary venous confluence does not connect normally into the atrium, it coalesces with other venous structures. The most common connection is to the common cardinal system, usually on the left. When this

occurs, the confluence joins behind the left atrium and usually ascends as a left vertical vein anterior to the left pulmonary artery, left mainstem bronchus, and aortic arch to join the left innominate vein and then the superior vena cava (Figure 7-8). Occasionally the vertical vein passes between the left pulmonary artery and the left mainstem bronchus, causing severe obstruction. Less commonly, the ascending trunk ascends the right side of the mediastinum and enters the back of the superior vena cava or the azygous vein. This is more commonly associated with mixed anomalous pulmonary venous drainage and other complex anomalies, such as right atrial isomerism.

The next most common connection is infradiaphragmatic, in which the pulmonary venous confluence descends below the diaphragm, anterior to the esophagus, and joins the umbilicovitelline venous system. This form of anomalous pulmonary venous connection is almost always obstructed at birth, because the pulmonary venous return must enter the relatively small portal system as the ductus venosus closes. Since the pathophysiology and clinical presentation of obstructed pulmonary venous return differs significantly from the defects that cause excessive pulmonary blood flow, infradiaphragmatic anomalous pulmonary venous connection is discussed in Chapter 8.

The third most common site of connection is directly to the coronary sinus. In this case, the pulmonary venous confluence lies entirely within the pericardium and connects to the mid portion of the coronary sinus in the atrioventricular groove. This connection is rarely obstructed.

Lastly, the pulmonary veins may connect directly to the right atrium. This usually is not a single connection but there is mixed drainage with the right-sided pulmonary veins connecting to the right atrium and the left-sided pulmonary veins connecting to the left atrium. This form of anomalous pulmonary venous connection is commonly associated with left atrial isomerism.

Clinical Presentation
The newborn with total anomalous pulmonary venous connection without obstruction is not symptomatic at birth, although transient cyanosis may be recognized. The presence of mild arterial desaturation is becoming much more commonly appreciated because of the frequent use of pulse oximetry. Most newborns with unobstructed total anomalous pulmonary venous connection have supradiaphragmatic drainage of the veins (either via a left vertical vein or less commonly via the coronary sinus). In both of these situations, the fully saturated pulmonary venous

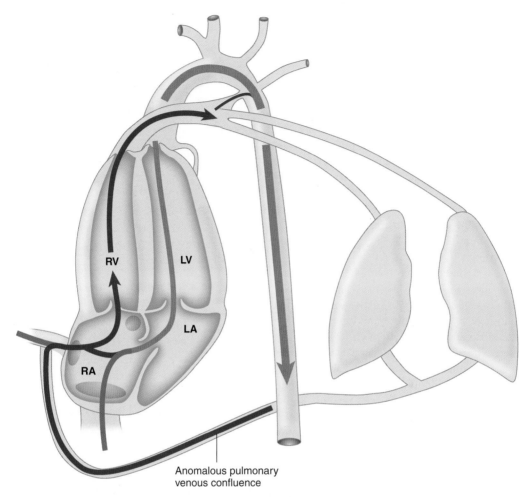

FIGURE 7-8. Total anomalous pulmonary venous connection above the diaphragm. In this defect, the fully saturated pulmonary venous blood returns via the left innominate vein to the superior vena cava and, along with systemic venous return from the upper body, preferentially crosses the tricuspid valve to the right ventricle and main pulmonary artery. The less saturated systemic venous blood from the inferior vena cava passes preferentially across the foramen ovale to the left atrium and then into the left ventricle and ascending aorta. Therefore, pulmonary arterial oxygen saturation is higher than ascending aortic oxygen saturation. If there is a patent ductus arteriosus, a small right-to-left shunt causes descending aortic oxygen saturation to be higher than that in the ascending aorta. Contrast this diagram with the idealized situation depicted in Figure 7-2 where complete mixing is assumed to occur in the right atrium. Abbreviations: LA, left atrium; LV, left ventricle; RA, right atrium; RV, right ventricle.

blood follows the path of superior vena caval flow, preferentially crossing the tricuspid valve into the right ventricle (Figure 7-8). The less saturated inferior vena caval blood preferentially crosses the foramen ovale to the left ventricle and ascending aorta. If the ductus arteriosus remains patent, a small right-to-left ductal shunt usually occurs because of the increased pulmonary blood flow. The right-to-left shunt causes the arterial oxygen saturation in the lower extremities to be higher than that in the upper extremities. The only other condition in which upper extremity saturation is less than that in the lower extremity is d-transposition of the great arteries. In d-transposition of the great arteries, however, upper extremity saturation is much lower than in total anomalous pulmonary venous connection. Thus, the finding of higher oxygen saturation by pulse oximetry in the lower extremity of a patient with mild cyanosis is pathognomonic of supradiaphragmatic total anomalous pulmonary venous connection.

If cyanosis is not appreciated at birth, the infant usually feeds well and often is discharged from the hospital without the defect being recognized. As pulmonary vascular resistance decreases, the right ventricle remodels and becomes more compliant. This increases pulmonary blood flow and systemic arterial saturation. Over time, symptoms of tachypnea and failure to thrive develop. The infant may be unnecessarily evaluated for pulmonary or gastrointestinal disease if the cardiac disease is not recognized.

On physical examination, the infant often appears thin and mildly tachypneic. Pulse oximetry usually shows oxygen saturations around 85% to 92%. Pulses and perfusion are generally normal, and the liver is mildly enlarged. The lungs are clear to auscultation although retractions are often present. The precordium is moderately hyperactive. The first heart sound is normal and the second heart sound is widely split with mild accentuation of the pulmonic component. An audible S_3 may be present. A murmur may be absent, which may contribute to the delay in diagnosis, but more often a soft systolic ejection murmur is heard best at the left upper sternal border and reflects increased pulmonary blood flow.

Ancillary Tests

Electrocardiography shows right ventricular hypertrophy with prominent R waves and upright T waves in the right precordium. Right atrial enlargement is suggested by tall-peaked P waves in lead II. The chest radiograph shows a normal-size heart with increased vascularity in the newborn, but if the diagnosis is delayed, cardiomegaly is present. A large vertical vein in the left upper mediastinum and enlargement of the superior vena cava in the right give the typical "snowman" appearance in cases of anomalous connection to the left innominate vein (Figure 7-9).

Echocardiography and color Doppler studies make the diagnosis of anomalous pulmonary venous connection much easier and more reliable. Because there is often a large pulmonary venous confluence behind the left atrium and the course of the pulmonary veins is normal, the recognition that the veins do not connect with the left atrium can be difficult. However, color Doppler can clearly

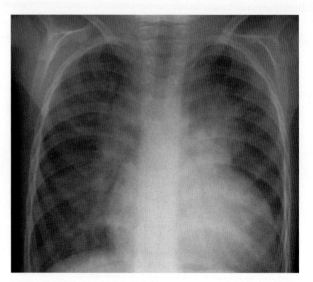

FIGURE 7-9. Chest radiograph in an infant with total anomalous pulmonary venous connection to the superior vena cava. A large vertical vein in the left upper mediastinum and enlargement of the superior vena in the right give the typical "snowman" appearance.

show whether the flow of blood from the pulmonary veins actually enters the left atrium or whether it travels anomalously (superiorly in supradiaphragmatic connection, or inferiorly if the confluent vein travels below the diaphragm to the portal system). When an anomalous connection is observed, it is important to assess the course of each pulmonary vein to ensure that the connection is not mixed, and to exclude associated heart disease. Cardiac catheterization can generally be avoided if all of the veins are defined. Magnetic resonance imaging can be extremely helpful in defining the extracardiac venous connections. The left ventricle often appears hypoplastic because right ventricular volume is so much greater than left. However, the left ventricle is always of adequate size, and coarctation of the aorta is not associated with this defect.

Therapeutic Considerations

Anomalous pulmonary venous connection is treated surgically. The specific approach depends on the details of the anatomy and course of the anomalous connections. In most cases, the pulmonary confluence behind the left atrium is anastomosed to the left atrium to allow pulmonary venous return to enter the left atrium. The vertical vein is generally ligated.

Single Ventricle Physiology Without Outflow Obstruction

Anatomic and Physiologic Considerations

A large number of congenital cardiovascular malformations are associated with complete mixing of systemic and pulmonary venous blood in a functionally single ventricular chamber. Of the patients with single ventricle physiology, only about one-third have unobstructed pulmonary and aortic outflow tracts. Most instead have pulmonary outflow obstruction and consequently present with cyanosis as the predominant manifestation of heart disease (Chapter 6). A smaller number have subaortic and aortic arch obstruction, and consequently present with decreased systemic perfusion as the predominant clinical problem (Chapter 7). In the remaining subset of infants with a single ventricle and unobstructed outflow, blood flows preferentially into the pulmonary artery and the predominant clinical manifestations are the result of excessive pulmonary blood flow.

The anatomy of these hearts is extremely variable. These defects are best described by their atrioventricular valve morphology, atrial-ventricular and ventricular-arterial connections, ventricular morphology, and associated defects. Two normal atrioventricular valves, atresia or straddling of one or the other atrioventricular valve, or a common atrioventricular valve may be present. The atrial-ventricular connections may be concordant, discordant, or double inlet (to the left ventricle). The ventricular-arterial connections may be concordant, discordant, or double outlet (to the right ventricle). Certain connections tend to track together. For example, the most common form of single ventricle physiology without outlet obstruction is l-malposition of the great arteries (ventricular-arterial discordance). When the great arteries are l-malposed and the physiology is that of a single ventricle, there are usually two normal atrioventricular valves, double-inlet left ventricle, and a subaortic outflow chamber of right ventricular morphology. In left atrial isomerism (sometimes called polysplenia, Chapter 6), an atrioventricular septal defect with a ventricle of uncertain morphology is often present, and there are many associated findings such as interrupted inferior vena cava with azygous continuation, bilateral superior vena cavae, abnormal pulmonary venous connection, a large atrial septal defect or common atrium, and bilateral left pulmonary arterial morphology.

Clinical Presentation

Independent of the precise anatomy, the clinical findings in infants with a single ventricle and unobstructed pulmonary blood flow are similar to those in infants with excessive pulmonary blood flow and bidirectional shunting caused by other types of structural defects. Growth is impaired, and oxygen saturation is modestly decreased. The liver and stomach positions should be evaluated for evidence of situs inversus or situs ambiguous, which can lead to specific cardiac diagnoses and noncardiac abnormalities. For example, a midline liver suggests the diagnosis of left atrial isomerism, which is associated with biliary atresia and intestinal malrotation. The precordium is active, and can be midsternal or located on either side of the sternum. The second heart sound is rarely heard to split because of the abnormal position of the pulmonary valve and the elevated pulmonary arterial diastolic pressures. Murmurs are often present, but their location, frequency, and characteristics depend on the specific anatomy, which can be quite variable.

Ancillary Tests

The electrocardiogram is variable, depending on the specific anatomic defects. The atrial forces should be evaluated to determine the axis of atrial conduction, paying particular attention to the presence of an inferior pacemaker with a superior axis (which occurs in left atrial isomerism). Atrioventricular conduction block should be carefully considered because it occurs commonly in left atrial isomerism and l-malposition of the aorta. The appearance of the chest radiograph is also very variable, but can be used to determine the size of the heart, its location within the thorax, the direction that the apex is pointing, the presence of symmetrical lungs, and the amount of vascularity. The echocardiogram is extremely useful for defining cardiac anatomy, function of the atrioventricular and semilunar valves, pulmonary arterial blood flow, and associated arterial and venous anomalies. In addition to echocardiography, an abdominal ultrasound should be performed because of the nearly universal finding of malrotation. Determining the anatomy of the gastrointestinal tract may help in the diagnosis of intestinal obstruction later. Liver function should also be assessed because of the association of biliary atresia.

Therapeutic Considerations

Regardless of the specific anatomic details, the general approach to these infants is similar. The ultimate goal is to separate the pulmonary and systemic circulations by use of a bidirectional Glenn shunt and modified Fontan operation

(Chapter 6). This is generally accomplished using a staged approach. In the neonate and young infant, aggressive medical and nutritional therapy is indicated to minimize symptoms and promote normal growth. In cases of severe refractory heart failure, early surgical intervention to reduce the amount of pulmonary blood flow becomes necessary. This can be accomplished by banding the main pulmonary artery (see following text). Alternatively, the pulmonary artery is surgically disconnected from the ventricle and a systemic-to-pulmonary artery shunt is placed.

Truncus Arteriosus

Anatomic and Physiologic Considerations

The most common defect with bidirectional shunting and excessive pulmonary blood flow is truncus arteriosus. The primary developmental defect in this defect is failure of septation of the aortopulmonary septum and the truncus arteriosus (Chapter 1). The failure of aortopulmonary septation results in a single arterial trunk from which arise the ascending aorta, the pulmonary arteries, and the coronary arteries (Figure 7-10). Failure of septation of the truncus

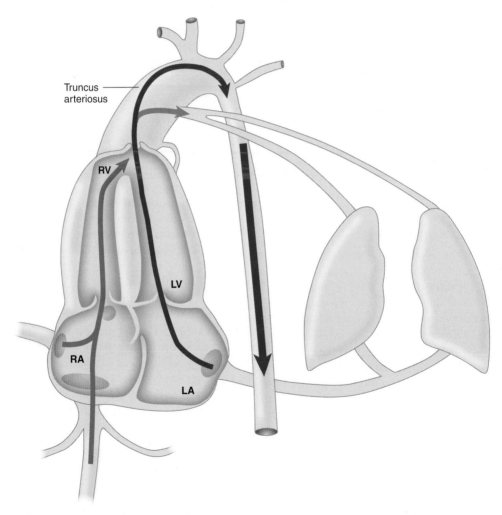

FIGURE 7-10. Truncus arteriosus. The right ventricle ejects the desaturated systemic venous blood posteriorly and to the left, whereas the left ventricle ejects the well-oxygenated pulmonary venous blood anteriorly and to the right. Because of these flow patterns, blood in the ascending aorta is somewhat more saturated than blood in the pulmonary arteries. Abbreviations: LA, left atrium; LV, left ventricle; RA, right atrium; RV, right ventricle.

arteriosus results in a single semilunar valve as the outlet for both ventricles. The truncal valve may have from one to six valve leaflets, though most commonly it is a tricuspid valve. The valve is frequently dysplastic and may be associated with significant insufficiency, or less commonly, stenosis.

Abnormal migration of ectomesenchymal cells derived from the cardiac neural crest has been implicated in the pathogenesis of this defect. This field defect is also associated with abnormalities in parathyroid and thymic function seen in microdeletion 22q11 (DiGeorge) syndrome. This syndrome occurs in approximately one-third of infants with truncus arteriosus and is more common when the aortic arch is right sided. These infants may be identified as having a microdeletion of the short arm of chromosome 22 (22q11 deletion syndrome). The ductus arteriosus is absent except when there is an interrupted aortic arch.

Truncus arteriosus is classified into various categories depending on the origins of the branch pulmonary arteries and the presence of an interrupted aortic arch. Most commonly, the two pulmonary arteries arise either as a single trunk (type I) or with a fine raphe separating them (type II) from the posterior and leftward side of the trunk. In this configuration, truncus arteriosus is not a complete mixing defect. Because the left ventricle ejects blood anteriorly and to the right and the right ventricle ejects blood posteriorly and to the left, the left ventricle will preferentially eject into ascending aorta and the right ventricle into the branch pulmonary arteries (Figure 7-10). Often, there is a separation in saturation of about 5% to 8% between the two vascular beds, with the ascending aortic saturation being higher. This is the reason that when systemic oxygen saturation measured by pulse oximetry is 94% to 95%, pulmonary blood flow is not actually 10 times that of systemic blood flow (as would be predicted if complete mixing is assumed). Usually, the systemic oxygen saturation is around 88% to 92% and pulmonary blood flow is about three to four times that of systemic blood flow. Clearly, this physiology is not associated with either visible cyanosis or metabolically significant systemic desaturation. Instead the infant will have symptoms of excessive pulmonary blood flow.

Clinical Presentation

On physical examination, cyanosis may only be observed in the first few hours or first day of life, while pulmonary vascular resistance is still relatively high. Because the shunt is both systolic and diastolic, the rapid fall in pulmonary vascular resistance results in arterial oxygen saturations in the range of 85% or higher very soon after birth. This feature makes cyanosis difficult to appreciate after the first few hours of life. Over time, the infant becomes more tachypneic with significant intercostal and subcostal retractions. Failure to thrive is almost universal, except when there is the rare occurrence of stenosis of the pulmonary arterial ostium. Tachycardia and diaphoresis are prominent. The facies of microdeletion 22q11 syndrome may be present, including a sloping forehead, hypertelorism, micrognathia, low-set and posteriorly rotated ears, and a small mouth. The pulses are bounding in all extremities except when the aortic arch is interrupted, in which case the infant presents with diminished systemic perfusion if the ductus arteriosus begins to close. However, it seems that ductal closure in infants with truncus arteriosus and interrupted aortic arch occurs less commonly than in other infants with heart disease. There is moderate hepatomegaly. The precordium is hyperactive though no thrill is present unless there is truncal valve stenosis, which may cause a suprasternal notch thrill. The first heart sound is normal and the second heart sound is single and loud because of the single semilunar valve. An important and extremely frequent finding is a systolic ejection click arising from the dysplastic truncal valve. There is usually a harsh systolic ejection murmur of mid to high frequencies around the midsternum. The systolic murmur radiates to the lungs and to the carotid arteries. An early diastolic murmur of truncal valve insufficiency should be carefully sought. Often, an apical mid-diastolic murmur is present, reflecting the very large pulmonary blood flow and increased inflow across the mitral valve.

Ancillary Tests

The electrocardiogram shows right and usually biventricular hypertrophy within the first weeks of life, and left atrial enlargement may also be evident. The chest radiograph shows generalized cardiomegaly with increased pulmonary vascular markings. A strong clue to the diagnosis is the presence of an abnormal structure in the left upper mediastinum, which represents the elevated takeoff of the left pulmonary artery (Figure 7-11).

The echocardiogram is diagnostic, showing the common trunk with the takeoff of the great arteries and the coronary arteries as it ascends. It is most important to evaluate the origin of both branch pulmonary arteries, the function of the truncal valve, associated muscular ventricular septal defects, the orientation of the aortic arch, and the presence or absence of aortic arch interruption.

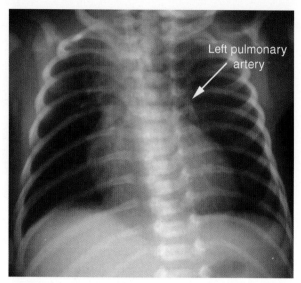

FIGURE 7-11. Chest radiograph in an infant with truncus arteriosus. The important findings are a left ventricle forming apex, a right aortic arch, and the high takeoff of the left pulmonary artery from the common trunk.

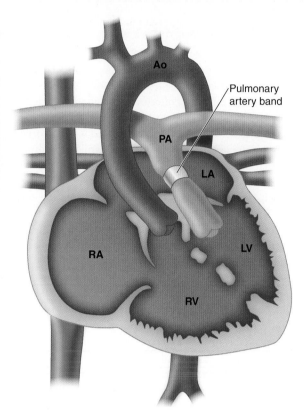

FIGURE 7-12. Pulmonary artery band. Ideally, the band should be placed in the mid-portion of the main pulmonary artery to avoid distortion of the pulmonary valve or origins of the right and left pulmonary arteries. Abbreviations: Ao, aorta; LA, left atrium; LV, left ventricle; PA, pulmonary artery; RA, right atrium; RV, right ventricle.

Therapeutic Considerations

Truncus arteriosus requires surgical repair, often in the neonatal period. Heart failure and failure to thrive can be severe, and unless there are compelling reasons that preclude surgical intervention, repair in the neonatal period is recommended. Several different surgical techniques are utilized, with the common goal of closing the ventricular septal defect in such a fashion that the left ventricle ejects across the truncal valve into the ascending aorta. The pulmonary arteries are disconnected from the common trunk and connected to the right ventricle using some type of conduit. Repair of truncus arteriosus in infancy requires additional surgical procedures in the future to replace the right ventricular to pulmonary artery connection as the child grows.

■ PULMONARY ARTERY BAND

If a patient has high pulmonary blood flow for a long period of time, congestive heart failure, failure to thrive, pulmonary hypertension, and pulmonary vascular disease are all possible complications. Generally, patients with defects such as a large ventricular septal defect or atrioventricular septal defect undergo open-heart repair before 6 to

12 months of age. Some patients are not candidates for open-heart repair because, for example, they have defects such as a functional single ventricle that are not amenable to repair. A pulmonary artery band (Figure 7-12) serves as reasonable palliation in these patients. Banding the pulmonary artery involves placing a ligature around the main pulmonary artery and tightening it so that an artificial obstruction is created. The degree of tightening requires critical judgment on the part of the surgeon; too little constriction will cause the patient to have too much pulmonary blood flow and too much constriction will result in the patient becoming too cyanotic either immediately or after a relatively small amount of growth. The band should be placed at the midportion of the main pulmonary artery; it should not be too close to the pulmonary valve or too close to the bifurcation of the pulmonary arteries. Bands

may migrate after placement. Improperly placed or migrated bands may damage the pulmonary valve or distort the origin of the right or left pulmonary artery. Because of the potential problems associated with pulmonary arterial bands, some advocate disconnecting the pulmonary artery from the heart and placing a systemic-to-pulmonary artery shunt to provide pulmonary blood flow.

SUGGESTED READINGS

General

Allen HD, Driscoll DJ, Shaddy RE, Feltes TF, eds. *Moss and Adams' Heart Disease in Infants, Children, and Adolescents Including the Fetus and Young Adult.* 7th ed. Philadelphia, PA: Lippincott Williams & Wilkins; 2008.

Hoffman JIE. *The Natural and Unnatural History of Congenital Heart Disease.* Oxford, United Kingdom: Wiley-Blackwell; 2009.

Park MK. *The Pediatric Cardiology Handbook.* 4th ed. Philadelphia, PA: Mosby Elsevier; 2010.

Rudolph AM. *Congenital Diseases of the Heart: Clinical-Physiological Considerations.* Chichester, United Kingdom: Wiley-Blackwell; 2009.

Left-to-Right Shunts

Anderson RH, Lenox CC, Zuberbuhler JR. The morphology of ventricular septal defects. *Perspect Pediatr Pathol.* 1984;8:235-268.

Fong LV, Anderson RH, Siewers RD, et al. Anomalous origin of one pulmonary artery from the ascending aorta: a review of echocardiographic, catheter, and morphological features. *Br Heart J.* 1989;62:389-395.

Kutsche LM, Van Mierop LH. Anatomy and pathogenesis of aorticopulmonary septal defect. *Am J Cardiol.* 1987;59:443-447.

McCurnin DC, Yoder BA, Coalson J, et al. Effect of ductus ligation on cardiopulmonary function in premature baboons. *Am J Respir Crit Care Med.* 2005;172:1569-1574.

McElhinney DB, Reddy VM, Tworetzky W, et al. Early and late results after repair of aortopulmonary septal defect and associated anomalies in infants <6 months of age. *Am J Cardiol.* 1998;81:195-201.

Nuutila M, Saisto T. Prenatal diagnosis of vein of Galen malformation: a multidisciplinary challenge. *Am J Perinatol.* 2008;25:225-227.

Tweddell JS, Pelech AN, Frommelt PC. Ventricular septal defect and aortic valve regurgitation: pathophysiology and indications for surgery. *Semin Thorac Cardiovasc Surg Pediatr Card Surg Annu.* 2006;147-152.

Van Overmeire B, Smets K, Lecoutere D, et al. A comparison of ibuprofen and indomethacin for closure of patent ductus arteriosus. *N Engl J Med.* 2000;343:674-681.

Bidirectional Shunts With Dominant Left-to-Right Shunt

Alton GY, Robertson CM, Sauve R, et al. Early childhood health, growth, and neurodevelopmental outcomes after complete repair of total anomalous pulmonary venous connection at 6 weeks or younger. *J Thorac Cardiovasc Surg.* 2007;133:905-911.

Butto F, Lucas RV, Jr., Edwards JE. Persistent truncus arteriosus: pathologic anatomy in 54 cases. *Pediatr Cardiol.* 1986; 7:95-101.

Karamlou T, Gurofsky R, Al Sukhni E, et al. Factors associated with mortality and reoperation in 377 children with total anomalous pulmonary venous connection. *Circulation.* 2007;115:1591-1598.

McElhinney DB, Driscoll DA, Emanuel BS, et al. Chromosome 22q11 deletion in patients with truncus arteriosus. *Pediatr Cardiol.* 2003;24:569-573.

Rajasinghe HA, McElhinney DB, Reddy VM, et al. Long-term follow-up of truncus arteriosus repaired in infancy: a twenty-year experience. *J Thorac Cardiovasc Surg.* 1997;113: 869-878.

Pulmonary Arterial Banding

Pinho P, Von Oppell UO, Brink J, et al. Pulmonary artery banding: adequacy and long-term outcome. *Eur J Cardiothorac Surg.* 1997;11:105-111.

Approach to the Infant With Inadequate Systemic Perfusion

- ■ INTRODUCTION
- ■ PATHOPHYSIOLOGY OF INADEQUATE SYSTEMIC PERFUSION

  Fetal Physiology and the Transition at Birth
- ■ LEFT HEART OBSTRUCTION

  Total Anomalous Pulmonary Venous Connection With Obstruction

Cor Triatriatum
Mitral Stenosis
Hypoplastic Left Heart Syndrome
Valvar Aortic Stenosis
Interruption of the Aortic Arch
Coarctation of the Aorta

- ■ SUGGESTED READINGS

■ INTRODUCTION

Inadequate systemic perfusion is the second most common manifestation of symptomatic heart disease in newborn infants. The infant often presents with moderate to severe respiratory distress in addition to signs of decreased systemic perfusion. Respiratory distress is caused by increased pulmonary venous pressure causing pulmonary edema. Pulmonary venous pressures are increased because (1) there is obstruction to the egress of blood from the lungs or from the left atrium into the left ventricle, or (2) the left ventricle cannot adequately eject blood. In some infants, the decrease in systemic perfusion is profound, with decreased to absent peripheral pulses, cool extremities, hypotension, and severe metabolic acidosis. In these cases, the compromise of systemic blood flow is life threatening and requires urgent diagnosis and therapy. In other infants, respiratory distress is the most impressive finding and the signs of decreased systemic

perfusion are subtle, often leading to the erroneous conclusion that the infant has primary pulmonary disease rather than heart disease. Signs of decreased systemic perfusion, which may be indicated solely by mildly decreased pulses or by a mild metabolic acidosis, should be carefully sought and considered in all infants with significant respiratory distress.

The two hemodynamic categories of cardiovascular pathophysiology that cause decreased systemic perfusion are left heart obstruction and cardiomyopathy. This chapter will review the various anatomic defects that cause left heart obstruction. Cardiomyopathies in newborn infants are reviewed in Chapter 9 and will not be discussed here.

■ PATHOPHYSIOLOGY OF INADEQUATE SYSTEMIC PERFUSION

The primary pathophysiologic abnormality in the infant with inadequate systemic perfusion is the inability of the heart to supply an adequate amount of oxygen to the tissues to meet metabolic needs. In this context, the onset is more acute and severe as compared with the chronic heart failure syndrome discussed in Chapter 11. Furthermore, in contrast to cyanotic infants (Chapter 6), oxygen saturation and content are usually normal in infants with decreased systemic perfusion. Instead, the overriding problem is inadequate systemic blood flow.

Fetal Physiology and the Transition at Birth

In the normal fetus, different ventricles perfuse the upper and lower portions of the body. The right ventricle supplies the lower body and the left ventricle supplies the upper body. During fetal life, obstruction to one ventricle, or a myopathic process isolated to that ventricle, does not lead to decreased systemic perfusion. Inflow can be diverted to the healthy ventricle via the foramen ovale, and a portion of the outflow of the healthy ventricle can be diverted to the other vascular bed via the ductus arteriosus (Chapter 3, Figure 3-5). Left-sided obstruction causes decompensation after birth because the postnatal changes in the circulation prevent the right ventricle from performing the work of the left ventricle. At birth, pulmonary blood flow increases greatly, causing the flap of the foramen ovale to close the atrial communication. In newborn infants in whom blood flow into or out of the left ventricle is critically obstructed, closure of the foramen ovale causes decreased systemic perfusion almost immediately after birth. Blood flow may cross the foramen ovale in a left-to-right direction, but this occurs at the cost of increased left atrial pressures. Thus, an early and important finding in these infants is pulmonary edema and severe respiratory distress.

Some infants have either a widely incompetent foramen ovale or have more distal obstruction (eg, coarctation of the aorta) which is not dependent on decompression through the foramen ovale. Adequate systemic perfusion in these infants depends on patency of the ductus arteriosus. In the infant with hypoplastic left heart syndrome or interruption of the aortic arch, adequate systemic blood flow depends on a *widely* patent ductus arteriosus. Thus, these infants develop symptoms within the first 72 hours of life as the ductus arteriosus begins to constrict. In contrast, infants with coarctation of the aorta do not require full patency of the ductus arteriosus but merely a large ductal ampulla to maintain flow around the coarctation site into the descending aorta. The ampulla, which is located at the aortic end of the ductus arteriosus, provides a pathway for blood to flow from the aortic arch past the

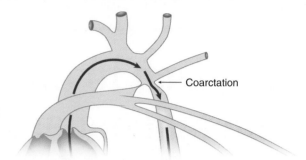

FIGURE 8-1. Coarctation of the aorta. Even when the ductus is fully closed in its mid-portion, the presence of an aortic ampulla allows for blood flow to bypass the coarctation site without significant obstruction to the descending aorta.

site of coarctation to the descending aorta (Figure 8-1). The ductus arteriosus constricts initially at its pulmonary end and only days later does the constriction progress to the aortic end. Thus, aortic obstruction and therefore, symptoms, may be delayed for several days or weeks after birth in infants with significant coarctation of the aorta.

■ LEFT HEART OBSTRUCTION

Left heart obstruction may occur either at the inflow of blood into the left atrium or ventricle, or at the outflow of blood from the left ventricle. The defects can be considered according to the anatomical site of obstruction, starting at the pulmonary veins and progressing through the left heart to the ascending and descending aorta (Table 8-1).

■ TABLE 8-1. Left-Sided Obstructive Defects

Anatomic level	Structural defect
Pulmonary veins	Total anomalous pulmonary venous connection with obstruction
Left atrium	Cor triatriatum
	Supravalvar mitral web/ring
Mitral valve	Atresia
	Stenosis (± parachute mitral valve)
Left ventricle	Hypoplastic left heart syndrome
	Subaortic stenosis
Aortic valve	Atresia
	Stenosis
Aorta	Supravalvar aortic stenosis
	Aortic arch hypoplasia
	Aortic arch interruption
	Coarctation of the aorta

Total Anomalous Pulmonary Venous Connection With Obstruction

Anatomic and Physiologic Considerations

The most proximal obstruction to filling of the left heart occurs at the level of the pulmonary veins. The embryonic pulmonary venous confluence is not part of the true left atrium but is a coalescence of the pulmonary veins from the five lobes of the lungs, which eventually connects to the left atrium. In total anomalous pulmonary venous connection, the confluence does not connect to the left atrium and instead it connects to various venous structures above or below the diaphragm. Pulmonary veins draining above the diaphragm usually have only modest pressure gradients associated with high flow through the venous channels. As discussed in Chapter 7, infants with supradiaphragmatic total anomalous pulmonary venous connection usually present with tachypnea secondary to high pulmonary blood flow rather than decreased systemic perfusion. An uncommon exception occurs when the superior course of a left vertical vein passes between the left pulmonary artery and bronchus rather than in front of both. This is termed a hemodynamic vise. As the left pulmonary artery and pulmonary veins fill with blood after birth, the vertical vein becomes compressed and the predominant signs are due to decreased systemic perfusion.

The most common anomalous pulmonary venous connection that is associated with postnatal pulmonary venous obstruction occurs when the pulmonary venous confluence coalesces below the diaphragm with the umbilicovitelline system. In this situation, the pulmonary venous confluence descends anterior to the esophagus and connects near the liver to the portal system or the ductus venosus (Figure 8-2). Because the ductus venosus is large in utero and pulmonary blood flow is small, the connection is unobstructed during fetal life. Immediately after birth, pulmonary blood flow increases greatly and the loss of placental blood flow is associated with constriction of the ductus venosus. These changes at birth result in increased flow through the anomalous venous channel, which is inadequate to provide unimpeded flow. The result is obstruction to egress of blood from the lungs, marked increase in pulmonary venous pressure and pulmonary edema.

Determining the location of the abnormal connection in a newborn infant with total anomalous pulmonary venous connection with obstruction may be possible at the bedside if the ductus arteriosus is patent. When pulmonary venous outflow is obstructed, pulmonary vascular resistance is high and right-to-left shunting occurs across the ductus arteriosus. If the veins drain superiorly, the pulmonary venous return preferentially descends with the superior vena caval flow toward the tricuspid valve, then into the right ventricle, main pulmonary artery, ductus arteriosus, and descending aorta. Consequently, oxygen saturation in the lower portion of the body is *higher* than that in the upper body. Conversely, if the veins drain below the diaphragm, pulmonary venous blood preferentially crosses the foramen ovale to the left atrium and ventricle and ascending aorta (Figure 8-2). In this situation, oxygen saturation in the lower portion of the body is *lower* than that in the upper body.

Clinical Presentation

The clinical presentation of the infant with obstructed total anomalous venous connection is dramatic and occurs shortly after birth. Moderate to severe respiratory distress with tachypnea, intercostal and subcostal retractions, nasal flaring, and grunting develop soon after birth. Oxygen saturation measured by pulse oximetry is usually modestly decreased, often in the mid-80s, but it may be much lower if obstruction is severe. As discussed earlier, a modest difference in oxygen saturation may be present between the upper and lower extremities if the ductus arteriosus is patent. The pulses are often mildly to moderately decreased in all extremities and perfusion may be similarly decreased. The blood pressure may show a narrow pulse pressure. The precordium is hyperactive with a prominent parasternal impulse because the right ventricle is ejecting much more blood than normal and is doing so at suprasystemic pressures. The first heart sound is normal and splitting of the second heart sound often is easy to hear because of the markedly increased pulmonary blood flow. A split second heart sound in the newborn infant with decreased systemic oxygen saturation is very unusual and strongly supports the diagnosis of total anomalous pulmonary venous connection. A nonspecific murmur associated with increase flow across the right ventricular outflow tract may be present, although this is less common when severe pulmonary venous obstruction is present.

This presentation is easily confused with persistent pulmonary hypertension of the newborn infant, another life-threatening condition with a similar early course of severe decompensation. Moreover, infants with total anomalous pulmonary venous connection with obstruction often have suprasystemic pulmonary arterial pressures, which further complicates differentiating between these two conditions. It is critically important to differentiate the two as

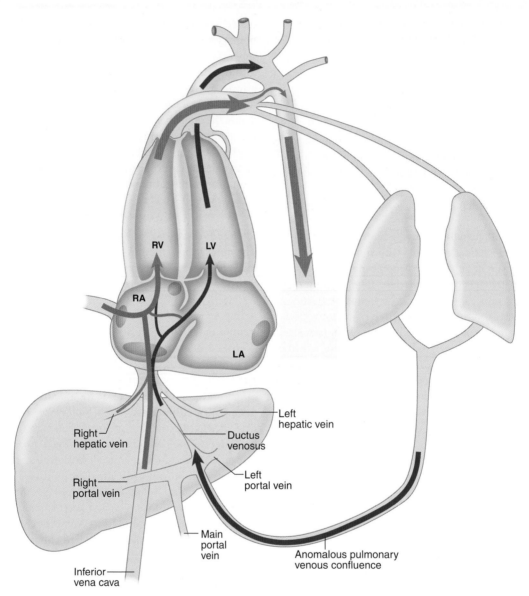

FIGURE 8-2. Total anomalous pulmonary venous connection below the diaphragm. Fully saturated pulmonary venous blood descends in the anomalous venous confluence below the diaphragm and inserts into to the portal venous system. At birth, pulmonary blood flow increases and the ductus venosus constricts, together increasing pulmonary venous pressures and causing pulmonary edema. As described in the text, there is preferential streaming within the atria so that if there is a patent ductus arteriosus (as shown in this diagram), a small right-to-left shunt causes descending aortic saturation also to be lower than that in the ascending aorta. Abbreviations: LA, left atrium; LV, left ventricle; RA, right atrium; RV, right ventricle.

soon as possible, because emergency surgery can be life-saving in the infant with total anomalous pulmonary venous connection. The prenatal course and delivery are usually benign in the infant with obstructed total anomalous pulmonary venous connection. In contrast, the infant with pulmonary hypertension frequently has a history of perinatal complications such as premature rupture of membranes, meconium in the amniotic fluid if not frank aspiration, low Apgar score, in utero growth retardation, or other findings consistent with perinatal distress. However, a high index of suspicion is critical if the correct diagnosis is to be made quickly. Because of the difficulty in differentiating the two conditions, every infant who is thought to have persistent pulmonary hypertension of the newborn should undergo echocardiography urgently, to evaluate the possibility that the pulmonary hypertension is caused by total anomalous pulmonary venous connection with obstruction.

Ancillary Tests

The electrocardiogram may be helpful in differentiating total anomalous pulmonary venous connection from pulmonary hypertension of the newborn. A "qR" pattern in the right precordial leads, which reflects severe right ventricular hypertrophy because of the markedly increased pulmonary arterial pressures, is frequently present in infants with anomalous pulmonary venous connection. Although persistent pulmonary hypertension of the newborn also may cause right ventricular hypertrophy, it is usually manifested as failure of inversion of the T waves in the first 2 weeks of life and not as a "qR" pattern in the right precordium. The chest radiograph in infants with anomalous pulmonary venous connection shows a small-to normal-sized heart and diffusely increased vascularity, with alveolar and interstitial edema. The markings are less coarse than those of meconium aspiration seen in the infant with persistent pulmonary hypertension, but this might be a subtle difference.

Echocardiography is diagnostic of total anomalous pulmonary venous connection, and should be performed on all infants suspected of having pulmonary hypertension of the newborn. Furthermore, echocardiography is indicated for all infants being considered for extracorporeal membrane oxygenation and in whom a definitive diagnosis has not been made. However, making the correct diagnosis and defining the precise pulmonary venous anatomy requires a skilled and experienced echocardiographer. Exclusive right-to-left shunting across the foramen ovale is

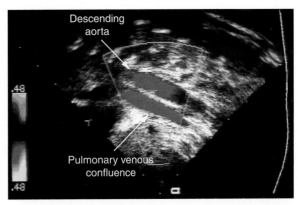

FIGURE 8-3. Echocardiographic still frame obtained from an infant with total anomalous pulmonary venous connection. Color Doppler study shows two large blood vessels, both with flow descending below the diaphragm. The posterior vessel is the descending aorta and the anterior vessel is the pulmonary venous confluence descending to connect to the portal venous system. Pulsed Doppler waveforms (not shown in this figure) can demonstrate that the posterior vessel has an arterial waveform and the anterior vessel has a venous waveform.

always found in patients with anomalous pulmonary venous connection. Color Doppler echocardiography has facilitated definition of venous anatomy (Figure 8-3). Color flow patterns can demonstrate the location of the obstruction, and pulsed wave Doppler can estimate its severity.

Therapeutic Considerations

Endotracheal intubation, positive pressure ventilation, and stabilization of the metabolic status of infants with obstructed anomalous pulmonary venous connection should be instituted immediately. Positive end-expiratory pressures may decrease alveolar edema and dramatically improve the ventilatory and cardiovascular status of the infant acutely. Prostaglandin E_1 should be administered to infants in whom obstructed total anomalous venous connection is suspected, without waiting for echocardiography to be performed. Prostaglandin E_1 may be helpful in dilating the ductus venosus and may be life-saving in other causes of left-sided obstruction, so delaying administration of this medication until a definitive diagnosis is obtained is contraindicated. Immediately following stabilization and definitive diagnosis, the infant with total anomalous pulmonary venous connection with obstruction should be taken to the operating room for repair.

Cor Triatriatum

Anatomic and Physiologic Considerations

Pulmonary venous return to the heart may be obstructed at the entrance to the left atrium. Discrete stenosis of one or more pulmonary veins may occur, but it is extremely rare and is generally untreatable although newer surgical techniques involving a "sutureless" repair are promising. More commonly, obstruction occurs between the pulmonary venous confluence and the primitive left atrium. The left atrium is effectively separated into two chambers, and the condition is therefore called cor triatriatum, meaning "heart with three atria." It is possible that the developmental mechanisms which result in anomalous pulmonary venous connection and cor triatriatum are similar, but in cor triatriatum the confluence comes in close enough contact with the atrium to create a single chamber but with incomplete coalescence. The pulmonary veins usually enter the accessory chamber that is connected to the left atrium by an opening of variable size (Figure 8-4). Although the anatomy may be variable, the more distal

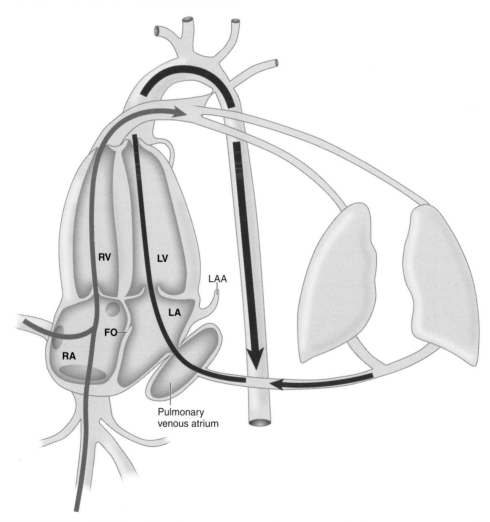

FIGURE 8-4. Cor triatriatum. The pulmonary venous confluence comes in close enough contact with the left atrium to create a single chamber but with incomplete coalescence. The pulmonary veins usually enter the accessory chamber that is connected to the left atrium by an opening of variable size. Although the anatomy may be variable, the more distal true left atrium usually communicates with the left atrial appendage and the foramen ovale.

true left atrium usually communicates with the left atrial appendage and the foramen ovale.

Clinical Presentation

The majority of infants with cor triatriatum are normal at birth, and present later with failure to thrive, recurrent lung infections, or signs of pulmonary hypertension. Occasionally, the obstruction is so mild that presentation is delayed for decades. When the pulmonary venous obstruction is severe at birth, the presentation is similar to that of obstructed total anomalous pulmonary venous drainage, except that the infant often has normal, or near normal pulse oximetry and the second heart sound is narrowly split. Thus, this condition also can be misdiagnosed as persistent pulmonary hypertension of the newborn.

Ancillary Tests

The electrocardiogram is usually normal at birth, but over time shows right ventricular hypertrophy. The chest radiograph shows diffuse, interstitial edema with a normal sized heart. Echocardiography shows a membrane within the left atrial cavity. The relationship between the membrane, and the left atrial appendage and foramen ovale should be defined, as well as the sites of entry of the pulmonary veins. The presence of turbulence in the mid-cavity of the left atrium is diagnostic, and signs of pulmonary hypertension are present. Doppler studies are helpful in defining the degree of obstruction.

Therapeutic Considerations

These patients should be referred for surgical resection of the membrane. The prognosis is excellent, even if prolonged pulmonary hypertension is present.

Mitral Stenosis

Anatomic and Physiologic Considerations

Critical mitral stenosis or mitral atresia usually leads to hypoplastic left heart syndrome, which will be discussed in the following text. However, other abnormalities of mitral inflow may be associated with inadequate systemic perfusion, particularly when associated with other defects. Supravalvar mitral rings or webs can increase left atrial pressure and cause alveolar edema, but these defects usually do not cause enough obstruction in a newborn infant to result in symptoms at birth.

A parachute mitral valve most commonly causes severe inflow obstruction, and is associated with complex outflow obstruction as well. The presence of a parachute mitral valve (with or without a supravalvar mitral ring), subvalvar and valvar aortic stenosis, and coarctation of the aorta is called Shone syndrome. The parachute mitral valve consists of a single papillary muscle to which chordae from both leaflets attach, causing the valve to open only partially, like a parachute. Other abnormalities of the mitral valve causing stenosis may occur at the annulus (hypoplasia), at the leaflets (commissural fusion or dysplasia), or at the chordae (shortened or absent chordae causing a mitral arcade).

Clinical Presentation

The clinical presentation of the infant with Shone syndrome is that of left ventricular inflow and outflow obstruction. The infant is tachypneic and is in moderate to severe respiratory distress, depending on the severity of the inflow obstruction. The pulses in the lower extremities may be normal immediately after birth, although within the first few days of life, the pulses decrease in conjunction with closure of the ductus arteriosus and development of obstruction at the coarctation site. Upper body oxygen saturations are nearly normal but lower body saturations may be decreased because of a right-to-left ductal shunt. The liver is enlarged. The precordium is active. The pulmonic component of the second heart sound is increased, but usually cannot be separated from the aortic component. A harsh mid- to high-frequency systolic murmur is heard best in the retrosternal area and radiates to the apex and to the neck. Despite the abnormality of the aortic valve, a systolic ejection click is rarely heard, likely because of the subaortic obstruction, the small aortic annulus, and the rapid heart rate. A mid-diastolic murmur is present at the apex and reflects mitral stenosis, although this may be difficult to hear in a neonate.

Ancillary Tests

The electrocardiogram evolves over time. During the first days of life it may be normal, but right ventricular hypertrophy develops rapidly; later, left atrial enlargement and, subsequently, left ventricular hypertrophy are present. The chest radiograph shows pulmonary edema and left atrial enlargement, sometimes with diffuse cardiomegaly if the coarctation is severe. Echocardiography defines the anatomy and the presence of obstruction at the mitral valve, subaortic area, aortic valve, and aorta. However, when multiple levels of obstruction are present, it is extremely difficult to ascertain the relative hemodynamic severity at each site of obstruction.

Therapeutic Considerations

The major decision in infants with Shone syndrome is whether a surgical approach can be designed to maintain two separate circulations perfused by separate ventricles. If not, a single ventricle palliation strategy or a heart transplant are the surgical options. If upper and lower body oxygen saturations are both normal in the presence of adequate systemic perfusion, the left ventricle must be providing all of the flow into the systemic arterial bed. In that case, once the obstruction is removed, the left ventricle should be sufficient for normal systemic output. In contrast, if the oxygen saturation in the lower portion of the body is decreased, part of the systemic flow to the lower body is being provided by the right ventricle through the ductus arteriosus. In that case, it is uncertain whether the left ventricle will be capable of supporting the systemic circulation after surgical repair. In either situation, however, careful consideration of other findings is necessary before making final recommendations regarding the most appropriate initial type of intervention.

Careful evaluation of the echocardiogram is very important. The mitral valve should be completely evaluated for the presence of a supravalvar ring, mitral annulus size, leaflet morphology, and chordae and papillary muscle anatomy and attachment. A hypoplastic mitral valve annulus precludes a two-ventricle repair, and a Norwood procedure is indicated (see following text). The Doppler velocity across the foramen ovale yields an approximate left atrial mean pressure (above right atrial mean pressure). The subaortic region should be evaluated for its size, and the site and cause of obstruction. The size of the left ventricle should be carefully measured. An abnormal mitral valve attachment causing subaortic obstruction is very difficult to approach surgically, and a very narrow left ventricular outflow tract may be an indication for a modified Konno procedure. In this procedure, the left ventricular outflow tract is enlarged by opening and enlarging the ventricular septum into the right ventricular outflow tract, and then a patch is used to augment the anterior outflow of the right ventricle. The degree of valvar aortic stenosis is extremely difficult to ascertain because of the proximal subaortic obstruction, but it is rarely severe. The aortic arch and isthmus are important to evaluate thoroughly to exclude a hypoplastic aortic arch and a coarctation of the aorta, both of which may require early surgical intervention. The presence of a large patent ductus arteriosus may make evaluation of the area of the potential coarctation difficult. Retrograde flow in the aortic arch during systole suggests that the left ventricle cannot supply even the upper body with adequate flow, and thus indicates that a two-ventricle repair is probably not possible.

Hypoplastic Left Heart Syndrome

Anatomic and Physiologic Considerations

Hypoplastic left heart syndrome is the most common and severe congenital heart defect that presents with inadequate systemic perfusion shortly after birth. In utero, the fetus develops normally because the right ventricle takes over the work of both ventricles by ejecting all of the combined venous return into the main pulmonary artery to perfuse the upper and lower portions of the body through the ductus arteriosus (Chapter 3, Figure 3-5). Normally, about one-third of combined ventricular output passes through the foramen ovale from the right to the left atrium. In the presence of hypoplastic left heart syndrome, a much smaller amount of blood, representing pulmonary venous return, passes from the left to the right atrium. Thus, the foramen ovale and the left atrium are relatively small structures, and restriction to flow through the left atrium to the right after birth may become apparent, as pulmonary blood flow increases greatly.

Rarely, the foramen ovale is restrictive in utero, which causes left atrial hypertension, increased pulmonary arteriolar muscle, pulmonary lymphangiectasia, and pulmonary venous thickening during fetal life. Abnormal pulmonary venous flow patterns are present in such fetuses characterized by significant flow reversal in the pulmonary veins. These fetuses may have hydrops fetalis, but if not, they are critically ill immediately after birth, showing signs of severe pulmonary arterial hypertension, pulmonary edema, and hypoperfusion. Their prognosis is extremely poor. Attempts at relief of the obstruction in utero with atrial septal dilation or stent placement, and postnatally with balloon atrial septostomy or atrial septectomy have met with limited success.

Clinical Presentation

Infants with hypoplastic left heart syndrome and a restrictive foramen ovale present within the first hours after birth with severe respiratory distress, cyanosis, and decreased systemic perfusion. Most infants, however, have an adequate foramen ovale after birth and therefore do not develop symptoms until the ductus arteriosus begins to close. Within hours or days of birth, tachypnea with respiratory distress become apparent, feeding is impaired, heart rate increases, the pulses become more difficult to palpate, and the infant appears pale and poorly perfused. The oxygen saturations are modestly decreased, usually in the high 80s to low 90s, because pulmonary blood flow is much higher than systemic blood flow. These clinical findings

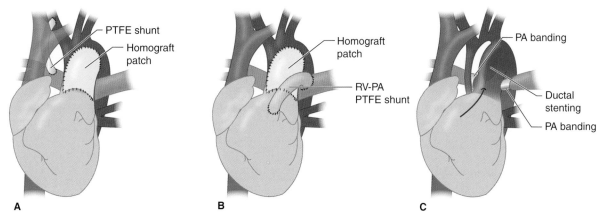

FIGURE 8-5. Various approaches to first-stage palliation of patients with hypoplastic left heart syndrome. **A** and **B**. In the surgical reconstructive approach the main pulmonary artery, augmented by a homograft patch, is sewn to the native hypoplastic ascending aorta creating the neo-aorta. Pulmonary blood flow is supplied by a modified Blalock-Taussig shunt in A, and by a right ventricle-to-pulmonary artery conduit in B. **C**. In this variant of the "hybrid" procedure, the ductus arteriosus is stented open using a direct approach via the main pulmonary artery and the bilateral branch pulmonary arteries are surgically banded. Abbreviations: RV, right ventricle; PA, pulmonary artery. *Reproduced with permission from* Pediatrics. *119(1):109-117, ©2007 by the AAP.*

are similar to those in infants with septic shock, which is often considered as the primary diagnosis. It is essential to consider the possibility of hypoplastic left heart syndrome in every neonate in whom sepsis is considered as the most likely diagnosis. As metabolic acidosis progresses in infants with hypoplastic left heart syndrome, the degree of tachypnea and tachycardia increases, the precordium becomes hyperactive, and hepatomegaly becomes apparent. The first heart sound is normal and the second heart sound is single. Murmurs are not an important component of the clinical findings, but a 2-3/6 medium-frequency murmur at the lower left sternal border of tricuspid regurgitation, or a soft axillary or infraclavicular murmur of the ductus arteriosus or pulmonary arterial flow, may be audible. Without appropriate treatment, blood pressure progressively falls, perfusion further decreases, and the infant usually dies within hours or days of presentation.

Ancillary Tests
The electrocardiogram shows decreased left-sided forces, with pure R waves in the right precordium, and no septal Q waves in the left precordium. Right ventricular hypertrophy does not often manifest until several days of age, when the normal inversion of the right precordial T waves does not occur. Occasionally, inversion of T waves is seen

across all precordial leads, thought to be related to inadequate perfusion of the right ventricular myocardium. P waves are often tall and peaked in limb leads II and III and in the right precordial leads, indicative of right atrial enlargement. The chest radiograph shows diffuse moderate cardiomegaly and increased vascularity, particularly in the hilar region due to pulmonary venous congestion. The echocardiogram usually is immediately diagnostic, most frequently showing a diminutive and fibrotic left ventricle with a very hypoplastic aortic valve. The ascending aorta is of variable size, often only a tiny vessel of 1 to 2 mm in diameter because it functions only as a conduit for the coronary arteries. Doppler interrogation demonstrates retrograde flow in the ascending aorta. Careful evaluation should be made for right ventricular dysfunction, the presence and severity of tricuspid insufficiency, and restriction of flow across the foramen ovale, ductus arteriosus, or aortic isthmus. The presence of pleural effusions should raise concern for the presence of Turner syndrome.

Therapeutic Considerations
Rapid intervention to stabilize these infants is required to prevent or reverse severe respiratory, hemodynamic, and metabolic decompensation. The infants require intubation, ventilation, and sedation to minimize the oxygen

consumption associated with their increased respiratory work and to resolve pulmonary edema. Immediate intravenous access must be obtained in order to infuse prostaglandin E_1 to maintain patency of the ductus arteriosus, inotropic agents if right ventricular function is impaired, and appropriate volume or vasodilator therapy. Adjustment of afterload to maintain adequate perfusion of the various organ beds is often a delicate balance because prostaglandin E_1 infusion tends to vasodilate the systemic arterial vasculature and thereby decreasing perfusion pressure so that volume infusion may be required. At the same time, right ventricular dysfunction and tricuspid insufficiency will improve by administration of an inodilator such as milrinone to decrease afterload. Lastly, any significant metabolic derangement must be corrected. Once stabilized, it is often possible to extubate the infant while awaiting intervention, but it is important to ensure a reasonable balance of systemic and pulmonary blood flow. Because of the low pulmonary vascular resistance and the relatively small ductus arteriosus and aortic arch, pulmonary blood flow is often excessively high at the expense of systemic blood flow which is low, even with a widely patent ductus arteriosus. To minimize this imbalance, the infant should not be in supplemental oxygen, and permissive hypercapnia may be necessary to increase pulmonary vascular resistance. In some cases, it is necessary to reduce the fraction of inspired oxygen below that of room air. In addition, the hematocrit should be maintained at a high level, at least 45%, to ensure adequate systemic oxygen delivery.

Surgical management of these patients requires a special approach because, unlike other lesions with only a single functional ventricle, they have a hypoplastic aortic valve and aorta. Thus, they cannot be managed initially with just a shunt or pulmonary artery band. The so-called stage I reconstructive palliation (Norwood procedure) offers a way to provide adequate systemic blood flow (Figure 8-5A and 8-5B). The main pulmonary artery is transected just below the bifurcation, opened longitudinally, and sewn together with the opened ascending aorta (often with homograft tissue augmentation). This enlarges the hypoplastic ascending aorta and establishes a connection between the proximal pulmonary artery and the descending aorta. There is usually a coarctation so the aortoplasty is extended distal to the area of coarctation. The area where the main pulmonary artery was attached to the branches is patched and then is reattached to the circulation either via a modified Blalock-Taussig shunt (Figure 8-5A) or via a right ventricle-to-pulmonary artery conduit (Figure 8-5B). An atrial septectomy is usually performed to ensure unobstructed blood flow from the pulmonary veins to the right ventricle. After this surgery, the systemic venous return enters the right atrium and then flows through the right ventricle and the old pulmonary valve (now the neo-aortic valve) to the neo-aorta. Some blood flows to the lungs through the shunt or conduit. The pulmonary venous return flows through the left atrium across a mandatory atrial septal defect to the right atrium and then to the neo-aorta. The coronary arteries are left connected to the original hypoplastic aorta and they are perfused in a retrograde manner from the main pulmonary artery.

These patients are always critically ill immediately after surgery. Particular attention should be focused on maintaining the correct balance between systemic and pulmonary blood flows. The modified Blalock-Taussig shunt provides continuous forward flow into the pulmonary arteries and is associated with diastolic retrograde flow in the descending aorta and coronary arteries. Because myocardial perfusion occurs primarily during diastole, this retrograde coronary blood flow ("coronary steal") may result in myocardial ischemia and circulatory instability. In contrast, coronary arterial flow patterns are not perturbed in patients with a right ventricle-to-pulmonary artery conduit. However, this approach also has potential disadvantages, including a negative impact on right ventricular function, arrhythmias or aneurysm formation related to the ventriculotomy, and decreased growth of the pulmonary arteries.

Outcomes in 555 infants randomized to either the modified Blalock-Taussig shunt or to the right ventricle-to-pulmonary artery conduit were evaluated in a trial conducted by the Pediatric Heart Network at 15 North American centers. Transplant-free survival 12 months after surgery was significantly higher for patients who received the right ventricle-to-pulmonary artery conduit than that for those who received the modified Blalock-Taussig shunt. However, the need for unintended interventions and complications were higher in the patients with the conduits. Additionally, intermediate-term data showed no significant difference in transplant-free survival between the two groups of patients beyond 12 months. Ongoing follow-up of these patients is necessary to determine if either shunt is superior in the long term.

Rather than this surgical approach which requires aortopulmonary bypass and aortic arch reconstruction, a "hybrid" procedure consisting of a combination of non-bypass surgery and interventional catheterization is performed in some centers, particularly when surgical risk is high because of associated defects or organ injury (Figure 8-5C). There are various modifications of the hybrid procedure but they all ensure unimpeded systemic blood flow by placement of stents in the ductus arteriosus and occasionally in the aortic isthmus, and control of pulmonary blood flow by the placement of bilateral pulmonary arterial bands. If the foramen ovale shows restrictive flow, a stent is also placed in the atrial septum. In these cases, reconstruction of the aortic arch is delayed until the second-stage surgery.

The second stage of this palliation is a superior cavopulmonary anastomosis. This is performed sometime between 4 and 8 months of age. The surgery usually consists of separation of the superior vena cava from the right atrium and its attachment to the proximal right pulmonary artery, and ligation of the azygous vein. The arch is reconstructed at this time if the patient previously underwent a hybrid procedure. The shunt or conduit is taken down at the time of the second stage to maximize volume unloading of the ventricle. The third stage of this palliation is a modified Fontan operation, performed typically at age 15 to 30 months (Chapter 6).

Rarely, the left ventricle is of reasonable size, almost apex forming. This occurs when the mitral valve is fairly well developed and there is patency of the aortic valve, representing a middle position in the continuum between hypoplastic left heart syndrome and critical valvar aortic stenosis (see following text). Indeed, there is now strong genetic evidence that hypoplastic left heart syndrome, valvar aortic stenosis, and bicuspid aortic valve without stenosis are levels of severity in the expression of the same genetic defect(s) (Chapter 1). In the situation in which the mitral valve and left ventricle are relatively well developed, it can be very difficult to decide whether or not to attempt a biventricular repair. Such an approach often necessitates a Ross-Konno procedure, in which the outflow tract is enlarged anteriorly into the right ventricle, the aortic valve is replaced with the native pulmonary valve, and a right ventricle-to-pulmonary artery homograft replaces the native pulmonary valve. A number of variables have been used in an attempt to determine whether the left ventricle will be capable of supporting systemic blood flow after surgery, but the important ones are the size and function of the mitral valve and the capacity of the left ventricle. In this regard, the function of the left ventricle cannot be evaluated adequately preoperatively because it is ejecting against an extremely high afterload imposed by the severely obstructed aortic valve. However, the presence of a very bright endocardium on echocardiography is of concern because it suggests fibrosis, which may not allow the left ventricle to fill under adequately low pressures after surgery. When uncertain, it is possible to perform a stage I palliation procedure in the newborn and later convert the infant to a two-ventricle circulation by takedown of the ascending aortic anastomosis with the main pulmonary artery and repair of the left ventricular outflow tract as described earlier.

Valvar Aortic Stenosis

Anatomic and Physiologic Considerations

A critically obstructed aortic valve in the presence of a normal mitral valve and normal-sized left ventricle is much less common than hypoplastic left heart syndrome. Valvar aortic stenosis is a relatively common isolated defect but it only occasionally presents as critical, or symptomatic, disease in the newborn infant. The majority of the stenotic valves are bicuspid rather than tricuspid. Most bicuspid aortic valves are not obstructive, at least until later years when the valve may become calcified. When the valve creates a critical degree of outflow obstruction in the newborn infant, it is usually very thick and dysplastic, and may be unicuspid. In critical aortic stenosis, a right-to-left shunt across the ductus arteriosus is necessary to maintain adequate systemic perfusion. A large left-to-right shunt across the foramen ovale is present because of the increased diastolic pressures in the obstructed left ventricle (Figure 8-6). This raises the oxygen saturation in the right ventricle and pulmonary artery greatly, and it is this relatively highly saturated blood that is shunted right to left through the ductus arteriosus.

Severe aortic stenosis is being diagnosed with increasing frequency in the fetus. It has been shown to progress to hypoplastic left heart syndrome as the fetus advances toward term providing further evidence that primary defects of the aortic valve represent a large continuum of clinical expression of the same genetic defect(s). Because of these findings, fetal intervention is being offered in some centers. Unfortunately, there is yet no evidence that it has a positive impact on outcome in the majority of infants (Chapter 4).

Clinical Presentation

The infant with critical aortic stenosis presents with tachypnea and respiratory distress caused by markedly increased left atrial pressure and resulting pulmonary

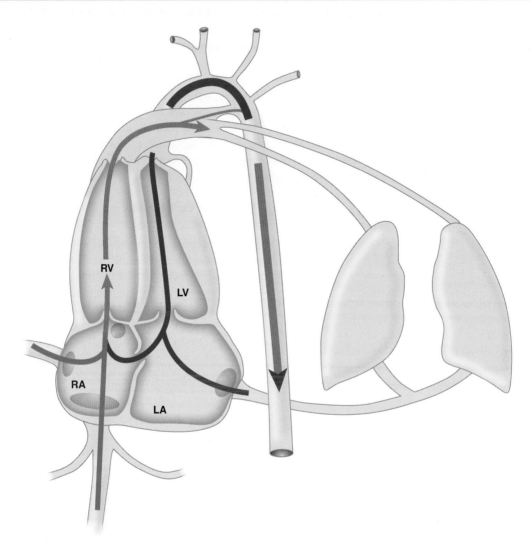

FIGURE 8-6. Critical valvar aortic stenosis. Because left ventricular end-diastolic pressure is very high, a large left-to-right shunt through the foramen ovale occurs. This shunt markedly increases right ventricular and pulmonary arterial oxygen saturation, which causes the descending aortic oxygen saturation to be relatively high despite a large right-to-left ductal shunt. Abbreviations: LA, left atrium; LV, left ventricle; RA, right atrium; RV, right ventricle.

edema. It may be difficult to clinically distinguish critical aortic stenosis from hypoplastic left heart syndrome. The pulses are decreased in all extremities, and perfusion is poor. The liver is often enlarged. The precordium is diffusely hyperactive, because much of the increased impulse is caused by the volume and pressure load on the right ventricle. The first heart sound is normal, and the second heart sound is often difficult to appreciate splitting because of the marked tachycardia. Despite the dysplastic aortic valve, an audible ejection click is rare because valve excursion is usually markedly reduced due to severe dysplasia and low-output across the valve. An S_3 gallop is frequently heard at the apex. A harsh systolic ejection murmur is heard best at the upper retrosternal area and radiates to the apex and the carotids. However, in patients with severe obstruction, the murmur may be absent or barely audible because of the very small amount of blood actually crossing the aortic valve. Pulse oximetry may distinguish patients with critical aortic stenosis from those with hypoplastic left heart syndrome. Pulse oximetry usually shows a higher saturation in the upper extremities as compared to the lower in critical aortic stenosis because the left ventricle is capable of ejecting blood to the upper body, whereas saturations are the same in all extremities in patients with hypoplastic left heart syndrome.

Ancillary Tests

The electrocardiogram usually shows left ventricular hypertrophy and diffuse ST-T wave abnormalities, either flattening or inversion, suggestive of subendocardial ischemia. Occasionally, dominant right-sided forces with right axis deviation are seen but unlike in hypoplastic left heart syndrome, a septal Q wave and R waves in the left precordium are present. Left atrial enlargement may also be present. The chest radiograph shows cardiomegaly, prominent vascular markings and venous congestion. The echocardiogram is used to define the size of the left ventricle, the degree of myocardial dysfunction, the presence of endocardial fibrosis, the size of the aortic annulus, and the anatomy of the valve. Patency of the ductus arteriosus is determined and the aortic arch is carefully evaluated for associated coarctation of the aorta though this rarely occurs. If the atrial communication is restrictive, the Doppler velocity can be used to approximate left atrial pressure.

Therapeutic Considerations

Supportive care is provided according to the degree of decompensation and impairment of systemic blood flow. An infusion of prostaglandin E_1 should be initiated to maintain ductal patency and flow from the pulmonary artery to the descending aorta As with hypoplastic left heart syndrome, a decision must be made whether it is possible to create a two-ventricle circulation. In the case of critical aortic stenosis, the problem is rarely the size of the ventricular cavity but instead the major concern is related to the function of the left ventricle. A ventricle that is severely fibrotic and if the left ventricle is unable to generate high pressures when obstructed, it may not be capable of supporting systemic blood flow even after the obstruction is relieved. Doppler studies can be helpful in this regard as the gradient across the aortic valve can be measured and an estimate of the peak left ventricular pressure can be obtained by measuring the peak velocity of a jet of mitral insufficiency.

Balloon aortic valvuloplasty is generally the preferred approach to alleviating the obstruction in most cases, but a surgical approach may also be considered. If the ventricle is contracting at infrasystemic pressures and cannot generate a peak systolic pressure gradient of more than about 20 mm Hg because of severe dysfunction, it likely will not be able to generate adequate pressure once the obstruction is relieved. In this situation, a staged palliative surgical reconstruction approach (eg, Norwood procedure) rather than a balloon aortic valvuloplasty may be warranted. If it is uncertain whether the left ventricle will be an adequate systemic ventricle, a hybrid approach (see earlier text) may be the best initial therapeutic approach as this is less invasive than the Norwood procedure and more easily converted to a two-ventricle circulation later in infancy.

The newborn infant with severe, but not critical aortic stenosis (ie, there is no hemodynamic decompensation and ventricular systolic function is normal) presents a therapeutic dilemma. The infant is hemodynamically stable but demands on the myocardium over the first weeks of life are large. In addition to the large increase in metabolic demand after birth, hemoglobin levels decrease in the first weeks of life, necessitating a further increase in output. Moreover, anemia causes systemic vasodilation, which decreases aortic diastolic pressure and causes tachycardia. The low-diastolic pressure, in association with tachycardia and the increased end-diastolic pressure of the hypertrophied ventricle, may further diminish coronary blood flow reserve. Late ventricular dysfunction may occur weeks after birth. If the ventricle fails because of myocardial ischemia, it may not recover adequate function when the obstruction is relieved. Thus, the decision as to whether a newborn infant should undergo a balloon aortic valvuloplasty or surgery at birth must be made not only in the infant with critical aortic stenosis but also in the infant with severe aortic stenosis. If therapy is delayed, it is extremely important that the infant be followed closely for any evidence of decompensation. Onset of even subtle symptoms should prompt intervention to relieve the aortic obstruction.

Interruption of the Aortic Arch

Anatomic and Physiologic Considerations

Interruption of the aortic arch occurs almost exclusively in association with other congenital heart defects, such as a posteriorly malaligned ventricular septal defect, an aortopulmonary window, or truncus arteriosus. The interruption occurs most frequently between the left carotid and left subclavian arteries (type B) and this is the type that occurs in association with ventricular septal defects and truncus arteriosus. It appears to be part of an embryologic abnormality in arch development and the majority of these infants have microdeletion 22q11 syndrome. In fact, interrupted aortic arch is more highly associated with a microdeletion of chromosome 22 than any other heart defect (Chapter 15).

Because interrupted aortic arch presents in association with many of the defects already discussed and because its impact on the presentation of the heart defect is similar to that of coarctation of the aorta, the clinical presentation will be discussed with coarctation of the aorta.

Coarctation of the Aorta

Anatomic and Physiologic Considerations

Coarctation of the aorta is a common congenital heart defect, occurring either in isolation or in association with other defects, most commonly a ventricular septal defect and/or a bicuspid aortic valve. Whether singly or in conjunction with another defect, the association of coarctation of the aorta and bicuspid aortic valve is extremely high (> 60%). Although coarctation of the aorta may occur as a part of a developmental defect in infants with embryological truncal and arch abnormalities, it seems that it is more often secondary to abnormalities of flow. For example, coarctation of the aorta is not only associated with a posterior malaligned ventricular septal defect, as is interruption of the aortic arch, but coarctation is also associated with muscular ventricular septal defects. In these cases, coarctation may result from decreased flow around the aortic isthmus caused by redirection of some of the output of the left ventricle to the right ventricle and main pulmonary artery in utero. With the increasing use of fetal echocardiography, it is apparent that there is a high incidence of ventricular septal defects during fetal life, and that many of these defects close spontaneously. It is possible that isolated coarctation of the aorta may not actually be isolated but may have been initially associated with a ventricular septal defect which subsequently closed in utero. Also, the high incidence of a bicuspid aortic valve may be a predisposing factor. The abnormal valve may cause a flow disturbance in the ascending aorta and aortic arch, and thus the area at the distal end of the aortic isthmus where ductal flow arises may be disrupted, causing a posterior shelf that becomes obstructive. Alternatively, bicuspid aortic valve may be associated with a diffuse aortopathy and it is possible that this aortopathy predisposes the fetus to develop a coarctation of the aorta.

Clinical Presentation

The timing of the clinical presentation of patients with coarctation of the aorta is quite different than that of hypoplastic left heart syndrome. Because the left ventricle and ascending aorta are normally formed in coarctation, symptoms of obstruction occur only when the distal part of the aortic isthmus (that portion of the aorta between the left subclavian artery and the origin of the ductus arteriosus) becomes critically obstructed. The ductus arteriosus closes initially at its pulmonary arterial end, and then closure progresses to the aorta (Figure 8-1). Thus, even functional closure does not necessarily cause significant obstruction. It is not until complete anatomic closure occurs that many infants with coarctation of the aorta present with decreased perfusion to the lower body. This may be delayed for 1 to 2 weeks, so it is important to be aware that a normal examination in the first few days of life does not preclude the presence of significant coarctation of the aorta.

The clinical findings depend on the severity of decreased systemic perfusion at the time of presentation. Ideally, the diagnosis is made during the first few days of life when the infant is found to have decreased pulses in the lower extremities. Dorsalis pedis and posterior tibial pulses are generally easy to palpate in infants because these arteries are superficially located and are easily felt over the underlying bones. In contrast, femoral pulses are often difficult to feel in the newborn infant because the femoral arteries are deeper and the hips must be abducted. Because collateral vessels around a coarctation develop over months or years after birth, radio-femoral delay is not present in the newborn infant with a coarctation of the aorta. If there is any suggestion of decreased lower extremity pulses, blood pressures should be measured. It is best to measure the right arm and either leg systolic blood pressures simultaneously. If a blood pressure difference is not identified, but the lower extremity pulses seem decreased, it is important to consider the possibility of a right aortic arch, and then to measure the left arm pressure simultaneously with that in one leg. If these measurements are also equal, the possibility should be considered that the infant has a left aortic arch with an anomalous right subclavian artery, an anatomic variant that is even more common than coarctation with a right aortic arch. In this situation, a lack of a systolic pressure differential should lead the clinician to palpate the carotid arteries carefully; the carotid pulses should be very strong in the presence of decreased upper and lower extremity pulses in a patient with coarctation of the aorta and an anomalous right subclavian artery.

A blowing systolic murmur is frequently heard in the axilla and back, and a mid-diastolic murmur is audible at the apex, even in the absence of a mitral valve abnormality.

If a bicuspid aortic valve is also present, a systolic ejection click and a systolic ejection murmur may be heard at the base.

If lower body perfusion is decreased for several hours, metabolic acidosis will develop and the infant will become tachypneic. Although the newborn heart is relatively insensitive to acidosis, the left ventricle will eventually begin to fail as the acidosis progresses and afterload increases. At this point, left ventricular end-diastolic pressure begins to increase and pulmonary edema develops. The infant then becomes distressed, with intercostal and subcostal retractions, nasal flaring, and grunting. At this time, the lower extremities become cool and capillary refill is prolonged as perfusion decreases. Soon thereafter, further left ventricular dysfunction develops, and even the upper body pulses become decreased. It is at this point in the progression of the disease that the diagnosis may be missed, because the pulse and the blood pressure differentials become obscured. Resuscitative measures must be undertaken immediately without waiting for definitive diagnosis. Endotracheal intubation and assisted ventilation, inotropic support, correction of acidosis, and infusion of prostaglandin E_1 all must be started as soon as possible. Since infants with septic shock may present with the same clinical findings, cultures should be obtained and antibiotic therapy should be initiated. If the infant with aortic coarctation is managed rapidly and appropriately, the upper body pulses rapidly improve, and the diagnosis becomes more obvious.

Ancillary Tests

The electrocardiogram is normal within the first few days of life, but eventually the T waves fail to invert, indicating right ventricular hypertrophy. Diffuse ST-segment depression may be present and reflects myocardial strain. The right ventricle is hypertrophied because it is ejecting through the ductus arteriosus at the coarctation site initially, and because pulmonary arterial pressures remain increased. Within a week or two of life, left ventricular hypertrophy also develops because of increased afterload. Thereafter, left atrial enlargement becomes evident. Chest radiography may be normal initially, but cardiomegaly and venous congestion develop as the infant deteriorates. The definitive diagnosis is made by echocardiography but a high level of skill and experience are necessary to obtain adequate images of the aorta for diagnosis. It can be difficult to assess for coarctation in the presence of a widely patent ductus arteriosus. If the posterior shelf is not apparent, pulsed wave and color Doppler studies may demonstrate the accelerated, disturbed flow through the area, and a slow upstroke in the descending aorta. A right-to-left ductal shunt may also be apparent. It is important to carefully evaluate the head and neck vessels, particularly the origin of the right subclavian artery, and the aortic arch, which is often hypoplastic. The aortic valve, subaortic region and the ventricular septum also should be evaluated. In some cases, the anatomy is difficult to define completely by echocardiography. If so, magnetic resonance imaging can be used and is extremely helpful in defining the anatomy of the aorta, arch vessels, ductus arteriosus, and site of coarctation.

Therapeutic Considerations

Surgical repair of the aorta and other associated defects is always indicated. Infants who present with shock and metabolic acidosis because of coarctation of the aorta or interrupted aortic arch can be stabilized by administration of prostaglandin E_1 and other supportive care. These infants are likely to have sustained end-organ damage because of decreased systemic perfusion. Deferring surgery for several days to allow recovery of renal and hepatic function decreases surgical morbidity and mortality. The presence of aortic arch hypoplasia often requires extension of the surgical repair along the undersurface of the arch to the carotid artery using an anterior sternotomy approach rather than the usual left thoracotomy.

SUGGESTED READINGS

Akinturk H, Michel-Behnke I, Valeske K, et al. Stenting of the arterial duct and banding of the pulmonary arteries: basis for combined Norwood stage I and II repair in hypoplastic left heart. *Circulation.* 2002;105:1099-1103.

Allan LD, Sharland G, Tynan MJ. The natural history of the hypoplastic left heart syndrome. *Int J Cardiol.* 1989;25:341-343.

Allen HD, Driscoll DJ, Shaddy RE, Feltes TF, eds. *Moss and Adams' Heart Disease in Infants, Children, and Adolescents Including the Fetus and Young Adult.* 7th ed. Philadelphia, PA: Lippincott Williams & Wilkins; 2008.

Alphonso N, Norgaard MA, Newcomb A, et al. Cor triatriatum: presentation, diagnosis and long-term surgical results. *Ann Thorac Surg.* 2005;80:1666-1671.

Alsoufi B, Bennetts J, Verma S, Calderone CA. New developments in the treatment of hypoplastic left heart syndrome. *Pediatrics.* 2007;119:109-117.

Braverman AC, Guven H, Beardslee MA, et al. The bicuspid aortic valve. *Curr Probl Cardiol.* 2005;30:470-522.

Glatz JA, Tabbutt S, Gaynor JW, et al. Hypoplastic left heart syndrome with atrial level restriction in the era of prenatal diagnosis. *Ann Thorac Surg.* 2007;84:1633-1638.

Hoffman JIE. *The Natural and Unnatural History of Congenital Heart Disease.* Oxford, United Kingdom: Wiley-Blackwell; 2009.

Hornberger LK, Sahn DJ, Kleinman CS, et al. Antenatal diagnosis of coarctation of the aorta: a multicenter experience. *J Am Coll Cardiol.* 1994;23:417-423.

Marshall AC, van der Velde ME, Tworetzky W, et al. Creation of an atrial septal defect in utero for fetuses with hypoplastic left heart syndrome and intact or highly restrictive atrial septum. *Circulation.* 2004;110:253-258.

Moller JH, Hoffman JIE, eds. *Pediatric Cardiovascular Medicine.* Philadelphia, PA: Churchill Livingstone; 2000.

Morin FC. 3d: Prostaglandin E1 opens the ductus venosus in the newborn lamb. *Pediatr Res.* 1987;21:225-228.

Norwood WI, Kirklin JK, Sanders SP. Hypoplastic left heart syndrome: experience with palliative surgery. *Am J Cardiol.* 1980;45:87-91.

Ohye RG, Sleeper LA, Mahony L, et al. Hypoplastic left heart—shunt type in infants undergoing the Norwood Procedure. *N Engl J Med.* 2010;362:1980-1992.

Park MK. *The Pediatric Cardiology Handbook.* 4th ed. Philadelphia, PA: Mosby Elsevier; 2010.

Pearl JM, Cripe LW, Manning PB. Biventricular repair after Norwood palliation. *Ann Thorac Surg.* 2003;75:132-136.

Rudolph AM. *Congenital Diseases of the Heart: Clinical-Physiological Considerations.* Chichester, United Kingdom: Wiley-Blackwell; 2009.

Sano S, Ishino K, Kado H, et al. Outcome of right ventricle-to-pulmonary artery shunt in first-stage palliation of hypoplastic left heart syndrome: a multi-institutional study. *Ann Thorac Surg.* 2004;78:1951-1957.

Taketazu M, Barrea C, Smallhorn JF, et al. Intrauterine pulmonary venous flow and restrictive foramen ovale in fetal hypoplastic left heart syndrome. *J Am Coll Cardiol.* 2004;43:1902-1907.

Tworetzky W, Wilkins-Haug L, Jennings RW, et al. Balloon dilation of severe aortic stenosis in the fetus: potential for prevention of hypoplastic left heart syndrome: candidate selection, technique, and results of successful intervention. *Circulation.* 2004;110:2125-2131.

Vida VL, Bacha EA, Larrazabal A, et al. Hypoplastic left heart syndrome with intact or highly restrictive atrial septum: surgical experience from a single center. *Ann Thorac Surg.* 2007;84:581-585.

Cardiomyopathies

■ INTRODUCTION

The term cardiomyopathy is used to indicate myocardial dysfunction in the absence of an obstructive lesion or sustained hypertension. Cardiomyopathy is either an isolated abnormality (ie, confined to the heart) or is associated with a multisystem disorder. Neonates who have an unrecognized underlying cardiomyopathy may come to medical attention with a life-threatening response to an otherwise minor illness. Alternatively, evidence of cardiomyopathy may be noted on an echocardiogram performed for evaluation of an unrelated problem.

Mutations in genes encoding multiple proteins of the sarcomere, cytoskeleton, sarcoplasmic reticulum, nucleus, and cell membrane of the myocardial cell are now known to cause cardiomyopathy (Figure 9-1). More information regarding the structure and function of these proteins is available in Chapter 2.

Classification of cardiomyopathies is problematic and has evolved as new information has become available regarding causation. Classification based on phenotype (ventricular morphology and physiology) is practical in that this information is what is most readily available after initial evaluation of the patient (Table 9-1). Phenotypic

groups can be subdivided based on etiology (Tables 9-2, 9-3, 9-4). Some congenital heart defects or systemic hypertension can cause phenotypes that mimic various forms of cardiomyopathy and are included in text and tables as they need to be included in the differential diagnosis when evaluating patients. Phenotypic classification is certainly not perfect as it does not define causation; moreover, it may be misleading because some myopathic processes may be classified as more than one type or may change from one type to another during the course of the disease.

The most logical approach to an individual patient begins with a careful assessment of the disease phenotype (cardiac and extracardiac) and then proceeds in a logical manner to the elucidation of the etiology. Genetic defects and abnormal proteins have been identified for many forms of cardiomyopathy that were thought previously to be idiopathic. Identification of a specific cause may lead to specific therapy and possibly to prevention, and will also facilitate genetic counseling. This chapter reviews the varied clinical presentations and many associated disorders and provides a rational approach to the array of available diagnostic tests and biochemical assays. Many forms of cardiomyopathy do not present in the neonatal period; as such, they are included for informational

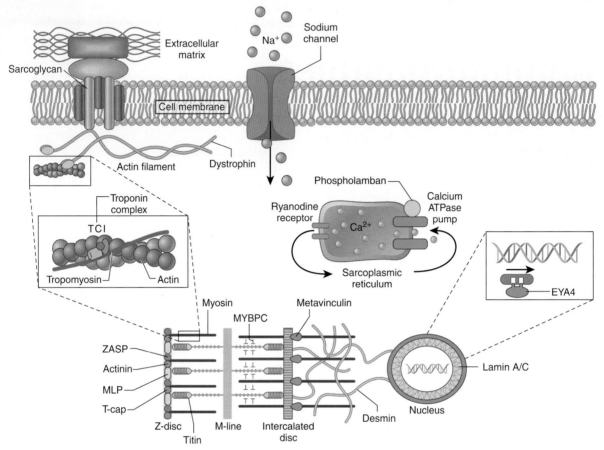

FIGURE 9-1. Myocyte cytoarchitecture. Various forms of cardiomyopathy may result from mutations in genes encoding multiple proteins within the cardiac myocyte. Different mutations in the same gene may cause different forms of cardiomyopathy. Abbreviations: EYA4, eyes absent homolog 4; MLP, cardiac LIM domain protein; MYBPC, myosin binding protein C; T-cap, telethonin; ZASP, muscle LIM-binding protein 3 (cypher). *Adapted from Olson TM, Hoffman TM, Chan DP. Dilated congestive cardiomyopathy, In: Allen HD, Driscoll DJ, Shaddy RE, Feltes TF, eds.* Moss and Adams' Heart Disease in Infants, Children and Adolescents. *7th ed. Philadelphia, PA: Lippincott Williams & Wilkins; 2008:1197.*

■ **TABLE 9-1.** Phenotypic Classification of Cardiomyopathy

Hypertrophic
Dilated
Restrictive
Arrhythmogenic right ventricular dysplasia[a]
Noncompaction

[a]This phenotype is not seen in neonates or young infants and is included only for informational purposes.

purposes in tables but are not discussed further. The reader is referred to several excellent recent reviews listed in *Suggested Readings*.

■ **HYPERTROPHIC CARDIOMYOPATHY**

Hypertrophic cardiomyopathy is characterized classically by a hypertrophic but nondilated left ventricle in the absence of systemic disease (eg, hypertension) or structural abnormalities (eg, aortic stenosis) capable of producing left ventricular hypertrophy. The left ventricular hypertrophy may be asymmetric affecting the interventricular septum more than the left ventricular free wall. In infants the right ventricle may also be involved.

In typical familial hypertrophic cardiomyopathy, histologic examination discloses cellular and myofibrillar disarray, interstitial fibrosis, and coronary arterial abnormalities. The genetic defect is heterogeneous; hundreds of different mutations, mostly missense, are described in more than 20 genes involving myofilament and Z-disc proteins (Table 9-2 and Figure 9-1). Defects in myofilament (sarcomeric) proteins show an autosomal dominant pattern of inheritance and account for about 60% of patients. Mutations in β-myosin heavy chain (25%-35%) and myosin-binding protein C (25%-35%) are most common. Expression within families is highly variable and is influenced by modifier genes and/or environmental factors.

Clinical genetic testing is available for nine genes and is primarily useful for diagnosis rather than for predicting outcome or for guiding therapy. Of those patients who undergo testing, a mutation is identified in 40% to 60% of sporadic and familial cases when testing is performed for these genes (http://www.genetests.org). However genetic testing may not be covered by an individual patient's health insurance plan, and of the 855 patients with hypertrophic cardiomyopathy in the Pediatric Cardiomyopathy Registry, 74% had no associated illness, no family history, and no defined genetic defect.

Left ventricular hypertrophy associated with familial hypertrophic cardiomyopathy is often not present until adulthood. Affected infants generally are identified by echocardiography and have severe hypertrophy that sometimes causes obstruction of right or left ventricular outflow. Many die within the first year of life usually because of congestive heart failure. Although congestive heart failure is present, positive inotropic agents are often contraindicated as these agents may increase outflow tract obstruction. By decreasing preload, diuretic therapy may also increase outflow tract obstruction. Administration of β-blocking agents is the most widely accepted therapy. Calcium channel blockers such as verapamil and nifedipine given orally are also sometimes beneficial.

The phenotype of ventricular hypertrophy may be present in many other conditions discussed in the following text, including inborn errors of metabolism usually involving multiple organs, genetic and malformation syndromes, and infants of diabetic mothers (Table 9-2). The age of presentation and clinical course are critically dependent on etiology.

■ **TABLE 9-2.** Conditions Associated with Phenotypic Appearance of Hypertrophic Cardiomyopathy

	OMIM
Familial, unknown gene	
Myofilament (sarcomeric) mutation	
Giant filament	
Titin	188840
Thick filament	
β-Myosin heavy chain	160760
α-Myosin heavy chain	160710
Ventricular regulatory myosin light chain	608758
Ventricular essential myosin light chain	608751
Intermediate filament	
Cardiac myosin-binding protein C	115197
Thin filament	
Cardiac troponin T	115195
Cardiac troponin C	613243
Cardiac troponin I	191044
α-Tropomyosin	115196
α-Cardiac actin	612098
Z-disc mutation	
Cardiac LIM domain protein (cysteine- and glycine-rich protein 3)	612124
Cytoskeletal protein mutations	
Vinculin/metavinculin	613255
Storage diseases (Table 9-7)	600858
Fatty acid oxidation disorders (Table 9-5)	
Respiratory chain disorders (Table 9-6)	
Neuromuscular disease	
α-Galactosidase (Fabry disease)[a]	
Malformation syndrome (Noonan, Beckwith Wiedemann, Costello, LEOPARD, cardio-facial-cutaneous)[a]	
Congenital heart disease associated with ventricular outflow tract obstruction	
Systemic hypertension	
Infant of diabetic mother	

[a]Indicates cardiomyopathy usually not present in infancy.

OMIM, Online Mendelian inheritance in man. Latest updates regarding gene(s) and loci can be obtained from this Web site: http://www.ncbi.nlm.nih.gov/omim. For an overview of the genetics of familial hypertrophic cardiomyopathy see 192600. See Chapter 2 for details of structure and function of listed proteins.

ZASP, Z-band alternatively-spliced PDZ motif-containing protein.

The Pediatric Cardiomyopathy Registry has published information regarding epidemiology and outcomes in groups of children with the phenotype of hypertrophic cardiomyopathy. Of the 855 patients from North America, 328 (38%) presented before 1 year of age. Of these, 14.6% had an inborn error of metabolism, 15.2% had a malformation syndrome, 0.9% had neuromuscular disease, and 69.2% were unclassified or idiopathic. Children with an inborn error of metabolism and malformation syndrome (mostly Noonan syndrome) presenting with hypertrophic cardiomyopathy before 1 year of age had a particularly poor prognosis, with a 5-year survival after diagnosis of 26% and 66%, respectively. The 1-year survival from the time of diagnosis in patients in the idiopathic group diagnosed at younger than 1 year of age was 86% compared with 99% in those diagnosed older than 1 year of age. However, no difference in annual mortality was observed between these age groups for those patients who survived beyond 1 year of age. Similar outcomes were reported in a registry of Australian patients.

■ DILATED CARDIOMYOPATHY

Dilated cardiomyopathy is characterized by dilation of the ventricles and decreased ventricular systolic function in the absence of abnormal loading conditions (eg, valve disease) sufficient to cause global systolic impairment. This is the most common morphologic type of cardiomyopathy and is also the most common reason for cardiac transplantation in children. According to data from the Pediatric Cardiomyopathy Registry, the incidence of dilated cardiomyopathy is higher in infants younger than 1 year of age than in older children (4.40 vs 0.34 per 100,000 per year; $P < .001$).

A number of conditions are known to cause dilated cardiomyopathy (Table 9-3). The etiology for 591 children younger than 1 year of age in the Pediatric Cardiomyopathy Registry was idiopathic in 78%, myocarditis in 11%, inborn error of metabolism in 5%, familial in 4%, malformation syndrome in 1.7%, and neuromuscular disease in < 0.1%.

Hereditary factors have been recognized recently to play a role in the etiology of idiopathic dilated cardiomyopathy in an increasing percentage of patients. In newly diagnosed adult patients, dilated cardiomyopathy can be identified in up to 20% to 50% of screened first-degree relatives. The pattern of inheritance is autosomal dominant in about 90% of adult cases. Penetrance and expression are frequently incomplete and age-dependent. For some mutations affected family members may show

different phenotypic patterns of cardiomyopathy. In some studies at least 80% of mutation carriers under the age of 20 years are clinically well. Familial disease is much less common in young infants but screening of all first-degree relatives by electrocardiography and echocardiography is recommended when the diagnosis is made.

Familial dilated cardiomyopathy is genetically heterogeneous and is caused by mutations in genes encoding proteins of the nucleus, sarcoplasmic reticulum, sarcolemma, mitochondria, and the cytoskeleton (Table 9-3 and Figure 9-1). In general, these mutations result in diminished force generation or alterations in mechanotransduction or myocyte signaling. None of the known mutations account for more than a few percent of cases and comprehensive screening of established genes is not available commercially. Of particular interest is the fact that different mutations in the same genes for sarcomeric proteins that are well known to be associated with hypertrophic cardiomyopathy have now also been associated with dilated cardiomyopathy. This is suggestive that the location of the mutation and the resulting consequences on protein structure and function play an important role in determining cardiomyopathy phenotype. The myofiber disarray seen in hypertrophic cardiomyopathy is absent in dilated cardiomyopathy caused by mutations in the same sarcomeric proteins. Interestingly, such mutations tend to increase calcium sensitivity of the cardiac myofilaments in hypertrophic cardiomyopathy, yet they tend to decrease calcium sensitivity in dilated cardiomyopathy. Further study is needed to understand the molecular mechanisms by which these mutations result in alterations in calcium sensitivity and the pathways that lead to a dilated or hypertrophic phenotype.

■ RESTRICTIVE CARDIOMYOPATHY

Restrictive left ventricular physiology is characterized by a pattern of ventricular filling in which increased stiffness of the myocardium causes ventricular pressure to rise excessively with small increases in volume. In general, ventricular systolic function is reasonably normal as is ventricular wall thickness. Ventricular volume is often reduced whereas atrial volume is usually markedly increased.

Multiple conditions are associated with restrictive physiology but endocardial fibroelastosis (EFE) is most common in infants (Table 9-4). EFE is a nonspecific reaction to endocardial stress and injury leading to deposition of collagen and elastic fibers within the endocardium of the left

■ **TABLE 9-3.** Conditions Associated With Phenotypic Appearance of Dilated Cardiomyopathy

	OMIM Number		OMIM Number
Familial, unknown gene		Intercalated disc protein mutations	612877
Myofilament (sarcomeric) mutations		Desmoglein-Z	
Giant filament		Sarcoplasmic reticulum mutations	
Titin	188840	Phospholamban	609909
Thick filament		Nuclear membrane mutations	
β-Myosin heavy chain	613252	Lamin A/C	115200
Thin filament		Emerin	310384
Cardiac troponin T	601494	Transcriptional coactivator mutations	
Cardiac troponin C	611879	Eyes absent homolog 2	605362
Cardiac troponin I	191044	Voltage-gated channel mutations	
α-Tropomyosin	611878	Cardiac sodium channel SCN5A	601154
α-Cardiac actin	102540	Fatty acid oxidation disorders (Table 9-5)	
Z-disc mutations		Respiratory chain disorders (Table 9-6)	
LIM domain-binding protein 3 (ZASP, cypher)	601493	Nonfamilial	
Telethonin	607487	Myocarditis	
α-Actinin 2	612158	Kawasaki disease[a]	
Cardiac LIM domain protein (Cysteine-		Thyroid disease[a]	
and glycine-rich protein 3)	607482	Drugs (anthracyclines, emetine, lead)[a]	
Nexilin	613122	Peripartum cardiomyopathy[a]	
Cytoskeletal gene mutations		Nutritional (thiamine, carnitine, selenium,	
Dystrophin	302045	hypophosphatemia, hypocalcemia)	
Desmin	604765	Tachycardia-induced cardiomyopathy	
Metavinculin	611407	Transplant rejection	
Sarcoglycan complex	606685	Myocardial insufficiency—ALCAPA, tachyarrhythmias	

[a]Indicates cardiomyopathy usually not present in infancy.

OMIM, Online Mendelian inheritance in man. Latest updates regarding gene(s) and loci can be obtained from this Web site: http://www.ncbi.nlm.nih.gov/omim. For an overview of the genetics of familial dilated cardiomyopathy see 115200. See Chapter 2 for details of structure and function of listed proteins.

ALCAPA, anomalous left coronary artery from the pulmonary artery; ZASP, Z-band alternatively-spliced PDZ motif-containing protein.

ventricle, aortic valve, mitral valve, and left atrium. Gross examination of the heart shows a thickened and smooth "pearly white" endocardium. EFE often accompanies abnormal increases in wall tension (provoked by chamber dilation) or markedly increased intracavitary pressure.

The endocardial thickening present in patients with EFE causes decreased ventricular compliance and diastolic dysfunction. Secondary EFE is associated with certain congenital heart defects such as aortic stenosis and metabolic disorders such as mitochondrial myopathies and Barth syndrome, but EFE also occurs as a primary diagnosis. Numerous etiologies including infectious agents, genetic mutations, and hypoxic injury have been proposed but remain unconfirmed. In some patients primary EFE appears to be an inherited condition with a varying pattern of inheritance but many cases are sporadic. Intrauterine anoxia and endocarditis are among the processes proposed as possible initiating events. Although EFE usually presents after the neonatal period in the first year of life, some infants develop congestive heart failure in the first weeks of life. The electrocardiogram typically shows prominent left ventricular forces and T-wave inversion over the left precordium (strain). On the echocardiogram EFE is seen as areas of echogenicity along the endocardial surface. Usually the left atrium and left ventricle are involved but sometimes the right ventricle is also involved.

■ **TABLE 9-4.** Conditions Associated With Phenotypic Appearance of Restrictive Cardiomyopathy

	OMIM Number
Familial, unknown gene	
Sarcomeric protein mutations	
Troponin I	115210
Troponin T	612422
Endocardial fibroelastosis	226600
Amyloidosis[a]	
Scleroderma[a]	
Desminopathy[a]	609578
Hemachromatosis[a]	
Glycogen storage disease (Table 9-7)	
Endomyocardial fibrosis	
Hypereosinophilic syndrome[a]	
Idiopathic[a]	
Chromosomal	
Drugs (serotonin, methysergide, ergotamine, busulfan)[a]	
Radiation toxicity[a]	

[a]Indicates cardiomyopathy usually not present in infancy.

OMIM, Online Mendelian inheritance in man. Latest updates regarding gene(s) and loci can be obtained from this Web site: http://www.ncbi.nlm.nih.gov/omim. For an overview of the genetics of familial restrictive cardiomyopathy see 115210.

The left ventricle is most often dilated. Systolic and diastolic ventricular dysfunction is present. Treatment is symptomatic (Chapters 11 and 12). The prognosis for affected infants is poor and many eventually will need cardiac transplantation.

■ NONCOMPACTION OF THE LEFT VENTRICLE

Noncompaction of the left ventricle describes a pattern of deep trabeculae with deep intertrabecular recesses involving most commonly the left ventricular apex and lateral wall. No consensus exists regarding the exact definition. This morphologic pattern is seen sporadically in association with a large number of disorders including mitochondrial myopathies, Barth syndrome, neuromuscular disease, and various forms of congenital heart disease. In newborn infants noncompaction is thought to be caused by a developmental arrest of unclear etiology resulting in insufficient compaction of the noncompacted myocardium during embryogenesis. The exact cause of the developmental arrest in some but not all patients with various genetic disorders is not clear and there may be multiple mechanisms. The morphologic pattern of noncompaction is acquired in some patients, especially in adults, and it has also been reported to disappear with time. These observations raise the possibility that this pattern is also a nonspecific response to various perturbations in myocardial function. Noncompaction is variably associated with ventricular hypertrophy, ventricular dilation, decreased systolic function, and arrhythmias. The prognosis is poor for patients presenting in infancy as many die before 1 year of age.

■ MULTISYSTEM DISORDERS ASSOCIATED WITH CARDIOMYOPATHY

Myocarditis

Myocarditis is an inflammatory disorder involving the myocardium and is characterized by lymphocytic infiltration of the myocardium often associated with myocyte necrosis. Myocardial injury is caused by direct pathogen-induced damage and an autoimmune response to myocytes transformed by viral infection.

Although rare in neonates, myocarditis should always be suspected in any infant with congestive heart failure in whom structural heart disease has been excluded. It is likely the most common cause of dilated cardiomyopathy in infants. Hepatitis and encephalitis may also be present. Overwhelming sepsis may be the initial diagnosis in many of these infants who are acutely ill. Almost any infectious agent can cause myocarditis. Enteroviruses, especially Coxsackie B and ECHO viruses, are the most common etiologic agents; however, disease secondary to adenovirus and toxoplasmosis also occurs. The initial symptoms are nonspecific and may include lethargy, poor feeding, emesis, and respiratory distress. Older infants may have had a preceding respiratory infection. Some infants come to medical attention having signs and symptoms of cardiovascular collapse. Congestive heart failure is present on physical examination and the chest radiograph shows cardiomegaly often with pulmonary edema. The electrocardiogram may show low-voltage QRS complexes and diffusely abnormal (often flat) T waves (Figure 9-2). Arrhythmias are common. Echocardiography shows ventricular dilation and decreased function. Hypertrophy is not present. Congenital defects, such as coarctation of the aorta and anomalous left coronary artery arising from the pulmonary artery, must be excluded.

Viral, bacterial, and fungal cultures should be obtained from nasopharyngeal and stool specimens. Serologic identification requires a threefold to fivefold increase in

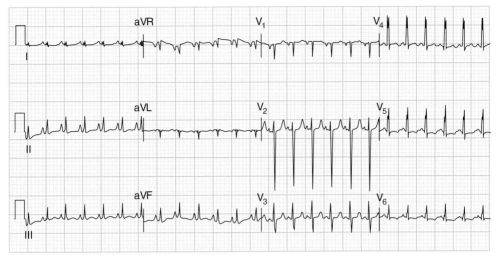

FIGURE 9-2. Electrocardiogram in a 10-month-old patient with acute myocarditis. Tachycardia, decreased QRS voltages, and diffuse ST-segment and T-wave abnormalities are present.

antibody titers but even this does not prove causation. Polymerase chain reaction is used to analyze nasopharyngeal specimens for specific viral sequences. This process allows identification of a presumptive etiologic virus in at least one-third of patients but also does not prove causation.

Supportive measures are the principle form of therapy (Chapters 11 and 12). Administration of intravenous immunoglobulin may be beneficial; however, efficacy has not been validated. Extracorporeal membrane oxygenation has been used with success especially in those patients who have malignant arrhythmias unresponsive to antiarrhythmic therapy. Nearly two-thirds of infants with myocarditis will recover substantially, some of the rest will die or need immediate cardiac transplantation, and the others will have chronic congestive heart failure and eventually need transplantation.

Myocardial Insufficiency

Perinatal Asphyxia

Severe perinatal asphyxia may occasionally cause ventricular dilation and dysfunction in newborn infants that is likely the result of myocardial ischemia. Myocardial oxygen delivery is impaired because cardiac output and arterial oxygen content decrease while oxygen demand is increased because of asphyxia-induced increases in pulmonary and systemic vascular resistances (afterload). The clinical features are variable and range from mild bradycardia to cardiovascular shock. These infants typically have low Apgar scores and metabolic acidosis at birth. Poor perfusion and poor pulses are present as are hepatomegaly and cardiomegaly. Sepsis must be excluded as well as other causes of neonatal cardiomyopathy and certain congenital heart defects, such as critical aortic stenosis.

Hypoxemia may be more prominent than shock in some asphyxiated infants. Tricuspid regurgitation, characterized by a systolic murmur at the lower left sternal border, is frequently present and may result from ischemia or even necrosis of the anterior papillary muscle of the tricuspid valve. Tricuspid regurgitation is exacerbated by pulmonary hypertension. The degree of hypoxemia is related to the amount of right-to-left shunting through the patent foramen ovale and/or ductus arteriosus. Cyanotic heart disease such as Ebstein anomaly of the tricuspid valve must be excluded.

The chest radiograph shows cardiomegaly. Typical electrocardiographic findings include ST-segment abnormalities and inversion of T waves. Echocardiography should exclude congenital defects and will often show ventricular dilation, global ventricular dysfunction, and tricuspid valve regurgitation. The laboratory tests routinely used to evaluate myocardial ischemia in adult patients are not always reliable in newborn infants. Both creatine kinase (CK)-MB isozyme and cardiac troponin T concentrations are higher in healthy neonates than in normal adults. Supportive care results in dramatic improvements in many of these infants over several days but those with extensive myocardial necrosis may not survive.

Anomalous Origin of the Left Coronary Artery

Anomalous origin of the left coronary artery from the pulmonary artery (ALCAPA) is an uncommon congenital defect that often results in severe congestive heart failure related to infarction of the anterolateral left ventricular free wall. During fetal life and at birth, desaturated blood flows from the pulmonary artery into the left coronary artery. As pulmonary vascular resistance and pulmonary arterial pressure decrease after birth, blood in the left coronary artery reverses direction and flows into the pulmonary artery. If collateral blood supply from the right to the left coronary artery is inadequate, myocardial ischemia and infarction may occur in early infancy. Collateral vessels between the abnormal left coronary artery and the normal right coronary artery gradually enlarge and eventually pulmonary to coronary arterial steal develops because blood in the collateral vessels flows preferentially into the pulmonary artery rather than into the higher resistance coronary arteries. This also may cause myocardial ischemia.

Episodic agitation especially during feeding or crying may be seen in affected infants and reflects myocardial ischemia. Other infants present with signs and symptoms of congestive heart failure and some are critically ill with cardiogenic shock. Physical examination may show a gallop rhythm and a murmur of mitral regurgitation. The chest radiograph shows marked cardiomegaly and often pulmonary edema. The electrocardiogram often shows findings compatible with an anterolateral myocardial infarction (Figure 9-3).

This anomaly can often be diagnosed by careful echocardiographic examination. The abnormal attachment of the left coronary artery to the pulmonary artery can be visualized in about 50% of patients by two-dimensional echocardiography alone. Color Doppler flow shows retrograde flow in the left coronary artery because flow passes from the coronary artery to the pulmonary artery rather than from the aorta to the coronary artery. This is an important differentiating point between patients with ALCAPA and those with dilated cardiomyopathies of other etiologies. In addition, diastolic turbulent flow is seen in the pulmonary artery at the site of the connection with the anomalous left coronary artery. The right coronary artery is often dilated. Global left ventricular dilation and dysfunction are present and mitral regurgitation is often seen. If the echocardiographic examination is not diagnostic, cardiac catheterization and coronary angiography are indicated in all patients who have clinical findings consistent with ALCAPA.

Most children with ALCAPA present in infancy and about 75% will die before age 1 year if not treated surgically. Various surgical procedures have been tried and for many years the mortality rate was relatively high, especially in infants who were critically ill. Direct reimplantation of the origin of the left coronary artery into the aorta is now the procedure of choice in most centers. The long-term results are encouraging. Ventricular function and mitral regurgitation improve dramatically and signs and symptoms of congestive heart failure resolve in many patients.

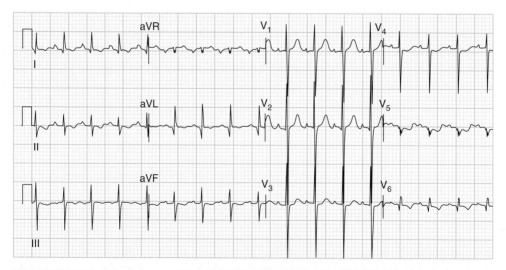

FIGURE 9-3. Electrocardiogram in a 5-month-old patient with anomalous origin of the left coronary artery from the pulmonary artery. Prominent Q waves are present in leads I and aVL.

Systemic Hypertension

Acute increases in systemic blood pressure may result in severe left ventricular hypertrophy and dysfunction in the neonate. In full-term infants, systolic pressures > 90 mm Hg and diastolic pressures > 60 mm Hg are cause for concern. Nomograms are available to facilitate interpretation of blood pressure measurements in premature infants. Causes of hypertension in neonates include renal and renovascular abnormalities, descending aortic thrombosis, and adverse effects of medications such as dexamethasone.

Symptomatic infants have gallop rhythms, poor peripheral pulses, and poor perfusion. Somewhat paradoxically the blood pressure is increased. Aortic coarctation must be excluded because some infants with this defect have upper extremity hypertension. Echocardiographic examination shows left ventricular hypertrophy and poor myocardial function. Angiotensin-converting enzyme inhibitors are often efficacious.

Arrhythmias

Certain sustained tachyarrhythmias and third-degree atrioventricular heart block may cause decreased ventricular function and congestive heart failure. These disorders are discussed in Chapter 10.

Metabolic

Inherited Errors of Metabolism

Mitochondrial disease

Disorders of fatty acid oxidation (Table 9-5). These disorders although relatively rare, can cause catastrophic complications including sudden death. Arriving at a correct diagnosis is imperative because the prognosis is often favorable once appropriate treatment is provided. A working knowledge of these disorders is essential for anyone caring for young infants because a high index of suspicion is often necessary to recognize patients who have these defects.

Pathophysiology. Fats are the most important source of fuel in the body and are the only substrate for oxidation during fasting or increased energy demand after depletion of hepatic glycogen. Decreasing blood glucose concentration causes lipid mobilization from fat stores. Stored fat is broken down into short, medium, long, and very long-chain fatty acids. Although skeletal and cardiac muscles metabolize fatty acids to generate ATP, the brain cannot metabolize fatty acids directly; ketone bodies synthesized by the liver are used for cerebral energy production.

The heart is critically dependent on energy generation. The fetal heart relies on anaerobic glycolysis and lactate as

■ **TABLE 9-5.** Disorders of Fatty Acid Oxidation Associated With Cardiomyopathy

	OMIM Number
Defects in carnitine-dependent transport of long- and very long-chain fatty acids	
Plasma membrane carnitine transporter deficiency (carnitine uptake defect) (D)	212140
Carnitine-acylcarnitine translocase deficiency (H)	212138
Infantile carnitine palmitoyltransferase (CPT) II deficiency (H)	608836
Defects in fatty acid β-oxidation	
Very long-chain acyl-CoA dehydrogenase (VLCAD) deficiency (H, D)	201475
Medium-chain acyl-CoA dehydrogenase (MCAD) deficiency	201450
Isolated long-chain 3-hydroxyacyl dehydrogenase (LCHAD) deficiency	609016
Multiple acyl-CoA dehydrogenase deficiency (glutaric acidemia type 2, electron transfer flavoprotein [ETF] component deficiency) (H,D)	231680

OMIM, Online Mendelian inheritance in man. Latest updates regarding gene(s) and loci can be obtained from this Web site: http://www.ncbi.nlm.nih.gov/omim.

D, dilated cardiomyopathy; H, hypertrophic cardiomyopathy.

energy sources. Among the many adjustments necessary during the transition to extrauterine existence is the use of fat as the main energy substrate for the heart. Up to 80% of the energy for cardiac function is produced by fatty acid oxidation in the mature heart.

Fatty acid oxidation, the process by which ATP is generated, occurs only within the mitochondria (Figure 9-4). A specific transporter facilitates movement of long- and very long-chain fatty acids across the cell membrane into the cytosol. Long- and very long-chain fatty acids are then activated by binding to coenzyme A (CoA) to form fatty acyl-CoA. This complex can then cross the outer mitochondrial membrane. At this point the enzyme carnitine palmitoyl transferase I (CPTI) catalyzes transfer of the fatty acid from CoA to carnitine forming acylcarnitine. The activity of this enzyme in the liver increases during fasting which preferentially directs fatty acids to the liver. Acylcarnitine is then transferred across the inner mitochondrial membrane by an enzyme called carnitine acyl translocase. Once inside the mitochondria the enzyme

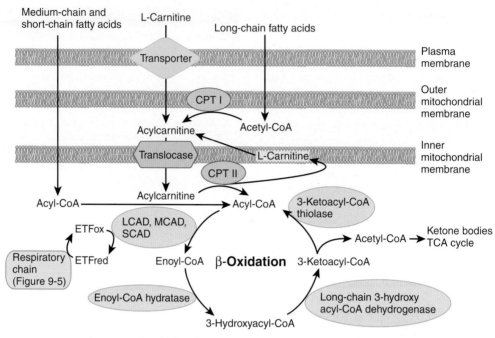

FIGURE 9-4. Oxidation of fatty acids. The trifunctional protein is composed of the enoyl-CoA hydratase, the long-chain 3-hydroxyacyl dehydrogenase (LCHAD) enzymes, and the 3-ketoacyl-CoA thiolase enzymes. Abbreviations: CPT, carnitine palmitoyl transferase; LCAD, long-chain acyl-CoA dehydrogenase; MCAD, medium-chain acyl-CoA dehydrogenase; SCAD, short-chain acyl-CoA dehydrogenase; TCA, tricarboxylic acid.

CPTII transfers the fatty acid from carnitine back to CoA. Short- and medium-chain fatty acids move across the plasma membrane (sarcolemma) and the outer and inner mitochondrial membranes without the aid of the carnitine-dependent transporter. Within the mitochondria all fatty acids undergo β-oxidation forming acetyl CoA (Figure 9-4). Acetyl CoA is metabolized by the tricarboxylic acid (Krebs) cycle producing electrons that pass through the respiratory chain generating ATP through oxidative phosphorylation (see following text). In fasting states when glucose is relatively unavailable, acetyl CoA is metabolized to ketone bodies in the liver. Ketone bodies then circulate in the blood where they are used preferentially by the brain for energy generation during fasting states.

Carnitine plays a pivotal role in fatty acid oxidation. Carnitine can be obtained from the diet but is it also synthesized from lysine and methionine in liver, kidney, and brain, but not in muscle. Carnitine is actively transported across the cell membrane by a carrier-mediated transport process. The carnitine concentration within the myocardial cell is 40 to 100 times above the concentration in plasma.

Disorders of fatty acid oxidation include abnormalities in carnitine-dependent transport or in mitochondrial β-oxidation of fatty acids. Defects may occur in any of the enzymes or transport proteins involved in fatty acid oxidation. Accumulation of substrates proximal to the specific enzyme defect explains many clinical findings in these patients:

- *Hypoketotic hypoglycemia*—Partial oxidation of fatty acids by the liver produces ketones. Patients who have these defects cannot produce ketones and therefore glucose becomes the only available fuel. During times of stress, for example, fasting, glycogen, and glucose stores become depleted and hypoglycemia develops.

- *Encephalopathy or Reye-like syndrome*—The brain is completely dependent on glucose and ketone bodies for energy generation. Neurological dysfunction results from failure to deliver these substrates to the brain during fasting.

- *Hepatic dysfunction and hyperammonemia*—Hepatic dysfunction results from the toxicity of accumulating metabolites and ammonia concentrations increase because acetyl CoA is required for hepatic synthesis of urea.

- *Organ steatosis*—The free fatty acids, which are released during fasting but cannot be metabolized, are often stored as triglycerides in various tissues. This may result in a hypertrophic or dilated cardiomyopathy, fatty liver, and/or lipid storage myopathy.

- *Abnormal urine organic acids*—Fatty acids within the mitochondria that cannot undergo β-oxidation can be diverted to the endoplasmic reticulum for omega oxidation which generates dicarboxylic acids and 3-hydroxydicarboxylic acids. These are excreted in the urine in an amount equal to or greater than the amount of ketones when the patient is fasting. Abnormal urine organic acids are generally not seen in patients who have defects involving the transport of fatty acids into the mitochondria.

- *Decreased plasma carnitine concentration*—Carnitine concentrations are decreased in patients with many of these disorders but this is a primary defect only in patients who have carnitine transporter deficiency. Carnitine concentrations are <5% of normal in these patients. In most other patients, carnitine deficiency (10%-50% of normal) is secondary. Free fatty acids that accumulate because of the metabolic block are toxic, so excess fatty acids usually are conjugated to carnitine and glycine. These acylcarnitines compete with free carnitine during reabsorption in the renal tubules. Free carnitine is excreted preferentially because the affinity of the renal carnitine transporter is higher for longer chain-length acylcarnitines. Thus decreased carnitine concentrations are secondary and the ratio of acylcarnitines to total carnitine usually is increased.

- *Cardiovascular dysfunction*—A large percentage of symptomatic patients show signs of cardiomyopathies, cardiogenic shock arrhythmias, and/or sudden death; these conditions are more common in patients who present at a younger age. The exact mechanisms by which these defects lead to the development of cardiovascular manifestations are unknown. As discussed earlier, excess fatty acids may be stored as triglycerides in the cytosol of the myocardial cells. In addition, an inadequate supply of ATP may result in contractile dysfunction and subsequent development of hypertrophic cardiomyopathy. Finally, accumulation of intermediary metabolites such as long-chain acylcarnitines may cause myocardial injury and rhythm disturbances.

Clinical features. All disorders of fatty acid oxidation are inherited in an autosomal recessive manner. Considerable

clinical heterogeneity exists within families. The estimated incidence of these defects is 1 in 6000 making these conditions among the more common of the inherited metabolic diseases.

These disorders usually become apparent during the first 2 to 3 years of life. The heart, skeletal muscle, and liver in particular are dependent on mitochondrial oxidation of fatty acids during periods of fasting. Thus clinical features of these disorders include hypoketotic hypoglycemia, encephalopathy, or Reye-like syndrome associated with increased transaminase concentrations and possibly hyperammonemia, cardiogenic shock, cardiac arrhythmias, and sudden death particularly during fasting stress. Cardiomyopathy, either dilated or hypertrophic, is present in about one-third of patients. Some infants show both ventricular hypertrophy and decreased systolic function. Skeletal lipid-storage myopathy is also seen. The pattern of symptoms in patients who have any specific defect, clinical course, and severity is often unpredictable. Symptoms often appear precipitously. Any situation which increases reliance on fatty acids for generation of ATP may precipitate heart failure or ventricular arrhythmias. In older infants and toddlers, an episode of infection such as gastroenteritis or pneumonia may precipitate acute decompensation. In other patients, cardiomyopathy and associated myocardial dysfunction may develop over time. Because these conditions are inherited as autosomal recessive traits, a family history of sudden death in siblings is relatively common.

An important proportion of patients who have these disorders experience hypoglycemia, hepatic failure, and severe metabolic acidosis within the first 48 to 72 hours after birth. Defects in fatty acid oxidation are estimated to cause about 5% of all cases of sudden infant death. A newborn infant who is breast-fed may be vulnerable until the mother's milk supply is plentiful. Breast-fed infants may receive very little nutrition during the first days of life, and this may result in significant and undue fasting stress, precipitating the acute and sometimes fatal presentation.

Specific defects (Table 9-5). More than 20 different specific defects have been described and those associated with cardiac pathology and/or sudden death in young infants, are described as follows:

DEFECTS IN CARNITINE-DEPENDENT TRANSPORT LONG- AND VERY LONG-CHAIN FATTY ACIDS.

PLASMA MEMBRANE CARNITINE TRANSPORTER DEFICIENCY (CARNITINE UPTAKE DEFECT OR SYSTEMIC CARNITINE DEFICIENCY). Impaired renal absorption of carnitine is present and plasma carnitine concentrations are 1% to 5% of normal. This defect is always associated with cardiomyopathy, usually dilated, and at times the clinical picture resembles endocardial fibroelastosis. Skeletal muscle weakness is also present. Acute hepatic encephalopathy superimposed on the cardiomyopathy has been associated with sudden death in infants. Serum carnitine may be normal in the early neonatal period because carnitine is transferred across the placenta; tandem mass spectrometry is more sensitive and specific. These patients respond very well to carnitine administration; complete reversal of cardiomyopathy is seen.

CARNITINE-ACYLCARNITINE TRANSLOCASE DEFICIENCY. This enzyme shuttles acylcarnitines and carnitines between the cytosol and the intramitochondrial matrix space. Most of these patients present in the newborn period with hepatic dysfunction, hypotonia, arrhythmias, and cardiomyopathy, often resulting in sudden death. This is a rare condition with a fairly high mortality. Administration of medium-chain triglycerides, which do not require carnitine for transport into the mitochondria matrix, may be beneficial. The efficacy of carnitine therapy, which is often recommended because of low-serum carnitine concentration, is not proven.

INFANTILE CARNITINE PALMITOYLTRANSFERASE II (CPTII) DEFICIENCY. Infants who have < 20% of normal enzyme activity present early in life with hypoketotic hypoglycemia, hepatic dysfunction, and cardiovascular collapse associated with hypertrophic cardiomyopathy often with decreased systolic function and arrhythmias. Life expectancy is very short. Extensive fatty infiltration of the heart, liver, and kidneys is seen at autopsy. These infants usually have null mutations which result in a complete lack of enzyme activity.

DEFECTS IN FATTY ACID β-OXIDATION. These patients often develop a Reye-like syndrome with associated hyperammonemia, cardiomyopathy, arrhythmias, and sudden death. Serum and urine concentrations of dicarboxylic acids usually are increased.

VERY LONG-CHAIN ACYL-COA DEHYDROGENASE (VLCAD) DEFICIENCY. The majority of these patients have cardiac disease characterized most commonly by hypertrophic cardiomyopathy. The specific gene defect is heterogeneous and results in variable loss of enzyme activity that is correlated with severity of disease. Patients with markedly decreased enzyme activity present in the newborn period with typical signs and symptoms and most die within a few

months. Some long-term survival has been reported in infants in whom the diet is strictly controlled.

MEDIUM-CHAIN ACYL-COA DEHYDROGENASE (MCAD) DEFICIENCY. This is one of the most common of the fatty acid oxidation disorders, especially in Caucasians from Northern Europe, in whom the predicted incidence (1:6500-1:17,000) is similar to that of phenylketonuria. This defect is associated with sudden death. Patients do not usually present with symptoms until just over a year of age but neonatal presentation in association with poor feeding after birth is described. Cardiomyopathy has not been described but various arrhythmias are reported. Fatty infiltration of the myocardium is seen at the time of autopsy. The prognosis is good with appropriate therapy once the diagnosis is established, especially if the condition is detected by newborn screening before the onset of symptoms.

MITOCHONDRIAL TRIFUNCTIONAL PROTEIN DEFICIENCY. Trifunctional protein is a multienzyme complex composed of four α units containing the enoyl-CoA hydratase and long-chain 3-hydroxyacyl dehydrogenase (LCHAD) enzymes and four β subunits containing the 3-ketoacyl-CoA thiolase enzyme. Mutations in any of the subunits can result in reduced activity of all three enzymes though this is much less common than isolated LCHAD deficiency (see following discussion). In addition to typical symptoms, sudden infant death is common in these patients, as well as cardiomyopathy and arrhythmias.

ISOLATED LONG-CHAIN 3-HYDROXYACYL DEHYDROGENASE (LCHAD) DEFICIENCY. This is one of the most severe fatty oxidation disorders. Affected infants are frequently growth retarded and delivered prematurely. They may present with profound liver failure. Cardiomyopathy, either hypertrophic or dilated, may result in severe myocardial dysfunction and death. Dietary management is effective. Isolated LCHAD deficiency in children (but not trifunctional protein deficiency) is associated with severe maternal liver disease during pregnancy with affected fetuses. Acute fatty liver of pregnancy also may occur during the third trimester and is characterized by anorexia, nausea, vomiting, abdominal pain, and jaundice. The HELLP syndrome (hypertension or hemolysis, elevated liver enzymes, and low platelets) is also reported. The mothers of these infants are obligate heterozygotes for the condition. It is speculated that abnormal fetal fatty acid metabolites may be toxic to the maternal liver. Offspring from pregnancies complicated by these conditions may benefit from screening for LCHAD deficiency.

MULTIPLE ACYL-COA DEHYDROGENASE DEFICIENCY. ETF dehydrogenase and ETF are enzymes involved in electron transport between the acyl-CoA dehydrogenase and the respiratory chain (Figure 9-4). Multiple acyl-CoA dehydrogenase deficiency (also known as glutaric acidemia type 2 and electron transfer flavoprotein [ETF] component deficiency) is the result of ETF dehydrogenase deficiency or deficiency of α or β subunits of ETF. Patients who have these defects excrete large amounts of organic acids including glutaric acid. Sudden death and arrhythmias have been reported. Neonatal onset disease may be associated with congenital anomalies including dysmorphic facies, enlarged or cystic kidneys, rocker bottom feet, and abnormal external genitalia. Cardiomyopathy is common and fatty infiltration of the myocardium is present. These infants, who are described as having an abnormal "sweaty-feet odor," are often severely symptomatic within 24 to 48 hours of life and usually do not survive the neonatal period. Another group of patients also has neonatal onset disease but do not have congenital anomalies. These infants also present with acute decompensation during the first few days of life and often have severe cardiomyopathy. Most of these patients die in infancy. A third group of patients who have mild or late-onset disease may not present until several months of age or possibly until adulthood. Riboflavin administration in addition to the usual supportive measures may improve the clinical course for these patients.

Diagnosis. Evaluation of multiple diagnostic criteria is necessary to diagnose a fatty acid oxidation disorder and consultation with a metabolic specialist knowledgeable about these disorders is essential. A protocol for evaluating patients suspected of having these disorders must rely on multiple independent factors. For example, the absence of fatty infiltration of the liver does not completely exclude these disorders. Routine laboratory evaluation should include serum glucose, electrolytes, liver function tests, lactate, ammonia, and creatine kinase as well as urine ketones. If possible, a complete metabolic evaluation needs to be obtained including plasma carnitine, acylcarnitine and free fatty acid concentrations, 3-hydroxy fatty acids, and urine organic acids and acylglycines. Metabolic abnormalities are often detected only during an acute crisis and biochemical screening may be uninformative when the patient is well. Thus, obtaining blood and urine samples at the time of the acute illness is very important. Tandem mass spectrometry is a powerful tool to diagnose some of these disorders. This technique can determine the concentration of many different fatty acids and fatty acylcarnitine compounds in a dried blood spot. Thus obtaining a portion of the blood spots collected for newborn screenings may be helpful for patients in whom no other samples are available. Metabolic flux studies by use of cultured skin fibroblasts and direct enzyme analysis may also be useful for some disorders. Direct analysis of DNA for mutations can be performed on blood cells, cultured fibroblasts, and liver or skeletal muscle.

A comprehensive autopsy must be done in all infants who die suddenly. Unfortunately, testing all infants who die suddenly for fatty acid oxidation disorders is not practical but the following patients certainly merit further attention: (1) those who are thought to be normal and die unexpectedly after a period of fasting; (2) those who have a family history of sudden death in an infant or young child; and (3) those in whom the autopsy shows fatty infiltration of the liver or other organs. Frozen postmortem liver specimens and samples of bile and urine are saved from all autopsies. Skin biopsies are obtained for fibroblast culture.

Newborn screening for many of these disorders has been implemented in many states. The National Newborn Screening and Genetics Resource Center Web site (http://genes-r-us.uthscsa.edu/index.htm) provides information regarding specific conditions screened and genetics programs in each state. Identification of presymptomatic newborns may allow prevention of sudden clinical deterioration and death. Early identification of affected individuals by expanded newborn screening using tandem mass spectrometry should improve understanding of the natural history of these disorders. The specificity and sensitivity of early detection as well as long-term benefits remains to be defined.

Therapy. Diet is the mainstay of therapy. In general, fat restriction and a high-carbohydrate diet are recommended. These patients must avoid prolonged fasting. Dextrose solutions must be administered intravenously when oral intake is poor. Infusion of glucose at 8 to 10 mg/kg/min (10% dextrose at 1.5 times greater than maintenance) will prevent mobilization of free fatty acids. Young infants should receive nighttime feedings. Older infants and children need to be fed frequent meals and a high-carbohydrate snack at bedtime, and be fed early in the morning. Cornstarch, which provides a sustained release source of glucose, can be added to the diet after 8 months of age when pancreatic enzymes are sufficient for full absorption. Supplementation of the diet with medium-chain triglycerides is often recommended but published studies demonstrating clinical benefit are limited. A minimum intake of long- and very long-chain triglycerides is necessary to prevent essential fatty acid deficiency.

Carnitine therapy clearly is indicated for those patients who have a defect in the carnitine transport protein. Treated patients show a dramatic reversal of cardiomyopathy. For patients who have other defects, therapy with carnitine has not shown consistent benefit.

Because these disorders are autosomal recessive, prenatal or presymptomatic screening needs to be done in siblings. Improved awareness, understanding, and treatment of fatty acid defects by clinicians should improve outcomes for patients and families.

Disorders of mitochondrial oxidative phosphorylation (Table 9-6).

Respiratory chain diseases. Although neuromuscular and ocular abnormalities usually predominate, all morphologic forms of cardiomyopathy may be present in patients with respiratory chain diseases and some defects are also associated with conduction disturbances. The frequency of cardiac involvement is 17% to 40%. Patients who present with cardiac manifestations have a poorer outcome.

PATHOPHYSIOLOGY. The respiratory chain is a series of five enzyme complexes within the mitochondria that produce ATP by a metabolic process called oxidative phosphorylation (Figure 9-5). Complexes I and II collect electrons generated from the metabolism of fats, carbohydrates, and proteins. These electrons are transferred sequentially to coenzyme Q (ubiquinone), complex III, and complex IV. The energy generated by these electron transfers is used by complexes I, III, and IV to pump protons from the mitochondrial matrix into the intermembrane space located between the inner and outer mitochondrial membranes. Complex V (ATP synthetase) then uses this proton gradient to generate ATP from ADP and inorganic phosphate.

Mitochondria are unique organelles in that they have their own DNA as well as nuclear DNA. Nuclear genes encode most of the mitochondrial proteins. Mutations in nuclear DNA show Mendelian inheritance and can cause abnormalities in:

■ **TABLE 9-6.** Disorders of Oxidative Phosphorylation Associated With Cardiomyopathy

	OMIM Number
Respiratory chain subunits	
Complex I (NADH-ubiquinone reductase) deficiency (D)	252010
Complex III (ubiquinone-ferrocytochrome c oxidoreductase) (H)	256000
Complex IV or cytochrome c oxidase (COX) deficiency (H)	220110
Cataracts and cardiomyopathy (Senger syndrome) (H)	212350
Abnormalities in mitochondrial lipids	
Barth syndrome (H,D,NC)	302060
Disorders related only to mitochondrial genome mutations	
Mitochondrial myopathy, encephalopathy, lactic acidosis and stroke-like episodes (MELAS) (H)[a]	540000
Myoclonus, epilepsy, and red-ragged fiber disease (MERRF) (H,D)	545000
Kearns-Sayre syndrome (H,D)[a]	530000
Pearson syndrome[a]	557000

[a]Indicates cardiomyopathy usually not present in infancy.

OMIM, Online Mendelian inheritance in man. Latest updates regarding gene(s) and loci can be obtained from this Web site: http://www.ncbi.nlm.nih.gov/omim. For an overview of the genetics of Leigh syndrome see 256000.

D, dilated cardiomyopathy; H, hypertrophic cardiomyopathy; NC, noncompaction.

- Respiratory chain subunits
- Ancillary proteins for respiratory chain subunits (abnormalities in proteins necessary to synthesize or direct assembly of respiratory chain subunits)
- Mitochondrial lipids
- Communication between the nuclear and mitochondrial genomes (abnormalities in control of mitochondrial replication, maintenance and translation)

Mitochondrial DNA genes encode several essential subunits of the respiratory chain complexes and the transfer and ribosomal RNAs responsible for their translation. Mutations in mitochondrial DNA, which are usually point mutations or small or long DNA deletions, can therefore cause abnormalities in respiratory chain subunits or in genes responsible for protein synthesis.

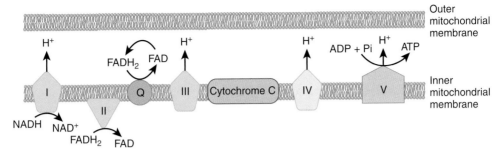

FIGURE 9-5. The mitochondrial respiratory chain. I, NADH: ubiquinone oxidoreductase (NADH reductase); II, succinate: ubiquinone oxidoreductase (succinate dehydrogenase); Q, ubiquinone (coenzyme Q_{10}); III, ubiquinol: ferrocytochrome c oxidoreductase (ubiquinol-cytochrome c reductase); IV, ferrocytochrome c: oxygen oxidoreductase (cytochrome c oxidase); V, ATP synthetase. NAD^+ and FAD are necessary for fatty acid β-oxidation.

The unique molecular and genetic properties of the mitochondrial genome account for some of the unusual features of mitochondrial disorders. The mitochondrial genome has a relatively high rate of spontaneous mutation and each cell contains many mitochondrial DNA copies which are distributed randomly among daughter cells during cell division. Mutant and normal DNA often occur together within cells (heteroplasmy). A minimum "mutation load" (usually > 80%) is necessary to cause mitochondrial dysfunction (threshold effect) and the resulting clinical disease. The proportion of mutant DNA per cell varies among tissues and may shift as the cells divide. This latter fact explains why clinical characteristics may change as the patient ages. Point mutations usually show a maternal rather than a mendelian pattern of inheritance because the mtDNA in the fertilized egg is derived from the oocyte. The disease will be expressed in both sexes but will show only maternal transmission. Large-scale rearrangements (single deletions, duplications, or both) are usually sporadic.

The precise mechanism for cardiomyopathy in these disorders is not defined. Cardiac hypertrophy may result from increased oxidative stress but this is speculative.

CLINICAL FEATURES. Disorders of oxidative phosphorylation may affect nearly every organ in the body because ATP is vital to cell function. Atypical clinical presentations with an unexplained association of symptoms and involvement of seemingly unrelated organ systems should prompt consideration of oxidative phosphorylation disorders. Brain, heart, and skeletal muscle are typically involved because of their relatively high energy demands. Severely affected infants present immediately after delivery or in the first few days of life.

Many neonates with respiratory chain disease are diagnosed with Leigh syndrome. Affected infants have severe psychomotor regression and lactic acidosis. Cerebellar and pyramidal signs are present. Magnetic resonance imaging shows focal symmetric lesions in the basal ganglia and brainstem. These findings are thought to be the result of damage to the developing brain because of impaired oxidative metabolism. Pathologic examination shows necrosis with gliosis and vascular proliferation. Leigh syndrome is genetically heterogeneous; mutations have been identified in mitochondrial respiratory chain complexes I, II, III, IV, and V and components of the pyruvate dehydrogenase complex. Although cardiomyopathy occurs in a few patients, the heart is not typically involved.

Some neonates present with cardiovascular collapse immediately after delivery. Other neonates may present with cardiomyopathy and skeletal myopathy, or isolated skeletal myopathy. Mutations in both mitochondrial and nuclear-encoded genes are reported. The cardiomyopathy is most often hypertrophic but dilated forms also occur. Arrhythmias, including ventricular tachycardia and more rarely, Wolff-Parkinson-White syndrome, occur less commonly. Apnea, poor feeding, vomiting, and hepatomegaly may also be seen.

Older children usually have generalized hypotonia and weakness, psychomotor retardation, lactic acidemia, and often cardiorespiratory insufficiency. The older patients most often come to attention because of a skeletal myopathy that results from the mitochondrial myopathy.

Classical histologic abnormalities include abnormal skeletal muscle fibers (ragged-red fibers) and abnormal mitochondria but this is not always present and is not required for diagnosis. The ragged-red fibers result from accumulation of abnormal mitochondria under the plasma membrane and may not be present in infants. Laboratory manifestations are variable but may include increased lactate to pyruvate ratio and normal serum glucose to ketone body molar ratio.

DESCRIPTION OF SELECTED DISORDERS. *Complex I (NADH-ubiquinone reductase) deficiency* may occur as an isolated defect or together with other respiratory chain defects. This complex consists of at least 36 nuclear-encoded and 7 mitochondrial-encoded subunits. Deficiency can be caused by mutations in several different nuclear or mitochondrial-encoded genes. The majority of cases are caused by mutations in nuclear-encoded genes. The fatal infantile form (lethal mitochondrial disease) is a multisystem disorder characterized by severe lactic acidosis, hypertrophic or dilated cardiomyopathy, hepatomegaly, apnea, and feeding difficulties. Severe cardiac dysfunction often results in death within a few weeks after birth. Muscle biopsies show ragged-red fibers. Measurement of enzyme activity in affected organs or cultured skin fibroblasts establishes the diagnosis.

Complex III (ubiquinone-ferrocytochrome c oxidoreductase) deficiency results in a multisystem disorder or in a myopathy. Infants who develop cardiomyopathy have severe hypertrophy and arrhythmias in which the myocytes appear to be replaced by large rounded cells resembling histiocytes (histiocytoid cardiomyopathy). Fatal arrhythmias have been reported.

Complex IV or cytochrome c oxidase (COX) deficiency can result in an encephalopathy (Leigh syndrome) or myopathy. Deficiency of this complex is caused by mutation in multiple nuclear-encoded and mitochondrial-encoded genes. Leigh syndrome usually does not present until after early infancy when psychomotor regression is noted. The fatal infantile myopathy (lethal mitochondrial disease or fatal cardioencephalomyopathy) is characterized by diffuse hypotonia associated with respiratory insufficiency, lactic acidosis, and hypertrophic cardiomyopathy and/or renal dysfunction. These patients do not respond to treatment and usually die from respiratory insufficiency. In contrast, the benign infantile form presents similarly but these patients do respond to aggressive supportive therapy and they improve spontaneously. Both lactic acidosis and ragged-red fibers gradually regress.

Sengers syndrome is characterized by abnormal mitochondria in cardiac and skeletal muscle, cataracts, and lactic acidosis. The exact cause of this disorder is not known. In the fatal neonatal form these findings are present at birth. These patients have severe hypertrophic cardiomyopathy that causes death within the first month of life. In the more benign form, cataracts may be the only symptom in childhood; cardiomyopathy develops during adult life.

Barth syndrome (cardioskeletal myopathy with neutropenia and abnormal mitochondria) is an example of a condition caused by abnormalities in the mitochondrial lipids. This is an X-linked disorder in which mitochondrial abnormalities are present in cardiac muscle, neutrophil bone marrow cells, and occasionally in skeletal muscle. Typical findings include cardiomyopathy often characterized by left ventricular noncompaction, cyclical neutropenia, skeletal myopathy, and growth retardation. Ventricular tachycardia is seen in about 10% to 20% of patients. Blood and urine concentrations of 3-methyl glutaconic acid are increased. Many patients die within the first few months to years of life from cardiac failure or sepsis but aggressive and proactive supportive care increases life expectancy.

This condition is caused by a mutation in the tafazzin gene (*TAZ*) which is located on the long arm of the X chromosome and encodes a phospholipid acyltransferase called tafazzin. Tafazzin is required for normal synthesis of cardiolipin, an acidic phospholipid that is the major component of the inner mitochondrial membrane. The respiratory chain complexes are embedded in this membrane; mutations in *TAZ* alter the concentration and composition of cardiolipin, leading to altered mitochondrial architecture and function. High-performance liquid chromatography-electrospray mass spectrometry shows decreased total cardiolipin and alterations in cardiolipin subclasses in fibroblasts from affected patients. *TAZ* mutation analysis establishes the diagnosis.

Disorders related only to mitochondrial genome mutations include *mitochondrial myopathy, encephalopathy, lactic acidosis, and stroke-like episodes* (MELAS) which is characterized by recurrent neurologic events. This condition is most often caused by a point mutation in the tRNA for leucine but other mitochondrial DNA point mutations have been described. *Myoclonus, epilepsy, and red-ragged fiber disease (MERRF)* is associated with a point mutation in the tRNA for lysine. These patients usually develop normally during the first few years of life, but neonatal onset has been reported. *Kearns-Sayre syndrome* is a sporadic condition that results from a large single deletion of mitochondrial DNA. Patients have progressive external ophthalmoplegia and frequently develop high-degree atrioventricular conduction defects in the second or third decade. They are usually asymptomatic as infants. However, some patients who have another manifestation of a large mitochondrial NA deletion, *Pearson syndrome* (sideroblastic anemia with pancytopenia and exocrine pancreatic insufficiency), eventually develop Kearns-Sayre syndrome.

DIAGNOSIS. The patient phenotype must be assessed carefully. A complete family history is important to determine whether mendelian or maternal inheritance is present. Standard metabolic testing including assay of blood and urine for organic acids and amino acids is done. A muscle biopsy is often necessary for histologic and biochemical analyses. Biochemical studies in particular are difficult because a variety of laboratory errors can produce false positive results. Genetic testing, including comprehensive mitochondrial DNA analysis, is also necessary if indicated. A fully-integrated multidisciplinary approach is necessary to reach a correct diagnosis. Consensus diagnostic criteria are available (see Bernier, et al in *Suggested Readings*).

THERAPY. Treatment of mitochondrial oxidative phosphorylation defects is difficult. Isolated publications report beneficial effects of cofactor substitution in a few cases but no accepted satisfactory therapy is available. Determination of whether a patient's phenotype is the result of abnormal nuclear DNA or mitochondrial DNA is important for genetic counseling of the family.

Storage disorders (Table 9-7).

Glycogen storage disease. Glycogen is present in large quantities in muscle and liver cells and serves as a reservoir for glucose. The glycogen storage diseases (GSD) comprise more than 10 different inherited disorders caused by abnormalities of the enzymes regulating the synthesis and degradation of glycogen but only a few of these affect the heart.

■ **TABLE 9-7.** Storage Disorders Associated With Cardiomyopathy

	OMIM Number
Glycogen storage disease	
Lysosomal	
Type II (Pompe disease, alpha-1,4-glucosidase [acid maltase] deficiency) (H)	232300
Non-lysosomal	
Type III (Cori disease, amylo-1,6 glucosidase, debranching enzyme deficiency) (H)	232400
Type IV (Andersen disease, branching enzyme deficiency) (D)	232500
Familial hypertrophic cardiomyopathy with Wolff-Parkinson-White syndrome (AMP-activated protein kinase)	600858
Other lysosomal storage disease	
Mucopolysaccharidoses	
Type I (Hurler, Hurler-Scheie, Scheie) (α-L-iduronidase) (H)	607014
Type II (Hunter) (iduronidase sulfatase) (D)[a]	309900
Type IVA (Morquio A) (galactosamine-6-sulfate-sulfatase) (D)[a]	253000
Type VI (Maroteaux-Lamy) (aryl-sulfatase B) (D)[a]	253200
Type VII (Sly) (β-glucuronidase) (H)	253220
Ganglioside degradation disorders	
G_{M1} gangliosidosis (β-galactosidase) (H)	230500
G_{M2} gangliosidosis (Sandhoff disease, hexosaminidase A/B deficiency) (H,D)	268800
Mucolipidosis, type II (I-cell disease, *N*-acetyl-galactosamine-1-phosphotransferase)	252500
X-linked vacuolar cardiomyopathy and myopathy (Danon disease, lysosome-associated membrane protein-2 [LAMP-2])[a]	300257
Fabry disease (α-galactosidase A)(H)[a]	301500
Congenital disorders of glycosylation, Type Ia (phosphomannomutase) (H,D)	212065

[a]Indicates cardiomyopathy usually not present in infancy.

OMIM, Online Mendelian inheritance in man. Latest updates regarding gene(s) and loci can be obtained from this Web site: http://www.ncbi.nlm.nih.gov/omim.

D, dilated cardiomyopathy; H, hypertrophic cardiomyopathy.

GSD II is caused by decreased activity of the lysosomal glycolytic enzyme alpha-1,4-glucosidase (acid maltase) and is transmitted as an autosomal recessive trait. The main purpose of this lysosomal pathway is to degrade the glycogen that is taken up in autophagic vacuoles during times of cellular turnover. The enzyme deficiency causes glycogen to accumulate in the lysosomes of cardiac, smooth, and skeletal muscle cells which results in cellular hypertrophy and lysosomal rupture.

Complete deficiency causes a severe infantile form of GSD II called Pompe disease. Pompe disease is unique among the GSDs because glycogen accumulates within the lysosomes (rather than in the cytoplasm) of tissues including the heart, liver, skeletal muscle, and central nervous system. Symptoms such as poor feeding, decreased spontaneous movement, failure to thrive and delayed development are frequently present. Physical examination shows hypotonia, macroglossia, and marked hepatomegaly. Cardiomegaly is always prominent. The electrocardiogram typically shows a short PR interval and markedly increased precordial voltages (Figure 9-6). The echocardiogram shows massive hypertrophy of the entire left ventricle, interventricular septum, and papillary muscles (Figure 9-7). The left ventricular cavity size is decreased as is ventricular function. The serum creatine kinase concentration is always increased. Muscle biopsy shows vacuoles filled with glycogen within all muscle fibers. With supportive care only, these patients usually die before 2 years of age because of impaired ventilation and heart failure. Enzyme replacement therapy with recombinant human alglucosidase alfa is currently being actively investigated. Preliminary results show decreased ventricular hypertrophy, improved motor skills, and prolonged ventilation-free survival. Antibody responses may decrease efficacy. It is reasonable to expect that therapy will be more efficacious if begun early in the course.

GSD III (debrancher deficiency, amylo-1,6-glucosidase, Cori disease) usually does not affect young infants but a rare infantile form occurs that is associated with severe hypertrophic cardiomyopathy.

A recently described glycogen storage disease, familial hypertrophic cardiomyopathy with Wolff-Parkinson-White syndrome, is caused by mutations in the *Prkag2* gene which encodes a regulatory subunit of an AMP-activated protein kinase. The activity of this enzyme is critical in regulating cellular glucose and fatty acid metabolic pathways. During times of increased energy demand in muscle, this enzyme promotes ATP repletion by facilitating cellular glucose uptake and oxidative metabolism. Mutations of this enzyme cause "gain of function" leading to excessive glucose uptake and pathological non-lysosomal glycogen storage disease in the heart.

Affected patients most commonly present in late adolescence with supraventricular tachycardia. Their electrocardiograms show ventricular preexcitation and may progress to advanced heart block. The echocardiograms

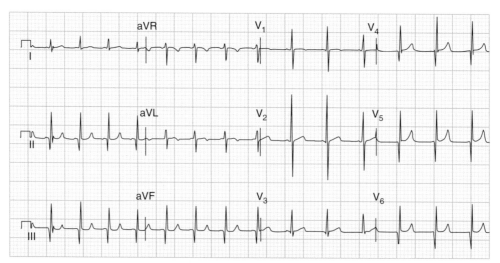

FIGURE 9-6. Electrocardiogram in a patient with Pompe disease. All leads are recorded at one-fourth standard (2.5 mm/V) because of the markedly increased voltage. The PR interval is short (80 ms).

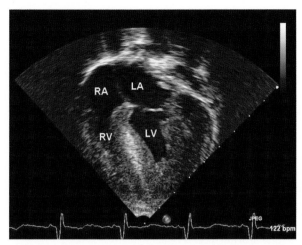

FIGURE 9-7. Echocardiogram from an infant with Pompe disease. Four-chamber view shows marked concentric left ventricular hypertrophy. Abbreviations: LA, left atrium; LV, left ventricle; RA, right atrium; RV, right ventricle.

often show varying degrees of ventricular hypertrophy that may progress to dilated cardiomyopathy. A much less common severe neonatal variant, previously attributed to deficiency of a cardiac variant of phosphorylase kinase, is thought to be related to a mutation in *Prkag2* that causes higher levels of enzyme activity than described for less severely affected older patients. These neonates show hypertrophic cardiomyopathy and ventricular preexcitation; they die of cardiorespiratory failure within a few weeks to months of birth. Interestingly, transgenic mice with mutations in this enzyme show that accumulating glycogen disrupts the normal development of the annulus fibrosis which explains the preexcitation.

Other lysosomal storage diseases. Lysosomal disorders, which include Pompe disease (discussed earlier), are the most common causes of metabolic cardiomyopathy in children. Lysosomes contain several hydrolytic enzymes and are primarily responsible for intracellular digestion of macromolecules. Lysosomal storage diseases are caused by genetic defects that affect one or more of these hydrolases which results in accumulation of undigested substrates within the lysosome. The severity of the condition depends in part on the number of enzymes affected.

Mucopolysaccharidoses. Glycosaminoglycans (muco-polysaccharides) are high molecular weight carbohydrate chains (eg, heparin, hyaluronic acid) located on the surface of the cell and in the extracellular matrix. These molecules are involved in cell communication, migration, and adhesion. Deficiencies in lysosomal enzymes involved in degrading glycosaminoglycans result in mucopolysaccharidoses (MPS). Excess glycosaminoglycans are stored in tissues and excreted in the urine. More than 10 different disorders have been described and they are transmitted as both autosomal and X-linked traits. In most cases valve dysfunction secondary to deposition of glycosaminoglycans develops. This is uncommon in neonates. Mitral valve regurgitation is most frequent but aortic valve regurgitation is also seen. Systemic hypertension is the result of arterial narrowing secondary to medial and intimal thickening. Myocardial ischemia is sometimes seen secondary to circumferential coronary arterial narrowing that tends to occur throughout the length of the vessel rather than in a discrete region and is therefore more difficult to identify. Cardiomyopathy, specifically in a pattern of endocardial fibroelastosis, may be seen. These problems usually develop over the first two decades of life but a few patients who have Hurler (MPS I) and Maroteaux-Lamy (MPS VI) syndromes have been reported who developed dilated cardiomyopathy with congestive heart failure in infancy.

G_{M1} *gangliosidosis.* G_{M1} gangliosides (sphingolipid plus >1 sialic acid residue) accumulate in multiple tissues in patients with this disorder because of decreased activity of β-galactosidase, a lysosomal enzyme involved in degradation of gangliosides. Enzyme activity is absent in the severe infantile form. Affected infants resemble those with Hurler syndrome. Radiographic studies of the skeletal bones show typical abnormalities. Echocardiography shows hypertrophic cardiomyopathy with asymmetric septal hypertrophy and mitral regurgitation. These patients usually die before age 5 years.

Type II mucolipidosis (I-cell disease). I-cells are fibroblasts with multiple inclusion bodies composed of acid hydrolases that accumulate because of deficiency of *N*-acetyl-glucosamine-1-phosphotransferase. Patients who have this autosomal recessive disorder resemble those with Hurler syndrome. Cardiomegaly and congestive heart failure may occur in early infancy. Left ventricular hypertrophy is present and is associated with aortic and mitral valve stenosis secondary to thickened valve leaflets. Cytoplasmic inclusions are seen in myocardial cells. Death occurs before age 5 years.

X-linked vacuolar cardiomyopathy and myopathy (Danon disease). This condition was previously classified as a glycogen storage disease but is no longer classified as such because intracellular glycogen is not always increased. This is an X-linked dominant condition caused by a defect in the gene encoding lysosome-associated membrane protein-2 (LAMP-2). Skeletal myopathy, cardiomyopathy, conduction defects, and mental retardation are common. Males often develop symptoms in childhood or adolescence and females may not present until adolescence or adulthood. These patients show ventricular preexcitation and cardiomyopathy that is most commonly hypertrophic in males and dilated in females. Histopathology shows clusters of vacuolated myocytes suggestive of impaired autophagy.

Congenital disorders of glycosylation. Congenital disorders of glycosylation (CDG) are a genetically heterogeneous group of autosomal recessive disorders caused by enzymatic defects in the synthesis and processing of asparagine (N)-linked glycans. Glycans are important components of cell membranes and play critical roles in metabolism, cell recognition, and adhesion. Multiple disorders have been described but CDG 1A is the most common and is the only one with cardiac manifestations. The most severe form presents in neonates and is characterized frequently by nonimmune hydrops fetalis, dysmorphic features, including inverted nipples and abnormal subcutaneous fat distribution, hypotonia, seizures, liver dysfunction, and coagulation abnormalities. Pericardial effusions and cardiomyopathy, often hypertrophic but sometimes dilated, may be present.

Propionic acidemia. This disorder results from a defect in propionic-CoA carboxylase. Neonates have poor suckling, respiratory distress, emesis, and hypotonia. Some patients have cardiomyopathy and/or arrhythmias and some have died from congestive heart failure or sudden death. Liver transplantation has been reported to reverse cardiomyopathy in isolated case reports. Laboratory abnormalities include metabolic acidosis with an increased anion gap, ketosis, and hyperammonemia. Urine organic acid analysis confirms the diagnosis.

Infants of Diabetic Mothers

Cardiorespiratory distress is common in infants born to diabetic mothers. This may be the result of congenital heart defects and/or a transient form of severe ventricular hypertrophy that has an echocardiographic appearance very similar to that of hypertrophic cardiomyopathy. This is the most common etiology of marked ventricular hypertrophy in newborn infants; true hypertrophic cardiomyopathy is much less common. The incidence of congenital heart defects is about three to five times higher in infants born to diabetic mothers than that in the general population. Of note, structural defects are likely the result of an embryopathy in long-standing diabetic mothers with increased hemoglobin A1c in the first trimester, whereas ventricular hypertrophy is more commonly seen in infants of mothers with gestational diabetes who have persistent hyperglycemia later in gestation.

Pathophysiology. Maternal hyperglycemia results in fetal hyperinsulinism that likely leads to high birth weights and enlarged viscera. The mechanism responsible for the congenital heart defects is undefined.

Clinical features. These large for gestational age infants are nearly always plethoric and edematous. Tachypnea and cyanosis are seen in symptomatic infants. Systolic murmurs may indicate defects such as ventricular septal defects, tetralogy of Fallot, or left ventricular outflow tract obstruction related to hypertrophic cardiomyopathy. Hepatomegaly is common. Hypoglycemia, hypocalcemia, and polycythemia may be present.

Ventricular hypertrophy with marked thickening of the interventricular septum is seen frequently. This may be relatively mild in asymptomatic infants but if more severe hypertrophy is present, diastolic dysfunction secondary in part to poor ventricular compliance results in heart failure. Ventricular hypertrophy can result in right ventricular outflow tract obstruction thereby causing cyanosis. Alternatively and more frequently, left ventricular obstruction causes left heart failure with poor pulses and perfusion.

Noninvasive evaluation. Cardiomegaly is present in up to 30% of infants and is more common in symptomatic infants. In one study the degree of cardiomegaly was not related to echocardiographic findings including ventricular chamber diameter or wall thickness. This may be explained in part by the fact that hypoglycemia, hypocalcemia, and polycythemia, which are also present frequently in these infants, may cause cardiomegaly. Evidence of pulmonary venous congestion may result from impaired left ventricular filling.

Generally, a consistent relationship between hypertrophy on the electrocardiogram and echocardiographic findings is not present. The electrocardiogram may be normal but right ventricular or biventricular hypertrophy

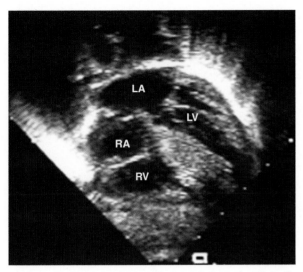

FIGURE 9-8. Echocardiogram from an infant of a diabetic mother. Subcostal four-chamber view shows marked left ventricular hypertrophy (septum greater than the left ventricular free wall). Abbreviations: LA, left atrium; LV, left ventricle; RA, right atrium; RV, right ventricle.

is seen frequently. The ST segments and T waves are normal for age.

An echocardiogram will define congenital heart defects if present and is essential for evaluating ventricular hypertrophy and ventricular outflow tract obstruction. All ventricular walls are usually thickened but disproportionate enlargement of the interventricular septum is often seen (asymmetric septal hypertrophy) (Figure 9-8). Left ventricular outflow tract obstruction is seen less frequently. Asymptomatic infants have milder degrees of hypertrophy.

Natural history. Even when hypertrophy is severe and causes symptoms in the newborn, it always resolves, usually within the first 6 months of life.

Management. Asymptomatic infants should receive usual neonatal care. Routine screening echocardiograms are not indicated. Symptomatic infants benefit from supportive care including aggressive management of hypoglycemia, hypocalcemia, and polycythemia. Mechanical ventilation may be necessary. Digoxin and intravenous positive inotropic agents are contraindicated unless the echocardiogram shows poor systolic function (eg, associated with concomitant perinatal asphyxia). These agents, as well as afterload-reducing agents, may decrease end-systolic ventricular cavity size and thereby cause or worsen left or right ventricular outflow tract obstruction. Although these infants appear edematous and have large livers, this does not often indicate excess total body water. Diuretics must be used cautiously if at all as decreased intravascular volume may also adversely affect ventricular output. β-Adrenergic antagonists reportedly have been administered to a few severely symptomatic patients.

Reversible Metabolic and Electrolyte Abnormalities
Hypocalcemia may cause decreased ventricular function and congestive heart failure in neonates. The electrocardiogram shows prolongation of the corrected QT interval. Cardiomyopathy is reversed with administration of calcium.

Hypoglycemia may also cause cardiomegaly, decreased ventricular function, and congestive heart failure in neonates. This is most frequently seen in infants of diabetic mothers but also occurs in low-birth-weight infants, critically ill infants, and in infants who have certain metabolic disorders. Ventricular function usually normalizes after administration of glucose.

Polycythemia is also sometimes associated with cardiomegaly and decreased ventricular function in neonates. Often concomitant electrolyte abnormalities are present (eg, in infants of diabetic mothers), so cause and effect are sometimes difficult to define. Treatment results in resolution of cardiac abnormalities.

Cor Pulmonale

Cor pulmonale is characterized by right ventricular dysfunction related to increased right ventricular afterload caused by hypoxic pulmonary vasoconstriction. Chronic lung disease and upper airway obstruction are the most common causes of hypoxic pulmonary vasoconstriction in neonates.

Clinically these infants may have hepatomegaly and peripheral edema related to right heart failure. The chest radiograph shows cardiomegaly. The electrocardiogram may show right axis deviation, right atrial enlargement, and/or right ventricular hypertrophy. Echocardiography first shows right ventricular dilation and then right ventricular hypertrophy often associated with pulmonary arterial hypertension. Tricuspid regurgitation occurs in more advanced cases. Severe right ventricular dilation and hypertrophy may adversely affect left ventricular function because of ventricular interdependence.

Aggressive treatment of chronic lung disease and/or upper airway obstruction is the most important component of therapy. Exacerbations of chronic lung disease are often associated with increased right heart failure. Adequate oxygenation and pH must be maintained. In some infants polysomnography is useful for assessing obstructive and central apnea, seizures, hypopnea, etc. Diuretics are frequently used in patients who have chronic lung disease. These agents alleviate pulmonary interstitial edema and fluid overload related to right heart failure. No studies show that digoxin is beneficial. Cor pulmonale may improve if lung disease resolves but chronic pulmonary artery hypertension and associated sequelae are a cause of long-term morbidity. The benefit of therapies known to be efficacious in older patients including intravenous epoprostenol, aerosolized prostacyclin, oral endothelin receptor blockers, and sildenafil remains to be defined in this population.

■ CLINICAL PRESENTATION AND DIAGNOSTIC APPROACH

Many disorders are associated with cardiomyopathy in infancy. As such, the list of possible diagnostic tests and biochemical assays is lengthy (Table 9-8).Clues from the history and physical examination should assist in focusing the diagnostic evaluation.

Those infants who have dilated forms of cardiomyopathy usually have signs and symptoms of congestive heart failure because of systolic and diastolic ventricular dysfunction. The initial findings may be subtle but some infants become acutely ill within a short period of time. The differential diagnosis includes structural heart disease, bacterial or viral sepsis, respiratory infection, and arrhythmias. Patients with hypertrophic forms of cardiomyopathy may have symptoms related to right or left ventricular outflow tract obstruction as well as from diastolic dysfunction.

A careful history must be taken and this should include information regarding prenatal and perinatal events. A complete family history, including history of recurrent fetal loss, parental consanguinity (as a marker for a recessively-inherited condition) must be obtained to assess for the presence of familial inheritance.

In addition to evaluating cardiorespiratory status, the infant is examined for signs of systemic disorders associated with cardiomyopathy. Dysmorphic features are often distinctive for certain malformation syndromes and

■ **TABLE 9-8.** Available Diagnostic Tests for Infants With Cardiomyopathy[a]

General
  Chest radiograph
  Electrocardiogram
  Echocardiogram
  Cardiac catheterization
  Endomyocardial biopsy
  Skeletal muscle biopsy
  Skeletal bone x-ray studies
  Magnetic resonance imaging of the head
  Nasopharyngeal and stool for viral cultures, PCR for viral genome
  Skin fibroblast culture for enzyme assays
  Ophthalmologic examination
Laboratory
  Blood
    Electrolytes, Ca^{2+}, Mg^{2+}, PO_4^{-2}
    Arterial blood gas (pH, anion gap)
    Liver function tests
    Ammonia
    Lactate, pyruvate
    Glucose, ketones
    Insulin
    Creatinine, blood urea nitrogen
    Carnitine, acylcarnitine profile
    Cholesterol
    Uric acid
    Creatine kinase and myocardial specific enzyme (CK-MB)
    Troponin I
    Lactate dehydrogenase
    Amino acids
    Free fatty acids
    Complete blood count
    Erythrocyte sedimentation rate
    C-reactive protein
    Viral serologies
    Blood for cell lines
    Cytogenetics
    Genetic testing
Urine
  Urinalysis
  Amino acids
  Organic acids
  Acylglycines

[a]Testing must be guided by clinical presentation and initial screening laboratory data.
PCR, polymerase chain reaction.

■ TABLE 9-9. Abnormal Features Found in Patients With Genetic Disorders Associated With Cardiomyopathy[a]

Organ system	Feature	Disorder
Growth	Short stature	Noonan syndrome
		Multiple lentigenes
		Mucopolysaccharidoses
	Macrosomia/overgrowth	Beckwith-Weidemann syndrome
		Costello Syndrome
Facies	Distinctive	Noonan syndrome
		Cardio-facio-cutaneous syndrome
		Monosomy 1p36 syndrome
	Coarse	Mucopolysaccharidoses
		Pompe disease
		Costello
Other craniofacial	Cataracts	Sengers syndrome
	Macroglossia	Beckwith-Weidemann syndrome
		Costello syndrome
	Neck webbing	Noonan syndrome
Skeleton	Hemihypertrophy	Beckwith-Weidemann syndrome
		Proteus syndrome
	Kyphoscoliosis	Noonan syndrome
		LEOPARD
		Mucopolysaccharidoses
	Pectus	Noonan syndrome
Skin/hair	Sparse curly hair	Cardio-facio-cutaneous syndrome
		Naxos disease
	Hirsutism	Mucopolysaccharidoses
	Hyperkeratosis/ichthyosis	Cardio-facio-cutaneous syndrome
	Lentigines	LEOPARD
		Naxos disease
	Cutislaxa, loose skin	Costello syndrome
	Deep palmar and plantar creases	Costello syndrome

[a]Online Mendelian Inheritance in Man (http://www.ncbi.nlm.nih.gov/omim/).

other genetic disorders associated with cardiomyopathy (Table 9-9). Hypotonia is present in several disorders (Figure 9-9). Encephalopathy associated with cardiomyopathy is suggestive of a mitochondrial oxidative phosphorylation disorder or a defect in fatty acid oxidation and appropriate laboratory investigation must be done.

The chest radiograph often shows cardiomegaly. Evidence of pulmonary venous congestion and possibly pulmonary edema are also often present.

The electrocardiogram frequently shows tachycardia and left ventricular hypertrophy. ST-segment and T-wave abnormalities are also fairly common but are relatively nonspecific. Some electrocardiographic features are relatively specific for certain diseases (Table 9-10). Arrhythmias are seen but are much less common than in older children and in adults.

The echocardiogram provides important information. First, structural heart disease must be excluded. For some lesions such as ALCAPA, careful scanning must be done by persons knowledgeable about congenital heart disease. The ventricles are evaluated for dilation and hypertrophy and the cardiomyopathy is classified as dilated,

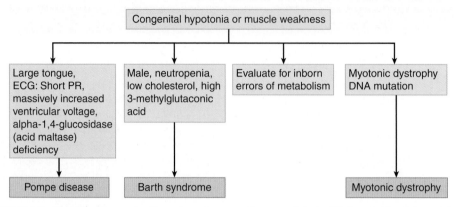

FIGURE 9-9. Algorithm for evaluation of cardiomyopathy associated with hypotonia. *Adapted from Schwartz ML, et al. Circulation. 1996;94:2021.*

hypertrophic, or restrictive. In patients with dilated cardiomyopathy, the left atrium and left ventricle are dilated. Mitral regurgitation may be present. Left ventricular function is decreased. Patients with hypertrophic cardiomyopathy may have hypertrophy of the left ventricle, right ventricle, and/or interventricular septum. The left and right ventricular outflow tracts are assessed for obstruction. Right ventricular outflow tract obstruction is common in neonates. Mitral regurgitation may be present. Measures of left ventricular dimension and wall thickness must be normalized for body surface area. Other findings such as isolated asymmetric hypertrophy of the interventricular septum, left ventricular noncompaction, and endocardial fibroelastosis are also suggestive of cardiomyopathy.

Signs and symptoms of multiple organ dysfunction may reflect profound cardiovascular insufficiency but inborn errors of metabolism should also be considered. The presence of hypoglycemia, metabolic acidosis with an increased anion gap, or hyperammonia is consistent with metabolic disorders and further evaluation is necessary (Figures 9-10 and 9-11). At times metabolic abnormalities are detected only during an acute clinical decompensation so blood and urine samples need to be obtained at the time of the acute illness and saved for analyses as indicated.

In most centers, cardiac catheterization is reserved for those patients in whom the echocardiographic diagnosis is uncertain and those being considered for cardiac transplantation. Myocardial biopsy is done in some cases but interpretation of results is complicated by frequent sampling error and specificity. For this and other reasons the role and value of the information obtained are not clear. For patients suspected of having metabolic myopathy, a skeletal muscle biopsy is equally informative and is less invasive. Skin fibroblasts can be obtained for enzyme assays as indicated.

Genetic testing is available for some disorders as discussed earlier (http://www.genetests.org) (Chapter 15).

■ **TABLE 9-10.** Specific Electrocardiographic Findings

Finding	Disorder
Short PR interval, massively increased precordial activity, inverted T waves left precordium	Glycogen storage type II (Pompe)
Ventricular preexcitation	X-linked vacuolar cardiomyopathy and myopathy (Danon disease) Familial hypertrophic cardiomyopathy with Wolff-Parkinson-White syndrome
Prominent Q waves in leads I and aVL	Anomalous origin of the left coronary artery from the pulmonary artery
Low-voltage QRS complexes (< 5 mm total amplitude) in limb leads, diffuse T-wave abnormalities	Myocarditis

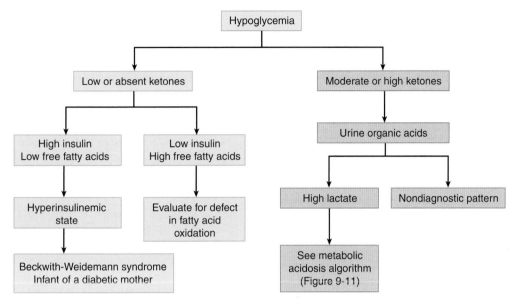

FIGURE 9-10. Algorithm for evaluation of cardiomyopathy associated with hypoglycemia. *Adapted from Schwartz ML, et al. Circulation. 1996;94:2021.*

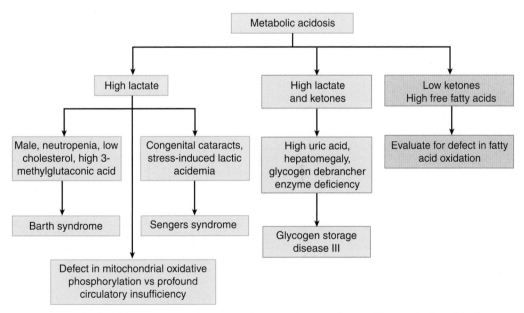

FIGURE 9-11. Algorithm for evaluation of cardiomyopathy associated with metabolic acidosis and an increased anion gap. *Adapted from Schwartz ML, et al. Circulation. 1996;94:2021.*

SUGGESTED READINGS

Hypertrophic Cardiomyopathy

Bos JM, Towbin JA, Ackerman MJ. Diagnostic, prognostic, and therapeutic implications of genetic testing for hypertrophic cardiomyopathy. *J Am Coll Cardiol.* 2009; 54(3):201-211.

Colan SD, Lipshultz SE, Lowe AM, et al. Epidemiology and cause-specific outcome of hypertrophic cardiomyopathy in children: findings from the Pediatric Cardiomyopathy Registry. *Circulation.* 2007;115(6):773-781.

Nugent AW, Daubeney PE, Chondros P, et al. Clinical features and outcomes of childhood hypertrophic cardiomyopathy: results from a national population-based study. *Circulation.* 2005;112(9):1332-1338.

Dilated Cardiomyopathy

Carballo S, Robinson P, Otway R, et al. Identification and functional characterization of cardiac troponin I as a novel disease gene in autosomal dominant dilated cardiomyopathy. *Circ Res.* 2009;105(4):375-382.

Daubeney PE, Nugent AW, Chondros P, et al. Clinical features and outcomes of childhood dilated cardiomyopathy: results from a national population-based study. *Circulation.* 2006;114(24):2671-2678.

Jefferies JL, Towbin JA. Dilated cardiomyopathy. *Lancet.* 2010;375:752-762.

Menon SC, Olson TM, Michels VV. Genetics of familial dilated cardiomyopathy. *Prog Pediatr Cardiol.* 2008; 25:57-67.

Morimoto S. Expanded spectrum of gene causing both hypertrophic cardiomyopathy and dilated cardiomyopathy. *Circ Res.* 2009;105(4):313-315.

Left Ventricular Noncompaction

Finsterer J. Cardiogenetics, neurogenetics, and pathogenetics of left ventricular hypertrabeculation/noncompaction. *Pediatr Cardiol.* 2009;30(5):659-681.

Klaassen S, Probst S, Oechslin E, et al. Mutations in sarcomere protein genes in left ventricular noncompaction. *Circulation.* 2008;117(22):2893-2901.

Disorders of Fatty Acid Oxidation

Bennett MJ. Pathophysiology of fatty acid oxidation disorders. *J Inherit Metab Dis.* Published online, October 2009 (DOI 10.1007/s10545-009-1294-6).

Exil VJ, Boles MA, Atkinson J, et al. Metabolic basis of pediatric heart disease. *Prog Pediatr Cardiol.* 2005;20:143-159.

Hill KD, Hamid R, Exil VJ. Pediatric cardiomyopathies related to fatty acid metabolism. *Prog Pediatr Cardiol.* 2008;25:69-78.

Rinaldo P, Matern D, Bennett MJ. Fatty acid oxidation disorders. *Annu Rev Physiol.* 2002;64:477-502.

Strauss AW, Andersen BS, Bennett MJ. Mitochondrial fatty acid oxidation defects. In: Sarafoglou K, Hoffman GF, Roth KS, eds. *Pediatric Endocrinology and Inborn Errors of Metabolism.* New York, NY: McGraw-Hill; 2009:51-70.

Disorders of Mitochondrial Oxidative Phosphorylation

Bernier FP, Boneh A, Dennett X, Chow CW, Cleary MA, Thorburn DR. Diagnostic criteria for respiratory chain disorders in adults and children. *Neurology.* 2002;59(9): 1406-1411.

DiMauro S, Schon EA. Mitochondrial respiratory-chain diseases. *N Engl J Med.* 2003; 348(26):2656-2668.

Gibson K, Halliday JL, Kirby DM, Yaplito-Lee J, Thorburn DR, Boneh A. Mitochondrial oxidative phosphorylation disorders presenting in neonates: clinical manifestations and enzymatic and molecular diagnoses. *Pediatrics.* 2008; 122(5): 1003-1008.

Haas RH, Parikh S, Falk MJ, et al. Mitochondrial disease: a practical approach for primary care physicians. *Pediatrics.* 2007;120(6):1326-1333.

Spencer CT, Bryant RM, Day J, et al. Cardiac and clinical phenotype in Barth syndrome. *Pediatrics.* 2006;118(2): e337-e346.

Yaplito-Lee J, Weintraub R, Jamsen K, Chow CW, Thorburn DR, Boneh A. Cardiac manifestations in oxidative phosphorylation disorders of childhood. *J Pediatr.* 2007;150(4): 407-411.

Storage Diseases

Burwinkel B, Scott JW, Buhrer C, et al. Fatal congenital heart glycogenosis caused by a recurrent activating R531Q mutation in the gamma 2-subunit of AMP-activated protein kinase (PRKAG2), not by phosphorylase kinase deficiency. *Am J Hum Genet.* 2005;76(6):1034-1049.

Kishnani PS, Corzo D, Leslie ND, et al. Early treatment with alglucosidase alpha prolongs long-term survival of infants with Pompe disease. *Pediatr Res.* 2009;66(3): 329-335.

Levine JC, Kishnani PS, Chen YT, Herlong JR, Li JS. Cardiac remodeling after enzyme replacement therapy with acid alpha-glucosidase for infants with Pompe disease. *Pediatr Cardiol.* 2008;29(6):1033-1042.

Maron BJ, Roberts WC, Arad M, et al. Clinical outcome and phenotypic expression in LAMP2 cardiomyopathy. *JAMA*. 2009;301(12):1253-1259.

Muenzer J, Wraith JE, Clarke LA. Mucopolysaccharidosis I: management and treatment guidelines. *Pediatrics*. 2009; 123(1):19-29.

Staretz-Chacham O, Lang TC, LaMarca ME, Krasnewich D, Sidransky E. Lysosomal storage disorders in the newborn. *Pediatrics*. 2009;123(4):1191-1207.

Miscellaneous

Colan SD. Classification of the cardiomyopathies. *Prog Pediatr Cardiol*. 2007;23:5-15.

Romano S, Valayannopoulos V, Touati G, et al. Cardiomy-opathies in propionic aciduria are reversible after liver transplantation. *J Pediatr*. 2010;156(1):128-134.

Schwartz ML, Cox GF, Lin AE, et al. Clinical approach to genetic cardiomyopathy in children. *Circulation*. 1996;94(8): 2021-2038.

Webber SA. Primary restrictive cardiomyopathy in child-hood. *Prog Pediatr Cardiol*. 2008;25:85-90.

Arrhythmias

■ INTRODUCTION

Although certain arrhythmias are more common in neonates and young infants compared to older children and adults, all types of arrhythmias can occur. Many are benign and do not cause hemodynamic compromise. Others may compromise cardiac output and cause decreased blood pressure and decreased perfusion. Sustained tachyarrhythmias may eventually cause myocardial dysfunction, which is known as tachycardia-induced cardiomyopathy.

The purpose of this chapter is to review diagnosis and management of common arrhythmias in neonates and young infants.

■ MECHANISMS OF ARRHYTHMIAS

Normally the electrical impulse originates in the sinoatrial (SA) node. The atrioventricular (AV) node, His bundle, and bundle branches provide the only normal pathway for transmission of impulses between the atria and ventricles.

Generation of impulses from the SA node is modulated by many factors including body temperature, blood pressure, autonomic nervous system, and circulating catecholamines. Conduction through the AV node is slowed so that atrial contraction is complete before ventricular contraction occurs.

Abnormal Impulse Formation

Abnormalities in impulse formation result in sinus bradycardia and tachycardia, premature atrial and ventricular contractions, and ectopic or automatic rhythms from the atria, AV node, or ventricles. Automatic tachycardias are usually incessant meaning that they are almost always present. Increased automaticity occurs when atrial, nodal, or ventricular cells display autonomous repetitive depolarization at a higher rate than is normal. Sinus tachycardia, atrial ectopic tachycardia, junctional ectopic tachycardia, and the automatic form of ventricular tachycardia are all forms of automatic tachycardia. Onset and termination are often gradual rather than abrupt. The rate of automatic tachycardias is often sensitive to changes in autonomic tone. Therapies that produce only transient effects, for example, direct current (DC) cardioversion and administration of adenosine, do not terminate automatic tachycardias.

Abnormal Impulse Conduction

Block within the normal conduction system is the most obvious form of abnormal impulse conduction. Block can occur at any point but atrioventricular block is most commonly seen.

Reentry, the other form of abnormal impulse conduction, is an important mechanism underlying supraventricular tachycardia (SVT) in infants. The reentrant circuit involves two functionally distinct pathways that have different conduction velocities and refractory periods. Unidirectional block is present in one pathway, an electrical impulse traverses the other pathway and conduction is delayed enough so that the impulse is able to "reenter" the blocked pathway from the other direction thus completing the reentrant circuit. Reentry mechanisms usually cause paroxysmal tachycardias, which may start and stop multiple times in the course of the day. Reentrant tachycardias start and stop abruptly and they often terminate in response to interventions that produce only transient effects (eg, adenosine) because interruption of the reentrant circuit usually terminates the tachycardia.

■ SINUS ARRHYTHMIA

Sinus arrhythmia is a normal phasic variation in impulse formation from the SA node that is often in cycle with respiration (Figure 10-1). This is the most common cause of an irregular heart rate, especially in older infants. The P-wave axis is usually normal. If substantial slowing occurs, junctional tissue depolarizes first and junctional escape beats may be seen. Sinus arrhythmia is more common at slower heart rates and is therefore more frequent in sleeping infants and in any patient with increased vagal tone (Table 10-1). This rhythm is a normal variant and no special monitoring or intervention is indicated.

■ BRADYARRHYTHMIAS

Sinus Bradycardia

The definition of sinus bradycardia depends on the method used to record the rhythm. An infant is usually stimulated by placement of the leads for a standard

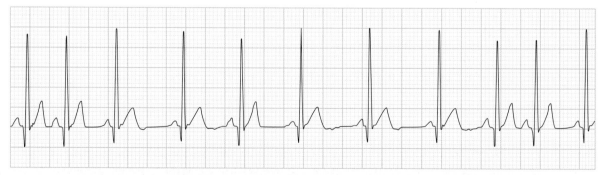

FIGURE 10-1. Sinus arrhythmia. The P-wave axis is normal and does not vary. The R-R interval varies from 400 to 700 milliseconds (86-150 beats/min).

■ **TABLE 10-1.** Causes of Increased Vagal Tone
Pharyngeal stimulation Gastric distention Upper airway obstruction Increased intracranial pressure Medication (including maternal, eg, bupivacaine) Valsalva during crying or straining

electrocardiogram (ECG), so bradycardia is usually defined as a heart rate < 100 beats/min. In contrast, the infant is much less stimulated during recording of a 24-hour electrocardiogram and sleeps during portions of the recording. During wakeful times, the average heart rate in young infants is 105 to 110 beats/min and the average minimum rate is in the low 90s. Based on these data, bradycardia in a neonate, defined as two standard deviations below the mean, is a heart rate of less than 80 beats/min while awake and less than 60 beats/min while asleep. This information has important implications for infants placed on apnea monitors. The alarm for low heart rate should not be set too high.

The most common cause of sinus bradycardia in neonates is increased vagal tone (Table 10-1). The next most common, especially in premature infants, is hypoxemia which may be related to apnea. Other causes of sinus bradycardia include hypothermia, drug therapy, and hypothyroidism. Infants with long QT syndrome often have slower heart rates so the QT interval corrected for heart rate (QTc) interval should be assessed carefully in all neonates with sinus bradycardia.

Rarely, infants with sinus bradycardia have familial bradycardia or tachycardia-bradycardia (sick sinus) syndrome.

These infants may need antiarrhythmic medication and/or pacemaker placement.

Atrioventricular (AV) Block

First-Degree AV Block

First-degree AV block is characterized by an abnormally long PR interval for age and heart rate. In neonates with normal heart rates, the upper limit of normal is 160 milliseconds on the first day of life and 140 milliseconds thereafter. According to these criteria, first-degree AV block is present in about 6% of normal newborn infants. First-degree AV block also results from decreased AV nodal conduction which is usually the result of medication (eg, digoxin) or from trauma/ischemia in patients who have had cardiac surgery. Treatment is not necessary, but further workup or monitoring may be required depending on the extent of first-degree AV block.

Second-Degree AV Block

Second degree AV block is defined as intermittent loss of AV conduction and is classified as Mobitz type I or Mobitz type II block. Mobitz type I (Wenckebach) block is characterized by gradual lengthening of the PR interval followed by a P wave without a subsequent QRS complex ("dropped beat"). This results in the typical "grouped QRSs" (Figure 10-2). Mobitz type I block is typically seen during sleep and in patients who have increased vagal tone (Table 10-1). No specific treatment is necessary.

Mobitz type II block is characterized by intermittent conduction of P waves and no prolongation of the PR interval before a dropped beat. Every other P wave is conducted in 2:1 block. Conduction may be lost for more than one P wave (eg, 3:1 block); this is called high-grade second-degree AV block and may progress to complete AV block.

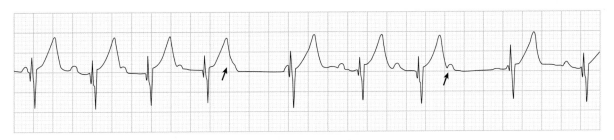

FIGURE 10-2. Second-degree atrioventricular block, Mobitz type I (Wenckebach block). Progressive lengthening of the PR interval is present before the nonconducted or dropped beats occur (arrows).

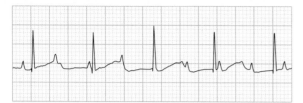

FIGURE 10-3. Electrocardiographic pattern of 2:1 AV block caused by prolonged ventricular refractoriness associated with a prolonged QT interval. Every other P wave is conducted to the ventricles. The corrected QT interval is 550 milliseconds.

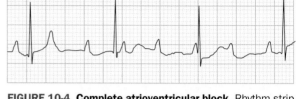

FIGURE 10-4. Complete atrioventricular block. Rhythm strip recorded in a neonate shows that P waves and QRS complexes are independent of each other. The atrial rate is 145 beats/min and the ventricular rate is 62 beats/min. The QRS complex is narrow.

This rhythm is uncommon in newborn infants and is thought to be related to block in the bundle of His. It can occur in infants born to mothers with connective tissue disease, in infants with congenital heart disease (eg, l-looped ventricles), and in infants who have had cardiac surgery. Mobitz type II block may progress to complete AV block, and for this reason, these patients must be observed closely. Patients with Mobitz type II block and a wide QRS complex should be considered for permanent pacemaker placement.

At times an electrocardiographic pattern of 2:1 AV block is associated with marked prolongation of the QTc interval and is caused by the very prolonged ventricular refractory period associated with the long QT interval (Figure 10-3). This can be caused by electrolyte disorders, especially hypocalcemia. Alternatively, although rare, patients may have congenital prolonged QT syndrome and will need aggressive treatment because the risk of sudden death is high even in asymptomatic patients.

Complete (Third-Degree) AV Block

Complete or third-degree AV block is characterized by failure of all atrial impulses to be conducted to the ventricle. Generally the atrial rhythm (P wave) is completely dissociated from the ventricular rhythm (QRS complex) (Figure 10-4). The atrial rate is normal for age and responds to chronotropic stimuli such as pain and arousal. The QRS complexes are regular and the heart rate, which varies little, is usually 60 to 80 beats/min in neonates. The QRS complexes may be narrow if the escape rhythm originates near the AV node and impulses flow down the normal ventricular conduction system, or wide if the escape rhythm originates from below the bundle of His. The onset of complete AV block in neonates is usually during fetal life and the condition is called congenital complete AV block

(CCAVB). If the heart is structurally normal, CCAVB is often associated with maternal collagen vascular disease such as systemic lupus erythematosus or Sjögren syndrome. Maternal autoantibodies to SSA/Ro and SSB/La proteins cross the placenta and interact with the developing conduction system. In addition to CCAVB, affected infants may show signs of neonatal lupus including discoid lesions, leukopenia, thrombocytopenia, and hemolytic anemia. Many mothers have no signs or symptoms so all mothers who have offspring with CCAVB and no structural heart abnormalities should be evaluated for connective tissue diseases. The incidence of CCAVB is 5% in offspring of mothers who have anti-Ro and Anti-La antibodies.

Newborns with CCAVB are often asymptomatic because stroke volume increases to compensate for the decreased ventricular rate and thus cardiac output is maintained. Infants with structurally normal hearts who are born with or develop congestive heart failure respond well to supportive therapy although the presence of hydrops fetalis and cardiac enlargement are risk factors for poor outcome. Inotropic agents such as isoproterenol and pacemaker placement are often necessary. Although rare, bradycardia may be severe at birth and produce signs and symptoms of inadequate cardiac output. In those cases, emergency pacing is necessary in the delivery room. This can be accomplished by placement of a temporary transvenous pacemaker or pacing by use of transcutaneous pacing electrodes until a permanent pacemaker is placed.

Criteria for pacemaker placement in neonates and young infants with CCAVB include congestive heart failure, cardiomegaly and/or ventricular dysfunction, premature ventricular contractions or ventricular tachycardia, prolonged QTc interval, and a wide complex (ventricular) instead of narrow complex (junctional) escape rhythm. Controversy exists as to whether a pacemaker should be placed in neonates solely because of a slow ventricular rate (< 55 beats/min). As many as 20% of those with CCAVB diagnosed during fetal life or shortly after birth may be at risk of developing dilated cardiomyopathy during childhood; the presence of maternal antibodies is likely a risk factor. Serial follow-up of ventricular function is important in these patients.

Heart disease including *levo-* or corrected transposition of the great arteries, heterotaxy syndrome (left atrial isomerism), and atrioventricular septal defects is present in about 50% of infants with CCAVB. These infants occasionally develop nonimmune hydrops. Despite aggressive treatment, the prognosis is poor in infants with complex heart disease and CCAVB.

Complete AV block may also occur after cardiac surgery especially in those patients with l-loop or in those who have had surgery involving the ventricular septum (eg, tetralogy of Fallot, ventricular septal defect, or atrioventricular septal defect). Permanent pacemaker placement is always indicated for postoperative patients in whom complete AV heart block related to cardiac surgery does not resolve within 10 to 14 days. Temporary pacing (transvenous, transcutaneous, temporary pacing wires) may be indicated and, rarely, isoproterenol infusion is necessary before a permanent pacemaker is placed. The threshold for the temporary pacer lead must be checked daily; a patient who has an inadequate underlying rhythm and high-pacing threshold should be considered for immediate permanent pacemaker placement.

■ TACHYARRHYTHMIAS

Sinus Tachycardia

Sinus tachycardia is characterized by a normal P-wave axis (upright in lead II) and a rate as high as 240 beats/min in neonates (Figure 10-5). Variability in the rate is common. Sinus tachycardia is usually caused by some other problem in neonates, for example, hypovolemia, fever, hypoxemia, sympathomimetic medications, anemia, pain, and inadequate sedation. When the heart rate is >170 to 180 beats/min, P waves may be difficult to see because they are superimposed on the preceding T wave. Sometimes vagal maneuvers (see following text) will transiently decrease the heart rate enough that sinus rhythm can be more easily identified. Neither vagal maneuvers, administration of adenosine, or DC cardioversion will terminate sinus tachycardia. Instead, treatment should address the underlying cause of tachycardia. For example, administration of analgesia to a postoperative patient in pain will decrease the heart rate and confirm sinus rhythm.

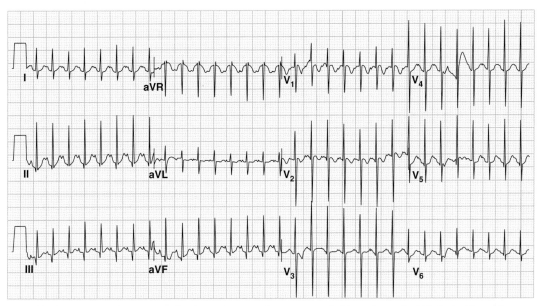

FIGURE 10-5. Sinus tachycardia. The electrocardiogram recorded in a 2-month-old infant with septic shock shows P waves in almost every lead. The heart rate is 230 beats/min. The P-wave axis is normal.

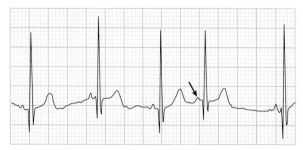

FIGURE 10-6. Premature atrial contraction (arrow).

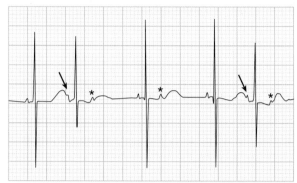

FIGURE 10-7. Premature atrial contractions. Lead II rhythm strip showing frequent blocked premature atrial contractions. P waves falling at the end of the T wave (arrow) are conducted to ventricles with aberration. The premature P waves falling within the ST segment or on the upstroke of the T wave are not conducted to the ventricles or blocked (*). The frequent blocked premature beats caused asymptomatic bradycardia in this neonate.

Premature Atrial Contractions

Premature atrial contractions (PAC) (supraventricular premature contractions) are early P waves (Figure 10-6). They are most commonly an incidental finding in infants who have been placed on cardiac monitors for other reasons. The morphology of the P wave may be different than that of the normal sinus P wave and reflects the ectopic origin of the impulse within the atrium. At times the P wave may be superimposed on the preceding T wave. Most often PACs are conducted normally to the ventricles and the QRS complex is normal. Occasionally there is conduction with aberrancy; a bundle branch pattern with a wide QRS complex is seen because the bundle branch is still refractory from the previous depolarization. If the premature P wave is very early, it will not be conducted to the ventricles because the AV node or proximal His bundle is refractory; this is called a blocked PAC. This will tend to slow the heart rate and frequent blocked PACs can cause bradycardia (Figure 10-7). Iatrogenic causes include endocardial irritation from an intracardiac catheter or extracorporeal membrane oxygenation cannula and effects of pharmacologic agents such as caffeine, theophylline, dopamine, epinephrine, and isoproterenol. Rarely, electrolyte or metabolic abnormalities, cardiac tumors, myocarditis, or structural heart disease is present. Possible predisposing conditions should be treated but a specific etiology is not determined in most cases. Even if frequent, PACs do not cause hemodynamic compromise and do not need to be treated. A healthy newborn infant who does not have any risk factors and who has a normal physical examination does not require further workup. PACs may occur in up to one-third of neonates and usually disappear within the first to third months of life.

Supraventricular Tachycardia: Reentrant

SVT is an abnormal tachycardia that requires atrial or AV nodal tissue for initiation and maintenance. This is the most common arrhythmia in infants and children and the incidence has been estimated to be as low as 1/25,000 and as high as 1/250 infants.

AV Reciprocating (Accessory Pathway-Mediated) Tachycardia

More than 75% of SVT in infants is related to an accessory AV pathway. Accessory pathways are anomalous bands of tissue that form an extra electrical connection between the atrium and the ventricle. Many accessory pathways will conduct from the atrium to the ventricle (antegrade) and from the ventricle to the atrium (retrograde). Patients in whom conduction occurs antegrade across the accessory pathway have preexcitation with a short PR interval and a delta wave. SVT and preexcitation is known as Wolff-Parkinson-White syndrome (WPW; Figure 10-8). Preexcitation may be difficult to perceive on the electrocardiogram in infants because of the rapid conduction through the AV node. In addition, up to one-third of patients with WPW show intermittent preexcitation, and thus some of their tracings may appear normal. The electrical impulse from the SA node passes through both the AV node and the accessory AV pathway. Impulses

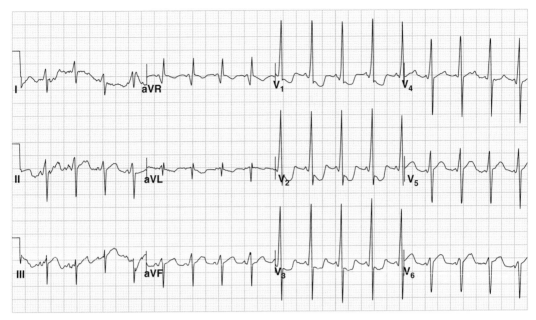

FIGURE 10-8. Wolff-Parkinson-White syndrome. The short PR interval (80 ms) and a delta wave are present in multiple leads which is consistent with preexcitation.

passing through the AV node are delayed as in normal conduction; the impulse passing through the accessory pathway is not delayed and thus the early ("preexcited") ventricular activation is reflected by the short PR interval and the slurred early QRS delta wave (Figure 10-9B). In other patients, the accessory pathway does not conduct in an antegrade manner. These patients have a normal ECG and what is known as a "concealed" accessory pathway (Figure 10-9C). This mechanism is responsible for more than half the SVT that occurs in infants. Most infants (60%-90%) will not have recurrent SVT beyond 1 year of age.

During an episode of abnormal tachycardia a reentry circuit forms between the AV node and the accessory pathway (Figure 10-9D). This is often triggered by a premature atrial contraction that travels normally through the AV node but is blocked in the accessory pathway. The impulse from the ventricle is then conducted retrograde in the accessory pathway back to the atrium, thus completing the reentrant circuit. The atrium is reactivated by the retrograde impulse and, in this manner, the reentrant circuit becomes self-perpetuating and thus sustains the abnormal tachycardia. The QRS complex is normal because the normal pathway is used for antegrade conduction, producing

the normal sequence of ventricular activation. The accessory pathway is used for retrograde conduction to maintain the reentry loop. This is the most common form of reentrant SVT and is called orthodromic reciprocating tachycardia (Figure 10-9D). When the impulse travels in the other direction, that is forward through the accessory pathway and retrograde through the AV node, the QRS is wide because of the abnormal sequence of ventricular activation. This is called antidromic reciprocating tachycardia and can be mistaken for ventricular tachycardia because of the wide QRS complex (Figure 10-9E).

AV Nodal Reentrant Tachycardia

The reentrant circuit in AV nodal reentrant tachycardia also involves two pathways but in this case one pathway is within the AV node and the other is a distinctly different pathway that may be within the AV node or a few millimeters outside the AV node (Figure 10-9F). The effective refractory period of one pathway is longer than that of the other pathway. This allows initiation of reentrant tachycardia when a premature atrial contraction is blocked in the pathway with the longer refractory period. This occurs rarely in infants but is the most common mechanism for SVT in adult patients.

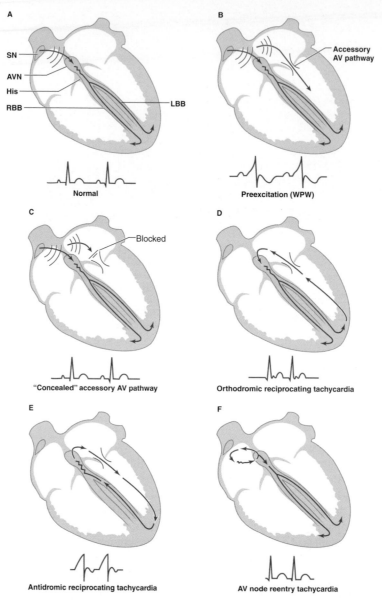

FIGURE 10-9. Mechanisms for conduction. A. Normal. Conduction in sinus rhythm. **B. Wolff-Parkinson-White (WPW) syndrome.** The impulse from the sinoatrial node passes through both the atrioventricular (AV) node and the accessory pathway. There is no delay within the accessory pathway so the early or "pre-excited" ventricular activation produces a short PR interval and the delta wave as seen on the ECG. **C. "Concealed" accessory AV pathway.** If the accessory pathway is blocked during sinus rhythm, the ECG is normal, because conduction is antegrade through the normal conduction system. **D. Orthodromic reciprocating tachycardia.** Normal antegrade conduction through the AV node results in a normal QRS complex. The reentrant circuit is completed by retrograde conduction through the accessory AV pathway which results in atrial activation shortly after ventricular depolarization (note the abnormal P waves just after the QRS complexes). **E. Antidromic reciprocating tachycardia.** Conduction is antegrade through the accessory pathway and retrograde through the AV node. The abnormal sequence of ventricular depolarization causes a wide QRS complex and P waves are often difficult to see on the surface ECG. This rhythm can be mistaken for ventricular tachycardia. **F. AV node reentry tachycardia.** Typically slow antegrade conduction occurs through a posterior "pathway" of atrial tissue (wavy line) and retrograde conduction travels via a "fast" pathway involving more anterior aspects of the AV node. The P waves are not seen; they are buried in the QRS complex because atrial and ventricular activation occur simultaneously. Abbreviations: AVN, atrioventricular node; His, His bundle; LBB, left bundle branch; RBB, right bundle branch; SN, sinoatrial node.

Permanent Junctional Reciprocating Tachycardia

In the permanent form of junctional reciprocating tachycardia (PJRT), the accessory pathway is concealed and conducts slowly in the retrograde direction. The rate is usually slower than typical SVT with rates of 180 to 200 beats/min in neonates. PJRT may be present as an incessant tachycardia during fetal life. The rate is more variable than most reentrant tachycardias because both limbs of the circuit are influenced by autonomic tone. Initially this tachycardia is fairly well tolerated because of the slower heart rate but eventually a tachycardia-induced dilated cardiomyopathy may develop. The ECG shows an abnormal superior P-wave axis, usually a negative P wave in lead II and an upright P wave in lead aVL. During tachycardia the interval from the R wave to the next P wave is relatively long; the P wave is located closer to the subsequent QRS complex than the previous one (Figure 10-10). This form of reentrant SVT responds less well to the usual medications (see following text). Flecainide and other medications may be efficacious in some patients, but others are refractory to medical management and will need to undergo ablation by a pediatric electrophysiologist.

Clinical Features

Typically the onset of reentrant tachycardia is sudden. If the tachycardia converts to sinus rhythm (either spontaneously or in response to therapy), there is an abrupt cessation of tachycardia, rather than a gradual slowing in heart rate. In infants, the heart rate is usually > 250 beats/min, and is often about 300 beats/min but it can be as low as 150 beats/min. Infants will generally tolerate these rapid heart rates initially, but after 36 to 72 hours signs and symptoms of heart failure develop. Cardiac output becomes compromised in part because the decreased duration of diastole interferes with coronary arterial flow to the myocardium. Infants with SVT rarely present in cardiogenic shock.

Patients with accessory bypass pathways typically have structurally normal hearts. However, 8% to 25% have structural heart disease, most commonly Ebstein malformation of the tricuspid valve or *levo-* or corrected transposition of the great arteries.

ECG Findings and Differential Diagnosis

The typical ECG shows a regular and narrow QRS tachycardia (Figure 10-11). P waves are often not visible. If visible, the P waves located just before the QRS complex are usually less prominent than normal and often are negative in leads II, III, and aVF (typical findings in PJRT). Retrograde P waves (seen within or just after the QRS complex) are also sometimes present (Figure 10-12). Sometimes the first few beats of SVT are wide because of aberrant conduction and then the QRS complex becomes narrow.

The most important differential diagnosis is sinus tachycardia. The maximal heart rate is usually < 240 beats/min in patients with sinus tachycardia. A normal P wave (upright in lead II) is suggestive of sinus tachycardia. Any patient with an increased heart rate should be evaluated for remediable causes of sinus tachycardia such as fever, anemia, pain, sympathomimetic medications, etc. Variability in the heart rate, for example, during crying or blood drawing, is consistent with sinus tachycardia. Sometimes administration of adenosine will transiently decrease the heart rate enough that sinus rhythm can be more easily identified. Other causes of narrow QRS tachycardia are discussed in the following text (Table 10-5).

Treatment

The AV node is an essential part of the reentry circuit in many patients with SVT and thus therapy directed toward slowing conduction through the AV node is often effective in breaking the tachycardia. Even if the AV node is not involved, slowing conduction through the AV node may

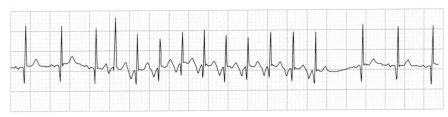

FIGURE 10-10. Persistent junctional reciprocating tachycardia. Rhythm strip shows intermittent narrow-complex tachycardia initiated by a premature ectopic beat. The RP interval is long (see text).

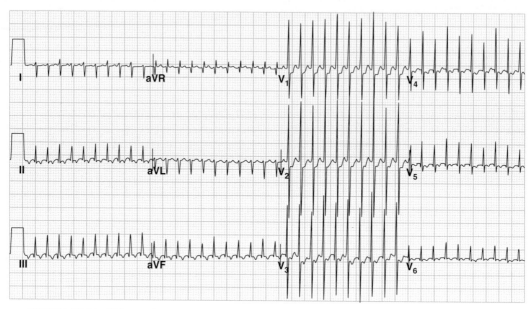

FIGURE 10-11. Atrioventricular reciprocating tachycardia (SVT). The QRS complex is normal. The heart rate is 315 beats/min.

decrease the ventricular rate thereby revealing the mechanism of the tachycardia. In either case, it is very important to record a rhythm strip during all attempts to break an episode of tachycardia.

Vagal maneuvers are the simplest, quickest, and safest way to break an episode of reentrant tachycardia. For patients < 12 months of age, application of an ice slurry to the forehead induces strong vagal stimulation (diving reflex). Ice and water are put in a glove or washcloth which is placed over the patient's forehead, eyes, and bridge of the nose. It is important not to cover the nose or mouth and not to press on the eyes. Contact between the ice slurry and upper face is maintained for 10 to 20 seconds. This may be repeated several times, but if this maneuver is performed correctly, it usually is effective on the first or second attempt. Repeated ice applications may cause skin burns in neonates, so care should be taken. Nasogastric stimulation or stimulation of a gag reflex may also be

effective but carotid massage is a much less effective vagal maneuver in young infants. Pressure should never be applied to the eyes because of the risk of retinal detachment.

Synchronized DC cardioversion is the treatment of choice for SVT in critically ill infants (very low or not measurable blood pressure, nonpalpable pulses, poor perfusion, and altered level of consciousness). The initial energy is 0.5 J/kg and this may be increased to 1 to 2 J/kg if there is no response to the first attempt. If however, this higher discharge energy is not effective, or tachycardia recurs immediately, DC cardioversion should not be repeated. Instead, pharmacologic therapy or overdrive pacing should be considered.

For infants in whom vagal maneuvers, adenosine, and/or cardioversion have resulted in only transient or no termination of the arrhythmia, drugs such as β-adrenergic blocking agents (eg, esmolol or propranolol), class I antiarrhythmic agents (eg, procainamide or flecainide), or class III agents (eg, sotalol or amiodarone) may be useful. Administration of intravenous verapamil is contraindicated in patients younger than 1 year of age (see following text).

Placing an electrode in the esophagus to record an atrial electrogram can be helpful in defining the precise mechanism of SVT and can also be used by a pediatric cardiologist to terminate SVT by overdrive pacing (pacing the atria

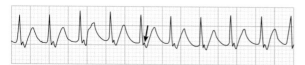

FIGURE 10-12. Atrioventricular reciprocating tachycardia. The rhythm strip shows retrograde P waves (arrow).

at a rate somewhat higher than the rate of the SVT for a brief period of time). This method of terminating SVT can be very effective while waiting for plasma concentrations of antiarrhythmic medications to become high enough to prevent reinitiation of tachycardia, and can be performed repetitively with low risk of adverse effect.

Prophylactic antiarrhythmic therapy is indicated for most infants with SVT because 20% to 30% will have more than one episode of SVT. Digoxin is commonly used in patients without evidence of preexcitation. In adults and older children with WPW (SVT and preexcitation) digoxin is contraindicated because it may increase conduction through the accessory pathway thereby permitting a very rapid ventricular rate during atrial fibrillation. Although atrial fibrillation is rare in newborns, some cardiologists prefer to use β-adrenergic blocking agents such as propranolol or atenolol as initial therapy for newborns with preexcitation. Some patients may require treatment with more than one agent. Digoxin and atenolol are very useful in patients who do not have preexcitation. Patient refractory to therapy may be treated with sotalol, flecainide, or amiodarone. All of these agents have important toxicities (see following text).

The recurrence rate of neonatal SVT after 6 to 12 months of age is less than 50%. Therefore, antiarrhythmic therapy may be discontinued after this time period in patients without signs of recurrence. In patients with recurrent SVT, oral medication is continued until they are older and the risks of ablation therapy are lower. Ablation therapy is only indicated for infants with symptomatic SVT refractory to medical management.

Atrial Flutter

Atrial flutter is a reentrant rhythm that is confined to the atrium. Atrial flutter is relatively rare in young infants and if it occurs in neonates, the heart is usually structurally normal. The flutter rate depends on the rate of conduction within the reentrant circuit and the length of the circuit, but is usually quite rapid (375-500 beats/min) in neonates and infants. The ventricular response is variable but 2:1 and 3:1 AV block are common. If the atrial rate and degree of block are such that the ventricular rate is ≥ 250 beats/min, congestive heart failure may occur. The typical ECG shows flutter waves that are P waves which give a sawtooth appearance to the baseline (Figure 10-13A). This may be difficult to discern in the presence of 2:1 AV block. A definite diagnosis can be made either by increasing AV block transiently, for example, by administering adenosine, or by performing transesophageal ECG recordings to facilitate visualization

of the flutter waves (Figure 10-13B). The R-R interval is constant except when the degree of AV block changes.

Although adenosine is sometimes helpful in establishing the diagnosis, this agent does not convert atrial flutter to sinus rhythm because the reentrant circuit does not involve the AV node. Neonates with structurally normal hearts and atrial flutter represent a special group of patients in that once flutter has been terminated, it rarely recurs, and long-term therapy is almost never needed. Atrial flutter in these neonates can be converted to sinus rhythm by use of overdrive pacing or DC cardioversion and no pharmacologic therapy is necessary. If pharmacologic therapy is preferred, digoxin is the first drug of choice because this agent decreases conduction through the AV node, thus increasing the degree of AV block and decreasing the ventricular rate. Digoxin often does not convert atrial flutter to sinus rhythm. To achieve this, overdrive pacing, DC cardioversion, or addition of procainamide may be necessary. Some neonates who have had atrial flutter subsequently develop supraventricular tachycardia. For older infants or those who have had cardiac surgery, digoxin or β-adrenergic blocking agents are administered to slow conduction of the flutter through the AV node. Overdrive atrial pacing from the esophagus usually terminates atrial flutter. DC cardioversion (initial dose 0.5-1 J/kg) is also therapeutic. Sotalol or amiodarone are used if necessary to prevent recurrence.

Supraventricular Tachycardia: Automatic

Atrial Ectopic Tachycardia

Rarely in infants, cells in the atrium undergo diastolic depolarization faster than the cells in the SA node. When this occurs, an incessant atrial ectopic tachycardia (AET) can develop. The P-wave morphology is often different from the normal sinus P wave because of the ectopic origin of the atrial impulse (Figure 10-14). In contrast to reentrant SVT, the onset and termination of AET are often gradual, and the rate is variable. AET may occur during fetal life and may cause hydrops fetalis. Neonates are not usually symptomatic immediately but this rhythm may cause a dilated cardiomyopathy and congestive heart failure after several months. AV block, such as that induced by adenosine, does not terminate this tachycardia, but can transiently slow the ectopic rhythm which may facilitate identification of the mechanism of the tachycardia. Intravenous infusion of the short-acting β-adrenergic blocking agent, esmolol, is often useful in controlling the heart rate acutely. It is usually impossible to eradicate this rhythm; a more reasonable goal of therapy is to decrease

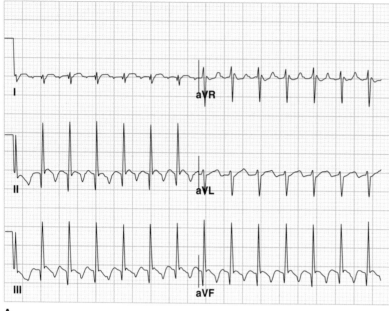

A

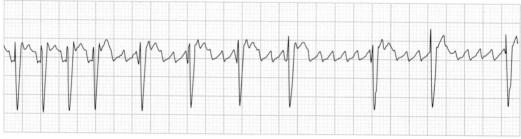

B

FIGURE 10-13. Atrial flutter. A. Negative flutter waves are present in lead II. The flutter rate is 400 beats/min and there is 2:1 AV block. **B.** Administration of adenosine increases AV block and facilitates visualization of the flutter waves. The flutter rate in this patient is 460 beats/min.

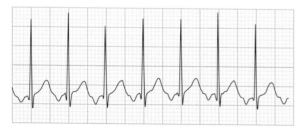

FIGURE 10-14. Atrial ectopic tachycardia. Negative P waves are present in this lead II rhythm strip.

the ventricular rate so that ventricular dysfunction associated with chronic tachycardia does not occur. A variety of oral agents including propranolol, atenolol, and sotalol are administered to patients with AET. Amiodarone is used in refractory cases. AET resolves spontaneously in many young patients. Definitive therapy involves catheter ablation of the ectopic focus, but because important long-term adverse effects may occur in small infants, this is reserved for those who do not respond to medical therapy. In surgical excision the ectopic focus has been reported.

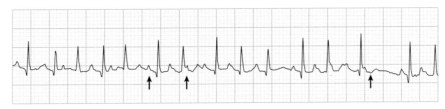

FIGURE 10-15. Chaotic atrial rhythm. Rhythm strip shows irregular P waves with differing morphologies consistent with. The R-R interval is irregular because of variable AV conduction.

Chaotic or Multifocal Atrial Tachycardia

Chaotic atrial tachycardia is a very rare tachycardia associated with three or more distinct P-wave morphologies (Figure 10-15). AV conduction is variable and so the QRS complexes are irregularly irregular. The onset and termination are gradual and the rate is variable. The exact mechanism of this arrhythmia is unknown; it may involve multiple ectopic foci or reentrant circuits. This arrhythmia may resolve spontaneously in infants and asymptomatic infants may not need therapy. Control of this arrhythmia is difficult and antiarrhythmic agents are not consistently beneficial, but rate control with digoxin, propranolol, or other agents can be useful if the infant develops ventricular dysfunction or is compromised by rapid ventricular response.

Junctional Ectopic Tachycardia

Junctional ectopic tachycardia (JET) is an automatic rhythm arising from the AV node or bundle of His. The QRS complex is narrow and JET is the only narrow QRS tachycardia in which the ventricular rate is higher than the atrial rate. The presence of AV dissociation confirms the diagnosis of JET (Figure 10-16).

JET is an incessant tachycardia and similar to AET. JET may cause tachycardia-induced cardiomyopathy. When

present during fetal life, JET may be associated with hydrops fetalis. Many cases are familial. Some patients eventually develop complete AV block. Congenital JET is very difficult to treat and does not respond to DC cardioversion, overdrive pacing, or routine medical therapy. Amiodarone is the most effective agent, although β-adrenergic blocking drugs or flecainide may control the heart rate adequately in some patients. Catheter ablation of the ectopic junctional focus is the best treatment available at the present time for patients who do not respond to pharmacologic therapy. Cryoablation is the preferred approach to minimize the risk of complete heart block (see following text).

Although JET is a rare rhythm in patients with structurally normal hearts, it may be seen in patients during the first few days after cardiac surgery. In patients who already have decreased cardiac reserve after surgery, the tachycardia combined with loss of the normal AV activation sequence often causes important hemodynamic compromise. Since this is an automatic tachycardia, treatment it is often difficult. Unfortunately, decreased blood pressure and perfusion which frequently occurs in the postoperative patient often causes caregivers to increase the doses of sympathomimetic medications which further predispose to JET.

For postoperative patients with JET, cooling the core temperature to 35°C is often effective in decreasing the rate. Decreasing the doses of sympathomimetic agents, correcting acidosis, normalizing electrolytes (including magnesium), and eliminating vagolytic agents (depolarizing muscle relaxants) may also be beneficial. Digoxin may also decrease the ventricular rate but benefit is often limited. If the ventricular rate is not too high, pacing the atrium at a slightly higher rate will restore AV synchrony and improve cardiac output. Intravenous amiodarone is efficacious in patients who are hemodynamically unstable. Procainamide is also sometimes effective. JET

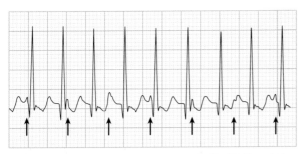

FIGURE 10-16. Junctional ectopic tachycardia. AV dissociation is present. P waves are indicated by the arrows. The atrial rate is 135 beats/min and the ventricular rate is 185 beats/min.

in postoperative patients is usually transient so control is necessary for only a limited period of time.

Premature Ventricular Contractions

A premature ventricular contraction (PVC) (ventricular premature beat) is a premature ventricular complex of different morphology from that of the sinus beat (Figure 10-17). It is not preceded by a P wave. In newborn infants, the QRS complex associated with a PVC may not be much wider than the normal QRS complex. PVCs with the same morphology are called uniform, and PVCs with different morphologies are called multiform. It is sometimes difficult to distinguish a PAC with aberrant conduction from a PVC. A fusion beat can result from near simultaneous activation of the ventricles from a supraventricular site (often the SA node) and an ectopic site in the ventricle; the morphology of the fusion beat is intermediate between the normal and the wide QRS. The presence of fusion beats confirms the ventricular origin of the premature beats. PVCs are relatively uncommon in newborn infants; PACs are much more common. Sometimes PVCs are related to administration of drugs such as caffeine, sympathomimetic agents, digoxin, or antiarrhythmic agents.

An infant with PVCs should be evaluated for metabolic abnormalities (hyperkalemia, hypokalemia, hypoxia, acidosis, hypoglycemia), the congenital long QT syndrome, myocarditis, cardiac tumors, and structural heart disease. Most often these studies are normal and no specific etiology is identified. No specific therapy is indicated for isolated uniform PVCs. There are no data suggesting that the morphology or frequency of PVCs influences outcome and they usually resolve over the first 2 months of life. Persistence of PVCs beyond 2 months of age should prompt additional investigation but may still have a benign prognosis. Multiform PVCs at any age require further investigation.

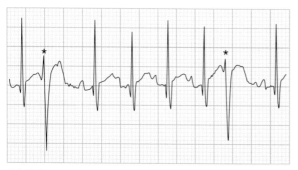

FIGURE 10-17. Premature ventricular contractions (∗).

Ventricular Tachycardia

Ventricular tachycardia is a wide-QRS complex rhythm usually resulting from reentry with the ventricle. In neonates the QRS complex may not appear as wide as in older children and adults. The QRS duration is between 60 and 110 milliseconds in patients who do not show much widening. Ventricular tachycardia should be recognized by altered QRS morphology during tachycardia when compared to the QRS complex during sinus rhythm. The rate should be at least 20% greater than the normal sinus rate; this distinguishes ventricular tachycardia from accelerated idioventricular rhythm. Additionally, abnormal repolarization causes the polarity of the T waves to be opposite that of the QRS complex (Figure 10-18). Nonsustained ventricular tachycardia is defined as a run of ventricular complexes lasting from three beats to 30 seconds and sustained ventricular tachycardia is a run lasting more than 30 seconds. Ventricular tachycardia with a uniform QRS complex morphology is described as "monomorphic." Polymorphic ventricular tachycardia is characterized by varying morphologies of the QRS complexes.

Ventricular tachycardia is sometimes difficult to differentiate from supraventricular rhythm, for example, SVT conducted with aberrancy. The presence of P waves which are dissociated from the QRS complexes usually confirms the ventricular origin of the tachycardia. However, retrograde ventricular-to-atrial conduction is often present in infants with ventricular tachycardia. The presence of intermittent sinus capture beats (dissociated sinus beats occurring at a time when conduction through the AV node to the ventricles is possible) or fusion beats with tachycardia is highly suggestive that the tachycardia is of ventricular origin.

Ventricular tachycardia is relatively uncommon in neonates. Causes include electrolyte and metabolic abnormalities, myocarditis, drug toxicity, prolonged QT syndrome, maternal cocaine and heroin abuse, CNS lesions, myocardial tumors, scarring from previous surgery, and ischemia, usually related to congenital heart defects such as anomalous origin of the left coronary artery from the pulmonary artery or severe aortic stenosis.

Incessant ventricular tachycardia (present 10%-90% of the day) in infancy is often difficult to treat. Most commonly pharmacologic therapy does not decrease the amount of time that the patient is in tachycardia. Tachycardia-induced cardiomyopathy can develop if the rate is not at least partially controlled. These infants often have associated myocarditis or myocardial fibrosis. Microscopic Purkinje cell tumors have been found in some

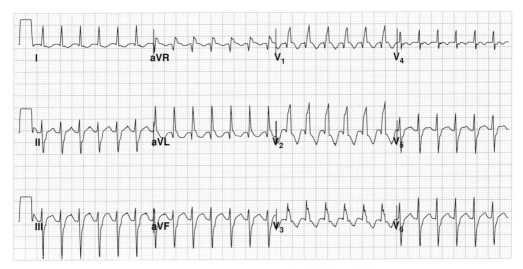

FIGURE 10-18. Ventricular tachycardia. The heart rate is 195 beats/min.

patients. These and other myocardial tumors may not be seen on an echocardiographic examination. MRI is sometimes helpful in visualizing tumors but often the diagnosis is confirmed only at the time of surgery. Some of these patients have undergone mapping and then excision and/or cryoablation of the tachycardia site.

Another form of ventricular tachycardia is an ectopic focus tachycardia often seen in infants called accelerated idioventricular rhythm. This is distinguished from more typical ventricular tachycardia by a slower rate which is about 10% above the sinus rate. Idioventricular rhythm is associated with sinus slowing and frequent transitions between sinus and ventricular rhythms are seen (Figure 10-19). This likely reflects increased automaticity of a ventricular focus. AV dissociation is typically seen. Although there is loss of the normal AV activation sequence, the rate is low enough that

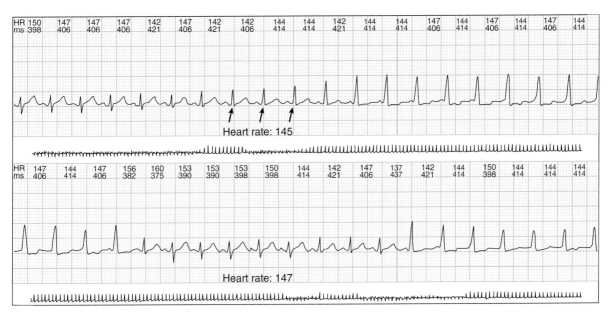

FIGURE 10-19. The rhythm strip shows sinus rhythm gradually transitioning to accelerated idioventricular rhythm. The rate is about the same as the sinus rate. Fusion beats are evident (arrows).

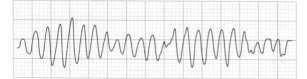

FIGURE 10-20. Torsade de pointes.

hemodynamic compromise does not occur. These infants are asymptomatic and specific therapy is not required. This arrhythmia usually resolves within a few months.

Torsade de pointes ("twisting of the points") is a particular form of ventricular tachycardia in which the morphology of the QRS complex is constantly changing such that it appears to spiral around the baseline (Figure 10-20). This rhythm is usually associated with underlying prolongation of the QT interval.

Treatment

Sustained ventricular tachycardia is a medical emergency. A brief history, vital signs, assessment of peripheral pulses and perfusion, laboratory studies, and a complete ECG should be obtained if the clinical situation permits. Reversible causes of ventricular tachycardia should be treated immediately. Medications that may cause ventricular tachycardia should be discontinued if possible.

Any patient who is hypotensive and unconscious should undergo immediate DC cardioversion with 1 to 2 J/kg. If the first shock is not successful, the energy should be doubled and repeated once or twice but not more.

If the patient is conscious and has reasonably stable vital signs, or if DC cardioversion is unsuccessful, intravenous amiodarone at 5 mg/kg should be administered as an infusion over 20 to 60 minutes. Procainamide at 15 mg/kg may be given instead, over 10 to 15 minutes. Esmolol may also be administered as necessary. Verapamil and digoxin are absolutely contraindicated for emergency treatment of ventricular tachycardia. Extracorporeal membrane oxygenation should be considered for ventricular tachycardia resistant to medical management. Magnesium sulfate infusion is the drug of choice for recurrent torsade de pointes. Administration of esmolol and overdrive pacing have reportedly also been effective.

A variety of agents are available for long-term suppression of ventricular tachycardia. β-Adrenergic blocking agents are the drugs of choice for patients with long QT syndrome. For other causes of ventricular tachycardia,

β-adrenergic blocking agents are often used in combination with other agents such as procainamide, mexiletine, sotalol, or amiodarone. Some asymptomatic infants, particularly those with accelerated idioventricular rhythm, do not need therapy.

Long QT Syndrome

The long QT syndrome is an abnormality of ventricular repolarization that is often inherited and is characterized by a prolonged QT interval on the electrocardiogram, polymorphic ventricular tachycardia (torsade de pointes), and sudden death. This syndrome is genetically heterogeneous and is caused most commonly by mutations in genes that encode various cardiac ion channels that regulate potassium, sodium, or calcium currents in the ventricle. These mutations can result in synthesis of nonfunctional channels or alter channel characteristics such that ion current is either increased or decreased (Table 10-2). Homozygous or compound heterozygous mutations in *KCNQ1* and *KCNE1* have a high lethality and are associated with congenital deafness. Hundreds of mutations in 10 genes have been described; each family tends to have their own "private mutation." About 30% of patients with long QT syndrome do not identify with one of the known loci and may have either novel loci or other conditions that manifest in a similar manner to long QT syndrome. In addition, phenotype does not always follow genotype. Some patients with gene mutations have neither symptoms nor abnormal electrocardiograms. The syndrome may become evident if these patients take drugs known to prolong the QT interval. Additionally, up to one-third of persons who carry an abnormal mutation do not have prolonged QTc on the ECG and about 5% of family members experience life-threatening arrhythmias or syncope despite having a normal QTc interval. Thus, certain mutations exhibit variable clinical expression that is mediated by genetic background, modifier genes, sympathetic nerve function, and environmental factors.

Clinical manifestations of long QT syndrome in neonates result from episodes of ventricular tachycardia and include syncope, seizures, and sudden death. A small percentage of infants whose deaths are attributed to sudden infant death syndrome (SIDS) also have mutations in ion channels associated with prolonged QT interval (see following text). Syncope and seizures correlate with episodes of nonsustained torsade de pointes whereas sudden death likely results from a prolonged episode. An electrocardiogram with careful manual measurement of

■ **TABLE 10-2.** Genetic Findings in Long QT Syndrome

LQTS type[a]	Chromosome	Gene	Protein	Ion current affected	Occurrence	Comment
1	11p15.5	KCNQ1	KvLQT1 (Kv7.1)	I_{Ks}	42%-54%	Heterozygous condition also known as Ward-Romano syndrome. Homozygous and compound heterozygous mutations are associated with congenital deafness (Jervell and Lange Nielsen syndrome)
2	7q35-36	KCNH2	HERG (Kv11.1)	I_{Kr}	35%-45%	
3	3p24-21	SCN5A	Nav1.5	I_{Na}	1.7%-8%	High lethality, cardiac events occur at rest or during sleep. Most common identified mutation in SIDS
4	4q24-27	ANK2	Ankyrin-B	I_{Na-K}, I_{Na-Ca}, I_{Na}	< 1%	Ankyrin B links ion channels to appropriate membrane microdomain
5	21q22	KCNE1	Mink	I_{Ks}	< 1%	Homozygous and compound heterozygous mutations are associated with congenital deafness (Jervell and Lange Neilsen syndrome) Clinical phenotype often relatively mild in heterozygous mutations
6	21q22	KCNE2	MiRP1	I_{Kr}	< 1%	Mild phenotype with low penetrance
7	17q23	KCNJ2	Kir2.1	I_{K1}	Rare	Anderson-Tawil syndrome, periodic paralysis, dysmorphic features
8	12p13.3	CACNA1C	Cav1.2	I_{Ca}	Rare	Timothy syndrome, Multisystem disorder including structural heart disease, syndactyly, dysmorphic features
9	3p25.3	CAV3	Caveolin-3	I_{Na}	< 2%	Caveolin-3 mediates interaction of signaling molecules within caveolae. Mutations found in SIDS
10	11q23.3	SCN4B	NaVβ4	I_{Na}	< 0.1%	
11	7q21	AKAP9	Yatiao	I_{Ks}	Rare	

[a]The current trend is to name the various long QT syndromes according to the affected gene rather than by LQTS number; these numbers are included here to facilitate reference to previous work.

LQTS, long QT syndrome; I_{Ks}, rectifier K[+] current, slow component; I_{Kr}, rectifier K[+] current, rapid component; I_{Na}, inward Na[+] current; I_{Na-K}, Na[+]-K[+] ATPase current; I_{Na-Ca}, Na[+]-Ca[2+] exchanger current; I_{K1}, inward rectifier K[+] channel; I_{Ca}, Ca[2+] current.

the QT interval should be obtained on any patient with unexplained seizures or syncope. In addition, electrocardiograms should also be done on relatives of patients in whom congenital long QT syndrome is diagnosed and on relatives of patients who experience sudden, unexplained death.

Identifying patients with long QT syndrome is often difficult. Genetic heterogeneity makes genetic testing difficult for many patients, although genetic testing is now commercially available. Diagnosis is generally based on the clinical characteristics of the individual patient and the family. Diagnostic criteria originally proposed in 1985 were revised in 1993 (Table 10-3). This algorithm assigns points to diagnostic criteria based on clinical significance.

Electrocardiographic abnormalities present in long QT syndrome include prolongation of the QTc interval, sinus bradycardia, T wave abnormalities, and episodic torsade de pointes. The QT interval is measured in leads II, V_5, or V_6 and is corrected for heart rate according to Bazett formula,

$QTc = QT/(R-R)^{1/2}$ (Figure 10-21). This measurement is often difficult even in adult patients because the measured QTc interval varies among the ECG leads, a prominent U wave may be present, and sinus arrhythmia can affect the QTc interval. The U wave is included when measuring the QTc interval if the amplitude of the U wave is at least 50% of the amplitude of the T wave. Measurement of the QTc interval in young infants is often additionally challenging because the more rapid heart rates make separating the T wave from the P wave more difficult. Findings consistent with long QT syndrome include relative sinus bradycardia, 2:1 AV block (related to prolonged ventricular refractory time), and T-wave alternans. Unsuspected nonsustained ventricular arrhythmias may be present.

When evaluating patients it is important that acquired causes of prolonged QTc interval be considered. Table 10-4 lists various medications and conditions associated with prolonged QTc interval.

The length of the QT interval is the most robust predictor of risk; QTc interval > 500 milliseconds confers an increased risk of cardiac events. Other factors associated with increased risk include aborted cardiac arrest in the first year of life, male gender in the first decade of life, female gender in adolescence and adulthood, and recent syncope. Interestingly, a positive family history of sudden cardiac death does not appear to be a predictor of outcome in childhood.

Therapy with β-adrenergic blocking drugs is considered standard of care for all patients in whom congenital long QT syndrome is diagnosed. Mexiletine may be considered in patients thought to have a sodium channel defect (SCN5A, LQT3). The importance of compliance must be stressed to parents and the medication dose must be increased as the infant grows. Affected individuals must avoid all medications known to prolong the QTc interval (http://www.azcert.org/medical-pros/drug-lists/list-03.cfm).

Pacemaker placement is indicated for those patients who have second-degree AV block. Pacemakers are also often needed in patients in whom baseline sinus bradycardia is exacerbated by treatment with β-adrenergic blocking drugs. Pacing may decrease pause-dependent ventricular arrhythmias.

High-risk patients are potential candidates for placement of an implantable cardioverter-defibrillator (ICD). Implantation of these devices clearly benefits high-risk adolescent and adult patients but indications for placement are controversial. The relatively large size of the

---

■ **TABLE 10-3.** 1993 Long QT Syndrome Diagnostic Criteria

	Points
ECG findings[a]	
A. QTc	
≥480 ms$^{1/2}$	3
460-470 ms$^{1/2}$	2
450 ms$^{1/2}$ (in males)	1
B. Torsade de pointes[b]	2
C. T-wave alternans	1
D. Notched T wave in three leads	1
E. Resting HR < second percentile for age	0.5
Clinical history	
A. Syncope[b]	
With stress	2
Without stress	1
B. Congenital deafness	0.5
Family history[c]	
A. Family members with definite long QT[d]	1
B. Unexplained sudden cardiac death	0.5
< 30 years among immediate family members	

Scoring: ≤ 1 point, low probability; 2 to 3 points, intermediate probability; ≥ 4 points, high probability.

[a]In the absence of medications or disorders known to affect ECG findings.

[b]Cannot count both torsade and syncope.

[c]Cannot count same family member in A and B.

[d]Defined by diagnostic score ≥ 4.

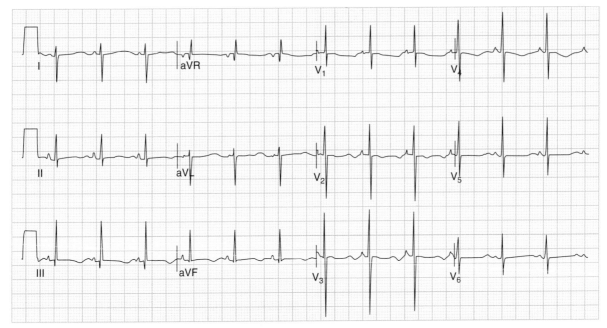

FIGURE 10-21. Long QT syndrome. Electrocardiogram from a 1-day-old infant with congenital long QT syndrome shows markedly prolonged QTc interval ($460/[670]^{1/2}$ = 562 ms) measured in lead III and bradycardia with a heart rate of 90 beats/min.

device and associated complications make this approach even more problematic in very young infants. Most commonly, ICDs should only be considered for those infants who fail medical therapy (not related to poor compliance). In contrast, ICD placement possibly should be considered early in patients with prolonged QT associated with congenital deafness (Jervell and Lange-Nielsen syndrome) because β-adrenergic blocking drugs have limited efficacy in this group.

Given the known adrenergic dependence of the arrhythmias, some advocate left cervicothoracic sympathetic ganglionectomy. The results have been variable and the procedure is controversial. In the future more precise genotype-phenotype correlation may improve diagnosis and management of these patients.

Sudden Infant Death Syndrome and Cardiac Arrhythmias

Sudden infant death syndrome (SIDS) is defined as unexpected death within the first year of life for which no cause is identified on postmortem examination. The peak incidence is between 2 and 4 months of age. The cause of SIDS is likely heterogeneous. In addition to abnormalities in brainstem respiratory control, developmental neurologic defects, dysautonomia, environmental factors, and cardiac arrhythmias (especially prolonged QTc syndrome) have been proposed to explain at least some cases of SIDS. Some investigators have identified important genetic variants in long QT syndrome genes in nearly 10% of children diagnosed with SIDS. Interestingly, half of the identified mutations occurred in the sodium channel gene, *SCN5A* (long QT 3). Defects in this gene, which are typically found in < 8% of patients with congenital long QT syndrome, are most often associated with ventricular arrhythmias occurring during rest or sleep. Despite these provocative findings, the vast majority of children with SIDS have normal QT intervals, no history of symptoms suggestive of an arrhythmia, and no family history of sudden death or prolonged QT interval. Although patients with congenital long QT syndrome have multiple episodes of ventricular arrhythmias, ventricular arrhythmias have been documented in only a very few patients at risk for SIDS despite extensive monitoring of these patients in the hospital and at home. Nevertheless, the finding of potentially disease-causing mutations has raised the question of whether routine neonatal ECG screening might identify infants at risk

■ **TABLE 10-4.** Causes of Acquired Prolonged QT Interval

Drugs[a]

  Antiarrhythmic agents (ibutilide, quinidine, procainamide, disopyramide, sotalol, dofetilide, procainamide, amiodarone [rare])

  Antibiotics (erythromycin, clarithromycin, azithromycin, sparfloxacin, chloroquine, pentamidine)

  Neuroleptics (phenothiazines, haloperidol, pimozide)

  Opiate agonist (methadone)

  Oral hypoglycemics

  Organophosphate insecticides

  Promotility agents (cisapride)

  Sedative (droperidol)

Electrolyte abnormalities (acute hypokalemia, chronic hypocalcemia, chronic hypokalemia, chronic hypomagnesemia)

Medical conditions

  Arrhythmias (complete AV block, severe bradycardia, sick sinus syndrome)

  Cardiac (myocarditis, tumors, cardiomyopathy, infarction)

  Endocrine (hyperparathyroidism, hypothyroidism, pheochromocytoma)

  Neurologic (dysautonomia, cerebrovascular accident, encephalitis, head trauma, subarachnoid hemorrhage)

---

[a] The Advisory Board at QTdrugs.org classifies drugs associated with prolonged QT interval as follows: (1) those associated with torsade de pointes; (2) those that may prolong the QT interval but are not associated with torsade de pointes; and (3) those that have been weakly associated with QT prolongation or torsade de pointes. Only those in the first group which are available in the United States are listed here. The complete list of drugs associated with prolonged QT interval is available at: http://www.azcert.org/medical-pros/drug-lists/bycategory.cfm.

for SIDS but this approach is problematic. The QTc interval is variable and often prolonged in the first few days of life. This is likely related to transient electrolyte abnormalities and/or to disturbances in autonomic control. The vast majority of infants with a prolonged QTc interval (> 440 ms) will not die from SIDS. In addition, a single QTc interval measurement on an electrocardiogram will not identify all infants with long QT syndrome. The low incidence of SIDS directly related to congenital long QT syndrome results in an extremely low positive predictive value (< 1%), which thus decreases the power of the ECG in identifying infants at risk for SIDS.

Recommendations from the American Academy of Pediatrics and the National Institutes of Health promoting supine or side positioning for sleeping have markedly decreased the incidence of SIDS in compliant populations. Further investigation is needed to find a balance between false positives and false negatives before implementing widespread newborn ECG screening programs.

Ventricular Fibrillation

Ventricular fibrillation is characterized by uncoordinated and ineffective ventricular depolarizations and inadequate cardiac output. The ECG shows low-amplitude oscillations instead of recognizable QRS complexes. The presence of ventricular fibrillation in an infant should raise the possibility of long QT syndrome, myocarditis, drug toxicity, or electrolyte abnormalities. Immediate DC cardioversion is indicated for all patients with ventricular fibrillation.

■ EVALUATION, ASSESSMENT, AND APPROACH TO DIAGNOSIS

Evaluation of Cardiac Rhythm

A 15-lead ECG (standard 12 leads and V_3R, V_4R, and V_6R) is invaluable for diagnosing arrhythmias. Caution should be used when looking at bedside monitors or even paper recordings from these monitors because wave morphology is highly dependent on lead placement. If P waves are difficult to discern on the ECG, an atrial electrogram can be recorded by positioning a flexible electrode catheter in the esophagus behind the left atrium. The amplitude of the atrial electrogram recorded transesophageally is much greater than the P wave recorded on the surface ECG. Recording the atrial electrogram and the surface ECG simultaneously often facilitates diagnosis of arrhythmias. For infants with intermittent arrhythmias, continuous monitoring on a telemetry unit or with 24-hour electrocardiography (Holter monitor) allows evaluation of the beginning and ending of arrhythmias as well as determination of minimum, maximum, and average heart rates.

Patients who have had cardiac surgery may have temporary epicardial wires in place. These are usually used for pacing if necessary. Electrograms recorded from the pacing wires can also be helpful in defining cardiac rhythms in postoperative patients.

Initial Assessment

A careful history including prenatal and perinatal events must be obtained for any infant with a suspected cardiac arrhythmia. The medication history is especially relevant. A careful family history, including history of heart disease, arrhythmias, syncope, seizures, stillbirths, and sudden unexpected deaths (including drowning and motor vehicle accidents), is also important.

The hemodynamic status must be assessed quickly and the infant classified as critically ill (very low or not measurable blood pressure, nonpalpable pulses, poor perfusion, and altered level of consciousness), seriously ill, or minimally ill to asymptomatic. If the clinical situation permits, laboratory evaluation (electrolytes, calcium, magnesium, phosphate, glucose, lactate, and arterial blood gas), chest roentgenogram, and 15-lead ECG should be obtained. Although these data are important, there should be no delay in administering therapy to a critically ill infant.

Rapid Classification of Arrhythmias and General Therapeutic Approach

All critically ill infants should be treated immediately. Infants with symptomatic bradycardia should be paced by use of a transvenous pacing catheter, epicardial leads, or transcutaneous electrodes, if the bradycardia is not associated with another condition, for example, hypoxia. Transesophageal pacing may be useful for treating infants with symptomatic sinus bradycardia but is unlikely to be effective in those with atrioventricular block. Intravenous atropine and isoproterenol should be administered if pacing is not immediately available. Once pacing is established, the etiology of the bradycardia can be determined.

Critically ill infants who have tachycardia should undergo DC cardioversion. For infants who are not critically ill, the tachycardia should be classified as narrow or wide QRS complex and a complete assessment should be done (see earlier discussion). The differential diagnosis of narrow QRS tachycardia is shown in Table 10-5. Induction of AV block by vagal maneuvers or by administration of adenosine will restore sinus rhythm in most reentrant tachycardias, and may assist in diagnosis of atrial flutter and automatic tachycardias. Careful examination of the ECG is essential.

A wide QRS tachycardia should always be treated as ventricular tachycardia until a definite diagnosis is made. An important caveat is that a conscious patient should never undergo emergent DC cardioversion. Time must be taken to completely assess a patient who is reasonably stable because these patients may not have ventricular tachycardia or may have the much more benign idioventricular

rhythm (Table 10-6). Elective cardioversion may be performed after the patient is deeply sedated. Amiodarone is efficacious for both SVT and ventricular tachycardia so this agent is a reasonable choice if the diagnosis is uncertain. Esmolol is also a good choice in these situations for infants who are only minimally symptomatic. This agent should be avoided in patients with poor ventricular function or hypotension.

■ PHARMACOLOGIC THERAPY

General Considerations

In contrast to older children and adults in whom catheter ablation (see following text) has decreased the need for pharmacologic management of arrhythmias, antiarrhythmic drug therapy remains very important in young infants because of the technical difficulties and increased risks of ablation in this age group. Pharmacokinetics differ in infants compared to older children (Chapter 11) and developmental changes in ion channels and the autonomic nervous system (Chapters 2 and 3) affect the responses of young infants to these agents. Despite these considerations, no controlled trials have been performed in young infants. Thus, therapy must be extrapolated from studies in adults.

Any rhythm disturbance should be documented as thoroughly as possible, preferably with a complete ECG, before therapy is begun. The rhythm should also be recorded continuously during any acute interventions and another complete ECG should be recorded after any change in the rhythm.

All patients receiving antiarrhythmic agents must be monitored carefully because many of these agents have the potential to produce arrhythmias other than those being treated (proarrhythmia). Serial ECG examinations are helpful in evaluating changes in response to various agents that may be proarrhythmic. Serum concentrations can be measured for most agents and should be monitored during initiation of therapy, with dose changes, and with administration of drugs that may affect metabolism of these agents. A steady-state concentration is usually reached after five times the drug's half-life. Proarrhythmia is most likely to occur soon after initiation of treatment but late proarrhythmic effects have been reported.

The Vaughan Williams classification of antiarrhythmic medications describes antiarrhythmic actions and is used traditionally. However, the usefulness of this scheme is somewhat limited from a clinical standpoint because

■ TABLE 10-5. Classification of Narrow-QRS Complex Tachycardias

Diagnosis	P waves	Onset and termination	Response to vagal maneuvers and to adenosine	Response to cardioversion	Comments
Reentrant tachycardias					
Accessory pathway-mediated SVT	P waves have abnormal axis and are not seen or follow QRS complex typically on upstroke of T wave	Abrupt	Terminate	Terminate	After termination, those with WPW syndrome have preexcitation
AV nodal reentry SVT	P waves usually not visible, superimposed on QRS complex	Abrupt	Terminate	Terminate	
Permanent form of junctional reciprocating tachycardia	P-wave axis abnormal and P waves precede QRS complex. Long RP interval	Incessant	Terminate	Terminate	
Atrial flutter	"Sawtooth" flutter waves	Abrupt	Continues in presence of AV block	Terminate	Rate up to 400-500 beats/min in newborn infants, variable block common
Atrial fibrillation (likely reentry)	Irregular and low amplitude	Abrupt	Continues in presence of AV block	Terminate	Irregularly irregular QRS complexes
Automatic tachycardias					
Sinus tachycardia	Normal P-wave axis, P wave before each QRS complex	Gradual	Continues in presence of AV block	None	Rate varies with autonomic tone
Atrial ectopic tachycardia	Abnormal P-wave axis, P wave before each QRS complex	Gradual	Continues in presence of AV block	None	No AV dissociation
Chaotic (multifocal) atrial tachycardia	Multiple P-wave morphologies	Gradual	Continues in presence of AV block	None	No AV dissociation
Junctional ectopic tachycardia	Normal P-wave axis with slower atrial than ventricular rate	Gradual	Continues in presence of AV block	None	May see AV dissociation and capture beats but no fusion beats

SVT, supraventricular tachycardia; WPW, Wolff-Parkinson-White.

■ **TABLE 10-6.** Classification of Wide-QRS Complex Tachycardias

Diagnosis	Comments
Ventricular tachycardia	AV dissociation is usually diagnostic of ventricular tachycardia but ventricular-atrial conduction common in young infants. Fusion beats diagnostic of ventricular tachycardia
SVT with aberration (rate-dependent bundle branch block)	AV dissociation not present. Aberration often resolves after first few beats of tachycardia
SVT with preexisting bundle branch block	AV dissociation not present. RBBB most common. Seen in patients who have had cardiac surgery. QRS complex morphology same as that in sinus rhythm
WPW syndrome with antidromic SVT	P waves seen before QRS complexes. QRS morphology similar to that of preexcited sinus rhythm
WPW syndrome with atrial fibrillation	Irregularly irregular QRS complexes

SVT, supraventricular tachycardia; WPW, Wolff-Parkinson-White.

several drugs have more than one effect, antiarrhythmic actions do not predict efficacy, and some useful agents, such as adenosine, do not fit into this classification. Recommended doses, pharmacokinetic details, and general indications are shown in Table 10-7.

Class 1A (Procainamide)

The 1A drugs decrease the upstroke velocity of the action potential by blocking sodium channels. This slows conduction time in the atrial and ventricular muscle cells, His-Purkinje cells, and accessory AV pathways. Automaticity is decreased. These agents also block potassium channels. The PR interval is prolonged, the QRS duration is increased and the QTc interval is prolonged. These agents are contraindicated in patients with long QT syndrome and should not be used with other drugs such as amiodarone that prolong the QTc interval. Because class 1A drugs have anticholinergic activity and so tend to increase AV node conduction, they should not be administered concomitantly with digoxin or β-adrenergic blocking agents.

Procainamide is administered intravenously but the patient must be monitored carefully for hypotension during the infusion. It is metabolized to *N*-acetylprocainamide (NAPA) which has class III actions. The risk of proarrhythmia, especially torsade de pointes, is moderate and not related to serum drug concentration. Procainamide causes mild depression of myocardial function.

Class 1B (Lidocaine, Mexiletine, Phenytoin)

These drugs block fast sodium channels thereby shortening action potential duration and the refractory period primarily in Purkinje fibers and in ventricular myocytes. Automaticity is decreased. Cells in the SA and AV nodes and autonomic tone are minimally affected. The ECG may show a slight decrease in QTc interval. Proarrhythmic effects are relatively uncommon with these agents. Lidocaine is given intravenously. High plasma concentrations depress myocardial function and toxicity often causes drowsiness, disorientation, muscle twitching, and seizures. Mexiletine is available for oral administration and is used in some forms of congenital long QT syndrome because of its effects on sodium channels. Phenytoin is used rarely and is generally restricted to the treatment of ventricular arrhythmias induced by digoxin toxicity.

Class 1C (Flecainide, Propafenone)

These agents markedly decrease the upstroke velocity of the action potential and decrease conduction in fast response cells. They do not affect autonomic tone. The PR interval is prolonged and the QRS duration increases. Flecainide is a particularly effective inhibitor of abnormal automaticity and reentry within atrial and ventricular muscle and in accessory AV pathways. It has been used successfully to treat many arrhythmias including SVT, persistent junctional reciprocating tachycardia, and ventricular tachycardia. The relatively high incidence of proarrhythmia,

■ TABLE 10-7. Antiarrhythmic Medications

Class	Drug	Dose	Half-life	Therapeutic concentration
IA	Procainamide (PA)	IV: 3-6 mg/kg over 5 min loading dose. May repeat every 10 min to maximum dose 15 mg/kg, then 20-80 µg/kg/min	1.7 h	PA 5-10 µg/mL PA + NAPA 10-30 µg/mL
IB	Lidocaine	IV: 1 mg/kg, may repeat every 5 min to maximum of 4 mg/kg, then 20-50 µg/kg/min	2-3 h	1-5 µg/mL
	Mexiletine	PO: 5-15 mg/kg/d divided q8h	12 h	0.5-2.0 µg/mL
	Phenytoin	IV: 3-5 mg/kg over 15 min, may repeat to maximum of 15 mg/kg over 1 h PO: 5-6 mg/kg/d divided q12h		10-20 µg/mL
IC	Flecainide	PO: 80-200 mg/m^2/d divided q8-12 or 2-6 mg/kg/d divided q8-12h	11-25 h	0.2-1.0 µg/mL
	Propafenone	PO: 150-600 mg/m^2 divided q8h IV: 2 mg/kg over 100 min then 4-7 µg/kg/min		
II	Propranolol	PO: 1-8 mg/kg/d divided q6h (start at 1 mg/kg/d, then increase as needed)	3-6 h	
	Esmolol	IV: 500 µg/kg loading dose then 100-200 µg/kg/min. May increase in 50-100 mg/kg/min increments as needed up to maximum of 1000 µg/kg/min	3-5 min	
	Atenolol	PO: 1-2 mg/kg/d q12-24h	8-10 h	
III	Amiodarone	PO: 10 mg/kg/d divided q12h for 5-10 d, then 5-7 mg/kg/d daily Decrease dose after several weeks to 2-5 mg/kg/d as tolerated IV: 5 mg/kg over 15-20 min, may repeat to maximum 15 mg/kg, then 10-15 mg/kg/d as continuous infusion	3-8 wk	1-2.5 µg/mL
	Sotalol	PO: 2-8 mg/kg/d divided q8-12h or 80-200 mg/m^2 divided q8-12h	10-20 h	
Other	Adenosine	IV: 0.1-0.2 mg/kg	7-10 s	
	Digoxin	PO: Total digitalizing dose (TDD): Premature 10 µg/kg, Term-1 mo: 20 µg/kg, > 1 mo: 20-30 µg/kg Schedule for TDD: $^1/_2$ TDD then $^1/_4$ TDD q8h twice. Maintenance dose = 5-10 µg/kg/d divided q12-24h IV: 75% of PO dose	18-45 h	1.0-2 ng/mL
	Magnesium sulfate	IV: 25-50 mg/kg over 10-20 min		

especially torsade de pointes, limits the use of flecainide in patients with structural heart disease but flecainide is useful for treating patients with SVT and structurally normal hearts who do not respond to β-adrenergic blocking agents and digoxin.

Propafenone blocks sodium channels but also has β-blocking effects and is a weak calcium channel antagonist. It is relatively effective in controlling reentrant and automatic tachycardias but should be used with caution in patients with structural heart disease because of the risk of proarrhythmia.

Class II (Propranolol, Atenolol, Esmolol)

These β-adrenergic blocking agents block binding of catecholamines which decreases automaticity and slows AV conduction. Direct membrane effects prolong action potential duration and effective refractory periods. Additionally, the threshold for ventricular fibrillation is increased. The slowing of AV conduction and suppression of premature beats that may initiate a reentrant circuit explain the efficacy of these agents in treating reentrant tachycardias. These agents are negative inotropes and must be used cautiously in patients who are hypotensive or who have decreased ventricular function.

Propranolol is a "nonselective" β-blocking agent. Oral administration is necessary every 6 hours. Intravenous propranolol is often associated with hypotension, bradycardia, and AV block. Given the relatively long half-life of propranolol, esmolol is now used when an intravenous β-adrenergic blocker is needed. Esmolol is a β_1-selective agent so bronchial constriction is less of a problem. Onset is rapid and the short duration of effect makes this agent relatively safe for therapeutic trials. Atenolol has minimal β_2 effects and has the advantage of requiring only twice a day administration in young infants. Fewer central nervous system effects occur with atenolol than with propranolol because atenolol does not cross the blood-brain barrier. These agents must be used with caution in patients with reactive airways disease.

Class III (Amiodarone, Sotalol)

These potassium channel blocking drugs prolong action potential duration by prolonging the plateau of the action potential. The upstroke velocity is not affected.

The pharmacologic effects of amiodarone are complex. Sodium, calcium, and the outward potassium channels are inhibited. The action potential duration is increased and the effective refractory period is prolonged in atrial and ventricular muscle, Purkinje fibers, and accessory AV pathways. The rate of automatic discharge for the SA and AV nodes is decreased. Amiodarone also has α- and β-blocking properties but does not depress myocardial function. Automaticity is decreased. Marked changes occur on the ECG including sinus slowing, prolongation of the PR interval, minimal widening of the QRS complex, and prolongation of the QTc interval. Proarrhythmic responses occur infrequently. This drug has toxicity in multiple systems; corneal microdeposits, hyper- or hypothyroidism, pulmonary interstitial fibrosis, hepatitis, peripheral neuropathy, and a slate-blue discoloration of the skin have been reported. These side effects are less common in pediatric patients than in adult patients. Baseline liver, renal, and thyroid function tests, ophthalmologic examination, and pulmonary function tests should be obtained before starting any patient on long-term therapy and then repeated every 6 months as long as the patient is taking this drug. Postoperative patients who have JET do not need these evaluations as the duration of amiodarone therapy will be short (see earlier text). Intravenous administration may cause hypotension. Amiodarone interacts with digoxin, phenytoin and warfarin and so the doses of these medications should be decreased and closely monitored when amiodarone is administered.

Sotalol is a nonselective β-adrenergic blocking agent at low doses but shows class III activity at higher doses. The QTc interval increases in a dose-dependent manner. Torsade de pointes occurs in up to 10% of pediatric patients usually within a few days of starting therapy. Close monitoring of the QTc interval on the ECG is recommended. Sotalol should not be administered with other drugs such as procainamide that also prolong the QTc interval.

Class IV (Verapamil)

Verapamil acts on the slow calcium current in SA and AV node cells thereby decreasing the rate of phase 4 automaticity and phase 0 depolarization and prolonging refractoriness and conduction time. Administration of intravenous verapamil is contraindicated in patients younger than 1 year of age because of the risk of precipitating cardiovascular collapse. This is likely the result of the increased dependence of the immature myocardium on extracellular rather than intracellular calcium for contraction.

Digoxin

Digoxin, the only antiarrhythmic medication that is a positive inotrope, directly affects cardiac cell membranes thereby decreasing the action potential duration and effective refractory period. Additionally, digoxin increases vagal tone causing slowing of SA node discharge and decreased AV node conduction. The ECG shows sinus slowing, prolongation of the PR interval, mild depression of the ST segment, and mild flattening of T waves.

Digoxin is used primarily for its effect on AV conduction and is therefore used to decrease the rate of ventricular response in atrial fibrillation, ectopic atrial tachycardia, etc. Digoxin is also effective in all reentrant arrhythmias in which the AV node is involved in the reentrant circuit. However, digoxin should not be used on an outpatient basis in patients with WPW syndrome because it may shorten the effective refractory period of the accessory AV pathway and thus allow very rapid ventricular response rates in patients with atrial fibrillation or flutter.

Cardiac toxicity caused by digoxin is characterized by sinus bradycardia, AV block, and ventricular ectopy. This is potentiated by hypokalemia and hypercalcemia. Life-threatening toxicity should be treated by intravenous administration of digoxin-specific Fab fragments. Temporary pacing is used for symptomatic AV block and phenytoin is recommended for treatment of digoxin-induced ventricular ectopy.

Adenosine

Adenosine is an endogenous nucleoside that has been considered as first-line medical therapy to terminate SVT since the late 1980s. This agent has a very short half-life and, when administered as a bolus dose, it causes AV conduction block. This will convert most reentrant tachycardias to sinus rhythm. Interestingly these effects are not seen when adenosine is administered as a continuous intravenous infusion; this is likely the result of reflex sympathetic stimulation. Thus, this agent must be given as a rapid intravenous bolus and then flushed in immediately. It is most convenient to employ a "two-syringe" technique. A syringe containing normal saline flush is connected to the intravenous line either through the same nipple introducer as the adenosine syringe or via a stopcock so that the saline can be flushed in immediately after the adenosine is administered. The most common reason for failure of adenosine to convert a patient to sinus rhythm is poor administration technique. If adenosine is not effective after 2 or 3 doses or it is effective but with rapid or frequent reinitiation of tachycardia, there is no reason to continue repeating the dose. If adenosine does not terminate tachycardia, other modalities should be considered because the tachycardia may not involve the AV node. At times, induction of AV block by adenosine allows flutter waves or P waves consistent with ectopic atrial tachycardia to be seen more easily on the ECG.

Magnesium

Magnesium, a cofactor in many enzymatic reactions, inhibits calcium channels. The resulting decreased intracellular calcium concentration likely explains the antiarrhythmic effects. In the past magnesium was used for many arrhythmias, but current data support administration only for torsade de pointes and documented hypomagnesemia.

■ DIRECT CURRENT CARDIOVERSION

DC cardioversion is indicated for any patient with severe hemodynamic compromise. The energy should always be synchronized to the QRS complex. This of course is not possible if the patient has ventricular fibrillation and may be difficult in patients with a rapid low-voltage QRS complex polymorphic ventricular tachycardia. Elective cardioversion should be performed under general anesthesia or deep sedation. Unsuccessful cardioversion must be distinguished from immediate arrhythmia reinitiation after successful conversion. If reinitiation occurs, medication should be administered to prevent reinitiation before further shocks are delivered. Failure of DC cardioversion to convert a tachycardia is highly suggestive of an automatic mechanism and other types of therapy, for example, overdrive pacing or pharmacologic agents, should be considered. Repeated DC cardioversion damages the myocardium.

■ OVERDRIVE PACING

Pacing at a rate greater than that of the intrinsic rhythm creates an area of refractory tissue within a reentrant circuit, thus interrupting the tachycardia. This will not be effective for automatic tachycardias. In young infants, overdrive pacing can be performed with a transesophageal pacing catheter. The esophageal catheter is positioned so that the maximum amplitude on the recorded atrial deflection is obtained. Pacing is begun at a rate 10% higher than the tachycardia rate and continued for 10 seconds. In contrast to DC cardioversion, overdrive pacing can be performed repeatedly without risk of myocardial damage.

■ CATHETER ABLATION

The development of radiofrequency ablation as a potentially curative therapy for many tachycardias has revolutionized care of older children and adults with these disorders. However, data from the Pediatric Electrophysiology Society Radiofrequency Catheter Ablation Registry show a higher complication rate in patients younger than 3 years of age compared to that in older patients. These complications involve sudden death within weeks of the procedure, coronary arterial ischemia, and pericardial effusion. Nevertheless, radiofrequency ablation is indicated for some infants with life-threatening arrhythmias refractory to medical management.

Cryothermal ablation is a useful addition to catheter-based ablation, especially in smaller patients. As compared to radiofrequency energy, cryotherapy takes longer to permanently destroy tissue. This allows creation of a reversible lesion during which the planned site of ablation can be evaluated for success as well as for adverse effects before completing the procedure. If adverse effects are noted, conduction will usually return when cryoablation is stopped. This has become the ablation method of choice when ablating tissue in close proximity to the AV node (eg, junctional tachycardia) to avoid the complication of complete heart block. Catheter stability due to tip adherence at cold temperatures is an added benefit. Despite the safety profile of cryothermal ablation, the indication to pursue an ablation procedure in lieu of antiarrhythmic therapy has not changed for infants.

SUGGESTED READINGS

General

Dick M. *Clinical Cardiac Electrophysiology in the Young.* New York, NY: Springer; 2009.

Walsh EP, Saul JP, Triedman JK. *Cardiac Arrhythmias in Children and Young Adults With Congenital Heart Disease.* Philadelphia, PA: Lippincott Williams & Wilkins; 2001.

Atrioventricular Block

Buyon JP, Clancy RM, Friedman DM. Cardiac manifestations of neonatal lupus erythematosus: guidelines to management, integrating clues from the bench and bedside. *Nat Clin Pract Rheumatol.* 2009;5(3):139-148.

Glatz AC, Gaynor JW, Rhodes LA, et al. Outcome of high-risk neonates with congenital complete heart block paced in the first 24 hours after birth. *J Thorac Cardiovasc Surg.* 2008;136(3):767-773.

Lopes LM, Tavares GM, Damiano AP, et al. Perinatal outcome of fetal atrioventricular block: one-hundred-sixteen cases from a single institution. *Circulation.* 2008; 118(12): 1268-1275.

Villain E, Coastedoat-Chalumeau N, Marijon E, Boudjemline Y, Piette JC, Bonnet D. Presentation and prognosis of complete atrioventricular block in childhood, according to maternal antibody status. *J Am Coll Cardiol.* 2006; 48(8): 1682-1687.

Wahren-Herlenius M, Sonesson SE. Specificity and effector mechanisms of autoantibodies in congenital heart block. *Curr Opin Immunol.* 2006;18(6):690-696.

Supraventricular Arrhythmias

Adamson PC, Rhodes LA, Saul JP. et al. The pharmacokinetics of esmolol in pediatric subjects with supraventricular arrhythmias. *Pediatr Cardiol.* 2006;27(4):420-427.

Chun TU, Van Hare GF. Advances in the approach to treatment of supraventricular tachycardia in the pediatric population. *Curr Cardiol Rep.* 2004;6(5):322-326.

Collins KK, Van Hare GF, Kertesz NJ, et al. Pediatric nonpostoperative junctional ectopic tachycardia medical management and interventional therapies. *J Am Coll Cardiol.* 2009;53(8):690-697.

Fish FA, Mehta AV, Johns JA. Characteristics and management of chaotic atrial tachycardia of infancy. *Am J Cardiol.* 1996;78(9):1052-1055.

Salerno JC, Kertesz NJ, Friedman RA, Fenrich AL, Jr. Clinical course of atrial ectopic tachycardia is age-dependent: results and treatment in children < 3 or > or =3 years of age. *J Am Coll Cardiol.* 2004;43(3):438-444.

Texter KM, Kertesz NJ, Friedman RA, Fenrich AL, Jr. Atrial flutter in infants. J Am Coll Cardiol. 2006;48(5):1040-1046.

Tortoriello TA, Snyder CS, Smith EO, Fenrich AL, Jr., Friedman RA, Kertesz NJ. Frequency of recurrence among infants with supraventricular tachycardia and comparison of recurrence rates among those with and without preexcitation and among those with and without response to digoxin and/or propranolol therapy. *Am J Cardiol.* 2003;92(9):1045-1049.

Long QT Syndrome/Sudden Infant Death Syndrome

Arnestad M, Crotti L, Rognum TO, et al. Prevalence of long-QT syndrome gene variants in sudden infant death syndrome. *Circulation.* 2007;115(3):361-367.

Berul CI, Perry JC. Contribution of long-QT syndrome genes to sudden infant death syndrome: is it time to consider newborn electrocardiographic screening? *Circulation* 2007; 115(3):294-296.

Collins KK, Van Hare GF. Advances in congenital long QT syndrome. *Curr Opin Pediatr.* 2006;18(5):497-502.

Goldenberg I, Moss AJ, Peterson DR, et al. Risk factors for aborted cardiac arrest and sudden cardiac death in children with the congenital long-QT syndrome. *Circulation.* 2008; 117(17):2184-2191.

Goldenberg I, Zareba W, Moss AJ. Long QT syndrome. *Curr Probl Cardiol.* 2008;33(11):629-694.

Morita H, Wu J, Zipes DP. The QT syndromes: long and short. *Lancet.* 2008;372(9640):750-763.

Richards JM, Alexander JR, Shinebourne EA, de Swiet M, Wilson AJ, Southall DP. Sequential 22-hour profiles of breathing patterns and heart rate in 110 full-term infants during their first 6 months of life. *Pediatrics.* 1984; 74(5):763-777.

Southall DP, Arrowsmith WA, Stebbens V, Alexander JR. QT interval measurements before sudden infant death syndrome. *Arch Dis Child.* 1986;61(4):327-333.

Southall DP, Richards J, Mitchell P, Brown DJ, Johnston PG, Shinebourne EA. Study of cardiac rhythm in healthy newborn infants. *Br Heart J.* 1980;43(1):14-20.

Spazzolini C, Mullally J, Moss AJ, et al. Clinical implications for patients with long QT syndrome who experience a cardiac event during infancy. *J Am Coll Cardiol.* 2009;54(9):832-837.

Triedman J. The meaning of lethal events in infants with long QT syndrome. *J Am Coll Cardiol.* 2009;54(9):838-839.

Van Hare GF, Perry J, Berul CI, Triedman JK. Cost effectiveness of neonatal ECG screening for the long QT syndrome. *Eur Heart J.* 2007;28(1):137-139.

Van Norstrand DW, Ackerman MJ. Sudden infant death syndrome: do ion channels play a role? *Heart Rhythm.* 2009;6(2):272-278.

Vincent GM, Schwartz PJ, Denjoy I, et al. High efficacy of beta-blockers in long-QT syndrome type 1: contribution of noncompliance and QT-prolonging drugs to the occurrence of beta-blocker treatment "failures." *Circulation.* 2009; 119(2):215-221.

Webster G, Berul CI. Congenital long-QT syndromes: a clinical and genetic update from infancy through adulthood. *Trends Cardiovasc Med.* 2008;18(6):216-224.

Pharmacologic Therapy

Moffett BS, Cannon BC, Friedman RA, Kertesz NJ. Therapeutic levels of intravenous procainamide in neonates: a retrospective assessment. *Pharmacotherapy.* 2006;26(12):1687-1693.

Saul JP, Scott WA, Brown S, et al. Intravenous amiodarone for incessant tachyarrhythmias in children: a randomized, double-blind, antiarrhythmic drug trial. *Circulation.* 2005; 112(22):3470-3477.

Catheter Ablation

Bar-Cohen Y, Cecchin F, Alexander ME, Berul CI, Triedman JK, Walsh EP. Cryoablation for accessory pathways located near normal conduction tissues or within the coronary venous system in children and young adults. *Heart Rhythm.* 2006;3(3):253-258.

Campbell RM, Strieper MJ, Frias PA, Danford DA, Kugler JD. Current status of radiofrequency ablation for common pediatric supraventricular tachycardias. *J Pediatr.* 2002; 140(2):150-155.

Chanani NK, Chiesa NA, Dubin AM, Avasarala K, Van Hare GF, Collins KK. Cryoablation for atrioventricular nodal reentrant tachycardia in young patients: predictors of recurrence. *Pacing Clin Electrophysiol.* 2008;31(9):1152-1159.

Kugler JD, Danford DA, Houston KA, Felix G. Pediatric radiofrequency catheter ablation registry success, fluoroscopy time, and complication rate for supraventricular tachycardia: comparison of early and recent eras. *J Cardiovasc Electrophysiol.* 2002;13(4):336-341.

McDaniel GM, Van Hare GF. Catheter ablation in children and adolescents. *Heart Rhythm.* 2006;3(1):95-101.

Morwood JG, Triedman JK, Berul CI, et al. Radiofrequency catheter ablation of ventricular tachycardia in children and young adults with congenital heart disease. *Heart Rhythm.* 2004;1(3):301-308.

Devices

Berul CI, Van Hare GF, Kertesz NJ, et al. Results of a multicenter retrospective implantable cardioverter-defibrillator registry of pediatric and congenital heart disease patients. *J Am Coll Cardiol.* 2008;51(17):1685-1691.

Stephenson EA, Batra AS, Knilans TK, et al. A multicenter experience with novel implantable cardioverter defibrillator configurations in the pediatric and congenital heart disease population. *J Cardiovasc Electrophysiol.* 2006; 17(1):41-46.

Walsh EP. Practical aspects of implantable defibrillator therapy in patients with congenital heart disease. *Pacing Clin Electrophysiol.* 2008;31 (suppl 1):S38-S40.

CHAPTER 11

Principles of Medical Management

■ INTRODUCTION

Providing medical care to a newborn with known or suspected heart disease can be daunting. Many practitioners are inclined to abdicate care to the pediatric cardiologist. This response is not only unnecessary, but also counterproductive to an integrated team approach to optimal care. An understanding of the pathophysiology of these conditions and the application of a few general principles will promote effective care and minimize the chance of iatrogenic misadventures. It is imperative that a concerted team approach is utilized, involving neonatology, cardiology, nursing, surgery, and anesthesiology. Effective and ongoing communication is essential for optimizing care and providing a uniform approach to the management of these complex medical patients.

This chapter reviews the diagnosis and management of infants with heart failure, infective endocarditis, and intracardiac and intravascular thrombi. In addition, nutritional support of infants with heart disease, an important but often overlooked problem, is discussed. Initial evaluation and treatment of newborns with heart disease are discussed in Chapter 5. Although much of the focus in this chapter is on the heart failure syndrome in neonates, it should be noted that compared to the plethora of data available in adults, far less information is available regarding heart failure in newborn infants. The roles of physiologic and neurohormonal compensatory mechanisms have been studied largely in chronic compensated states in adult patients and mature animal models. The causes of heart failure in neonates differ from those in older age groups. Furthermore, it is likely that normal developmental changes during the neonatal period impact upon the nature and magnitude of the compensatory physiologic responses and the responses to therapy. Lastly, there are marked differences in the psychosocial aspects of chronic disease and the impact of heart failure on growth, development, and quality of life.

■ HEART FAILURE

Overview

Heart failure in infancy is a syndrome that occurs as a consequence of the inability of the cardiovascular system to meet the metabolic and growth demands of the infant. It is a common feature of congenital heart disease presenting symptomatically in neonates. Heart failure in neonates and infants is most commonly caused by structural defects that result in decreased systemic output. The most common conditions associated with heart failure in infants are those in which there is a dominant left-to-right shunt with excessive pulmonary blood flow, reduced systemic blood flow, heart failure, and failure to thrive. Heart failure in neonates can also result from any structural defect that results in obstruction of systemic blood flow (eg, severe aortic stenosis) or by myocardial dysfunction (eg, dilated cardiomyopathy). Occasionally, heart failure occurs in situations in which the heart is structurally normal, but systemic output is very high and is associated with abnormal distribution of flow (eg, a large arteriovenous malformation), severe anemia, or excessive metabolic demands (eg, neonatal thyrotoxicosis).

Pathophysiology

The development and progression of heart failure results from a complex interplay of hemodynamic and neurohormonal factors. As illustrated in Figure 11-1, heart failure is viewed as a clinical syndrome that incorporates hemodynamics and compensatory neurohormonal responses in the overall conceptual framework. It should be noted that the roles of compensatory mechanisms that regulate cardiovascular function have been studied largely in chronic compensated states in adult patients and mature animal models. Although it is likely that developmental differences impact upon the compensatory physiologic responses and the responses to therapy that have been designed for adult patients, the general concepts are likely applicable to infants. Additional clinical and experimental studies are necessary to define the spectrum of pathophysiology of heart failure in preterm and term newborn infants.

Cardiac Dysfunction

Systemic output may be insufficient because of: (1) reduced ability to pump blood out of the ventricles due to either myocardial contractile dysfunction or to obstructed

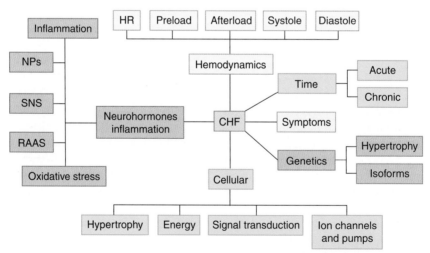

FIGURE 11-1. Interrelationships of various influences on the heart failure syndrome. Heart failure is a syndrome that occurs as a consequence of the inability of the cardiovascular system to meet the metabolic and growth demands of the infant. Compensation is achieved through the activation of physiologic and neurohormonal compensatory mechanisms, but heart failure occurs when these systems become overwhelmed or exhausted. Much of the theoretical and experimental framework for understanding the pathophysiology of heart failure has been developed in adults, but the general concepts are likely to be applicable (with modification) to infants. This schematic diagram is intended to illustrate the complexities involved in determining and modulating the responses to heart failure. Abbreviations: NPs, atrial natriuretic peptides; RAAS, renin-angiotensin-aldosterone system; SNS, sympathetic nervous system.

outflow (systolic dysfunction); (2) reduced ability of the heart to receive venous return caused by either myocardial diastolic dysfunction or to obstructed inflow (diastolic dysfunction); (3) abnormal distribution of cardiac output; or (4) combinations of the first three factors. Regardless of the primary etiology of heart failure, the interaction between the contractile (inotropic) and relaxation (lusitropic) properties of the heart are altered. At end-diastole, intraventricular pressure and volume are determined by preload (venous return), the lusitropic state of the myocytes, and the passive compliance of the non-myocyte elements of the ventricle. On the other hand, end-systolic ventricular pressure and volume are determined by central impedance and peripheral resistance (which together comprise the afterload against which the ventricle pumps) in combination with the inotropic state of the ventricular myocardium. These factors are interrelated and it is often difficult to separate the primary factors from secondary responses.

Systolic dysfunction. The fundamental problem in systolic dysfunction is impaired ventricular contractility. The healthy heart is able to increase its output in response to an increase in preload (the Frank-Starling relationship) and can maintain stroke volume in the face of an increase in afterload by increasing its contractile state. The heart with impaired systolic function is incapable of doing either. The ability to increase stroke volume with an increase in preload is diminished, and a small increase in afterload may lead to a marked decline in the output of a ventricle with systolic dysfunction. The corollary to this is that a small decrease in afterload may significantly improve cardiac output in a heart with systolic dysfunction. This forms the basis for the widespread use of vasodilator therapy for heart failure related to systolic myocardial dysfunction.

Afterload is determined primarily by the impedance of the aortic valve, aorta and the other central elastic arteries, and the resistance of the peripheral arterial vasculature. According to the LaPlace relationship, afterload (end-systolic wall stress) is proportional to both end-systolic pressure and end-systolic volume. As afterload increases, either because of an increase in central impedance (eg, aortic stenosis or coarctation of the aorta) or by an increase in peripheral resistance (eg, vasoconstriction caused by α-adrenergic stimulation), the ventricle with systolic dysfunction will not eject as much blood as a normal ventricle. Stroke volume will therefore decrease and end-systolic volume will increase.

Diastolic dysfunction. Diastolic dysfunction is characterized by decreased ventricular compliance. Consequently,

increased venous pressure is necessary to sustain adequate ventricular filling, and only small increases in venous return lead to large increases in venous pressure without concomitant increases in stroke volume. This is the basis of the concept of limited preload reserve in diastolic heart failure. That is, abnormal diastolic function may cause symptoms of inadequate cardiac output despite normal systolic function.

Abnormal distribution of cardiac output. Heart failure may be present in neonates despite normal (or near normal) systolic and diastolic cardiac function if systemic blood flow is inadequate. The most common scenario is a structural defect that results in a large left-to-right shunt (eg, large ventricular septal defect, single ventricle with unobstructed pulmonary blood flow, atrioventricular septal defect, large patent ductus arteriosus, or arteriovenous malformation). In this situation, combined ventricular output is high, but because of the large left-to-right shunt, there is excessive pulmonary blood flow and insufficient systemic blood flow. In this setting, which is common in infants with heart failure, compensatory neurohormonal mechanisms are activated and the heart failure syndrome develops despite normal cardiac pump function.

Neurohormonal Mechanisms
A variety of neurohormonal signaling pathways and physiologic mechanisms are involved in the normal maintenance and regulation of the cardiovascular system. When systemic output is reduced for whatever reason, a host of compensatory mechanisms are activated in an effort to maintain perfusion of vital organs. Most of the physiologic responses result from activation of the sympathetic nervous system and the renin-angiotensin-aldosterone system. In addition to the direct effects of increased sympathetic tone and increased levels of angiotensin and aldosterone, other responses include increases in vasopressin secretion and endothelin levels, and perturbations in nitric oxide signaling in the vasculature and myocardium. In the early stages of a reduced systemic output, these and other compensatory mechanisms help to maintain cardiac output and systemic blood flow, but with time and disease progression, these processes become deleterious (Figure 11-2).

The compensatory increases in neurohormonal activities initially result in an increase in myocardial contractility, selective peripheral vasoconstriction, sodium and water retention, and maintenance of blood pressure. A new state of cardiovascular homeostasis occurs (compensated heart

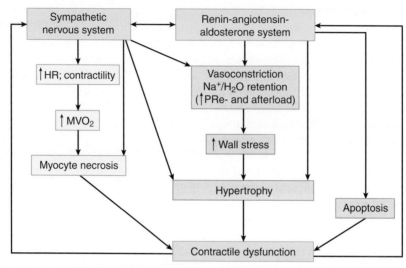

FIGURE 11-2. Compensatory neurohormonal mechanisms in heart failure. Contractile dysfunction (or impaired distribution of blood flow) results in activation of the sympathetic nervous system and the renin-angiotensin-aldosterone system. These systems produce an integrated physiologic response intended to provide compensatory support of the cardiovascular system. The potentially deleterious effects include hypertrophy and cell death that further contribute to cardiac contractile dysfunction, such that a cycle of progressive deterioration is established. It is essential to interrupt this cycle to provide optimal long-term management of the heart failure syndrome.

failure syndrome) at a higher baseline sympathetic output and increased activity of the renin-angiotensin-aldosterone system. However, when the heart failure state becomes chronic, the same responses that were beneficial in initially maintaining circulatory homeostasis may begin to accelerate myocardial cell death and exacerbate the hemodynamic abnormalities. Furthermore, excessive activation of vasoconstrictor systems is accompanied by a loss of counterregulatory vasodilator influences (nitric oxide, prostacyclin) that adds to the burden of the failing heart.

Enhanced sympathetic activity occurs in adult patients with systolic dysfunction even before clinical signs appear. A clear association exists between increased sympathetic tone, as reflected by increased plasma norepinephrine concentrations, for example, and increased mortality in adult heart failure patients. Increased plasma levels of norepinephrine and β-receptor down-regulation are also reported in the pediatric population.

Although activation of the sympathetic nervous system and renin-angiotensin-aldosterone system is quite effective for short-term compensation, the adverse consequences of continued activation of these systems eventually overcome the initial benefits. Myocardial oxygen consumption increases

due to increases in heart rate, contractility, and wall stress. If excessive, these oxygen demands may exceed oxygen delivery to the myocardium, particularly in the subendocardium.

Hypertrophy initially helps to compensate for an acute overload by decreasing wall stress and maintaining stroke volume. This occurs by activation of the hypertrophic response genes, which increases the number of functioning contractile elements within the myocytes, but does not increase myocyte numbers. These changes in gene expression also involve proteins external to the contractile elements that control myocardial calcium homeostasis. This may eventually diminish the ability to transport calcium to and from the contractile elements efficiently. Furthermore, hypertrophy increases the overall myocardial oxygen requirement.

Ventricular remodeling describes the structural changes in the myocardium that occur in response to changes in loading conditions. As indicated earlier, the myocyte compartment of the heart responds by hypertrophy. The nonmyocyte compartments of the heart also respond to autocrine and paracrine signals (eg, angiotensin II and aldosterone) independent of the hemodynamic status.

Aldosterone acts on fibroblasts and promotes collagen synthesis. Increased production of collagen decreases the proportion of the myocyte to non-myocyte compartment of the ventricular myocardium. This leads to increased stiffness of the ventricular wall and contributes significantly to diastolic dysfunction. Additionally, increased cardiac interstitial collagen deposition may contribute to reduced capillary density and increased oxygen diffusion distance. Other more direct effects of remodeling include activation of stretch-sensitive calcium channels. As a result of membrane deformation, resting intracellular calcium levels increase, which promotes activation of the hypertrophic gene response. Increases in loading conditions have also been associated with reexpression of fetal genes, early response genes (*c-fos, c-jun, c-myc*), and atrial natriuretic peptide, all early markers of cardiac hypertrophy.

In addition to the changes mentioned in the preceding discussion, activation of the sympathetic nervous system and renin-angiotensin-aldosterone system may be toxic to the myocytes. Myocyte necrosis occurs via a variety of cytotoxic mechanisms and may be observed in situations of both acute and chronic myocardial dysfunction. Microscopically, cellular swelling and inflammation characterize necrosis. In addition to necrosis, an increased rate of apoptosis appears to be a common feature of the heart failure syndrome. Apoptosis is an active process that involves activation (or lack of suppression) of genes encoding for programmed cell death. Although data are limited in adult human hearts, the intermediary factors responsible for apoptosis appear to be activated by angiotensin II. Apoptosis appears to be increased in the context of vascular remodeling, hypertension, ischemia-reperfusion states and other circumstances that promote ventricular remodeling. Both necrosis and apoptosis contribute to the progressive loss of myocytes that further diminishes the overall pumping capability of the heart and promotes perpetuation of the cycle of decompensation in heart failure (Figure 11-2).

Systemic Inflammatory Response in Heart Failure

Inflammation is a tightly regulated process that has been studied for many years. The same cascades that are operative in sepsis and autoimmune diseases are activated to varying degrees in the heart failure syndrome. Cytokines are central regulatory molecules involved in the systemic inflammatory response syndrome. Cytokines are produced by a variety of cells and can be categorized as "pro-inflammatory" or "anti-inflammatory." Pro-inflammatory cytokines such as interleukin-1, interleukin-6, and tumor necrosis factor-α depress myocyte contractile function, activate immune cells, and suppress production of anti-inflammatory cytokines. In contrast, anti-inflammatory cytokines (eg, interleukins-4, 5, and 10) reduce production of pro-inflammatory molecules and play a protective role in some disease states.

Although oversimplified, several clinical conditions such as septic shock are thought to result from an imbalance in these two systems with an unchecked pro-inflammatory response triggered by an inciting event (eg, bacterial infection). An emerging concept in heart failure is that similar immune system derangements contribute significantly to the pathophysiology and progression of the heart failure syndrome. The triggering mechanisms that initiate the systemic inflammatory response syndrome in heart failure and the potential of specific therapeutic strategies remain to be fully characterized. Additionally, nearly all of this work has been performed in adult patients and mature animal models and relatively little is known regarding the role of the systemic inflammatory response in neonates with heart failure.

Heart Failure Syndromes

As is evident from the preceding discussion, it is important to think of heart failure as a syndrome that is defined as a disorder of the cardiovascular system, not merely acute pump failure, resulting in inadequate oxygen delivery. Heart failure develops as a consequence of compensatory hemodynamic and neurohormonal mechanisms that become overwhelmed or exhausted in response to inadequate systemic blood flow. The signs and symptoms of heart failure result from these compensatory physiological responses and are related to the acuity of the disease process. Based on these concepts, the following definitions may provide a more useful framework for understanding and discussing heart failure syndromes in neonates.

Shock

Shock is defined as a state of acute circulatory dysfunction with completely overwhelmed and inadequate physiologic compensatory mechanisms. These infants are lethargic, exhibit poor perfusion, are often hypotensive and tachycardic, and generally appear quite ill. Blood pressure may be difficult to measure noninvasively in newborn infants. Additionally, blood pressure may be maintained at normal or near normal levels until the terminal stages of shock in infants. Thus, it is important to not rely solely on blood pressure as an indicator of the presence shock in newborns. However, confirmed hypotension in a neonate is an important finding and should prompt immediate intervention. Shock can result from a variety of noncardiac causes in neonates (eg, sepsis, severe anemia). However, cardiogenic shock may also be a presenting feature of left-sided obstructive lesions (such as critical aortic stenosis, interrupted aortic arch or hypoplastic left heart syndrome) and cardiomyopathies. Since the normal physiologic responses are inadequate to maintain circulatory homeostasis, shock must be treated emergently to avoid death.

Acute Heart Failure Syndrome (Decompensated State)

Acute decompensated heart failure occurs when physiologic and neurohormonal compensatory mechanisms are activated, but the responses are insufficient to maintain normal systemic circulation. The development of symptoms or the worsening of a previously compensated state marks the beginning of decompensation and onset of the acute heart failure syndrome. Additional myocardial injury, increased metabolic demands, or changes in loading conditions may trigger decompensation from a stable compensated state. Symptoms of fluid retention develop or progress because of peripheral vasoconstriction and sodium retention. Pulmonary congestion and hepatic distention related to fluid retention are common manifestations of decompensated heart failure syndrome in neonates. Infants with acute heart failure are symptomatic with restlessness, irritability, tachypnea, tachycardia, diminished peripheral perfusion, and decreased urine output. Without intervention, infants in a decompensated state will continue to deteriorate, often rather rapidly. It is important to recognize acute decompensated heart failure so that appropriate therapy can be provided urgently.

Chronic Heart Failure Syndrome (Compensated State)

The chronic heart failure syndrome is defined as a stable balance between diminished systemic blood flow and activation of compensatory hemodynamic and neurohormonal responses. These patients may exhibit few, if any, symptoms of "congestive" heart failure since activation of compensatory mechanisms, primarily the sympathetic nervous system and the renin-angiotensin-aldosterone system, maintain circulatory homeostasis. Often, the only noticeable finding in an infant is failure to thrive, because caloric intake is often reduced and metabolism is increased

because of enhanced sympathetic activity. This sustained activation of the sympathetic nervous system and the renin-angiotensin-aldosterone system ultimately contribute to progressive (and often silent) deterioration of myocardial function. Chronic heart failure is a common manifestation of many types of structural cardiac defects in neonates resulting from the abnormal distribution of blood flow or abnormal myocardial function.

Diagnosis of Heart Failure

Neonates represent a unique population in terms of cardiopulmonary function, clinical presentation, and approaches to management. It is important to have a firm understanding of these developmental differences to understand the pathophysiology of heart failure in neonates and age-appropriate approaches to therapy. Heart failure is a clinical syndrome that must be diagnosed by a comprehensive history and physical examination. No single test that can be performed to diagnose the presence of the heart failure syndrome. For example, an echocardiogram will not determine the presence or absence of heart failure. An echocardiogram can be very helpful in defining cardiac anatomy, ventricular function, and pulmonary artery pressure, but it does not provide a diagnosis of heart failure. An infant may have no clinical evidence of heart failure despite the presence of a large ventricular septal defect or echocardiographic evidence of decreased ventricular systolic function. Conversely, heart failure may be present in the setting of a structurally normal heart.

The pregnancy history may provide clues as to possibly acquired causes of heart failure, such as neonatal myocarditis or severe anemia caused by placental bleeding. However, the neonatal history is generally much more informative. The most prominent manifestation of the heart failure syndrome in newborn and young infants is related to the respiratory system. Infants with heart failure are almost always tachypneic, especially with feeding. The feeding history reveals decreased oral intake and prolonged feeding times often because of tiring during feeding and increased respiratory effort during oral feeding. Diaphoresis with feeding and emesis is frequently present. With chronic heart failure, infants generally exhibit failure to thrive with decreased growth velocity. Unfortunately, many other neonatal illnesses present similarly to heart failure and the signs and symptoms may be nonspecific. Poor feeding is a common manifestation of most neonatal medical problems (infection, metabolic diseases, etc). Consequently, the diagnosis of heart failure in infants is not always clear and straightforward.

Infants with heart failure often appear apathetic and uninterested in their environment. The physical examination generally shows tachycardia and tachypnea, even at rest. It is unusual to hear a gallop in newborn infants, even in the presence of severely depressed ventricular function. In infants with a left-to-right shunt, the presence of a diastolic inflow rumble indicates a large shunt with markedly increased pulmonary blood flow. Absence of a heart murmur does not exclude heart disease. For example, an infant with critical aortic stenosis may not have sufficient cardiac output to generate a murmur of aortic stenosis.

The lungs are usually clear to auscultation. With advanced heart failure, there may be diffuse inspiratory crackles. Neonates are more susceptible to atelectasis than older children and adults because of differences in pulmonary function. Functional residual capacity, or the volume of gas present in the lungs at the end of a normal expiration, is the balance between the inward recoil of the lung and the outward recoil of the chest wall. In neonates, the chest wall generates little outward recoil making the relaxation volume of the thorax smaller than that of the adult. Closing capacity, or the point at which small conducting airways begin to collapse, exceeds functional residual capacity, which results in the neonatal lung being more susceptible to atelectasis. Furthermore, failure to thrive, a common feature of chronic heart failure in infants, leads to respiratory muscle weakness that can compromise alveolar stability and pulmonary compliance.

The liver is usually enlarged and the size of the liver is used as a guide to the severity of fluid overload. The presence of hepatomegaly in a critically ill infant may differentiate heart failure from sepsis. Neonates rarely exhibit peripheral edema unless there is hypoproteinemia or renal failure. The extremities may be cool with diminished cutaneous perfusion if systemic cardiac output is markedly compromised.

Biomarkers

Given that heart failure is a dynamic clinical syndrome with involvement of neurohormonal, genetic, biochemical, and inflammatory mediators, a variety of biomarkers may provide useful information for the diagnosis, risk stratification, and monitoring of infants with heart failure. A clinically useful biomarker should be readily available at a reasonable cost, provide meaningful information that is not otherwise available from a standard clinical assessment, and the result should aid in medical decision making. Biomarkers of inflammation, oxidative stress, protease activity, neurohormonal activation, myocyte injury, and other pathways have been reported or are currently being studied in adults with heart disease. Most of the heart failure biomarkers that have been studied in adults have not been carefully characterized in neonates and young children. Two biomarkers that have been evaluated in children are norepinephrine and B-type natriuretic peptide (BNP). Norepinephrine levels correlate reasonably well with clinical assessments of heart failure severity in infants and children. BNP has been shown to be elevated in newborns with patent ductus arteriosus and other studies suggest that BNP levels can discriminate between heart disease and respiratory disease in children. However, additional studies are required to determine the utility of measuring levels of norepinephrine, BNP, or other biomarkers for risk stratification and monitoring the response to therapy in infants with heart disease.

Clinical Assessment of Heart Failure Severity

In most clinical settings, assessment of the severity of heart failure in neonates and infants is subjective and may vary among clinicians. For routine cases, a subjective assessment is adequate if the clinician pays careful attention to signs and symptoms of heart failure, including growth of the infant. However, in complicated cases and certainly for clinical trials comparing heart failure therapy, outcomes or quality of life, a more quantitative assessment of heart failure severity is necessary.

Heart failure severity in adults and adolescents is commonly graded according to the New York Heart Association classification, which uses functional capacity as a marker of heart failure severity. Because this approach is not applicable to infants, an alternative scoring system was developed by Ross and colleagues nearly two decades ago. The Ross classification has been used in several heart failure studies in infants and has been modified for use in older children. The New York University pediatric heart failure index was developed in an effort to further discriminate among early stages of disease and to detect more subtle changes in heart failure severity. However, neither the Ross classification nor the New York University pediatric heart failure index is considered to be sufficiently sensitive for early stages of disease. A staging system for adult heart failure advocated by a joint task force of the American College of Cardiology and American Heart Association has been modified for infants and children, but it remains to be validated. These three heart failure severity grading systems have been compared in only a single study in children. Although it was reported that the New York University pediatric heart failure index correlated better with radiologic, echocardiographic, and biologic assessment of heart failure, this study was performed in a small number of patients and did not include infants. Thus, additional work is necessary to develop a more accurate and sensitive method of measuring heart failure severity across a broad spectrum in infants.

Etiology of Heart Failure in Neonates

Heart failure in newborn and young infants may be caused by many different conditions. The age at onset may be helpful in narrowing the differential diagnosis. Table 11-1 provides guidelines to the most likely etiologies, based on the time of onset of the heart failure syndrome. It is important to formulate an appropriate differential diagnosis so that the evaluation can be focused on the most likely causes of heart failure, as this will expedite the diagnostic workup. Accurate diagnosis is essential for devising an appropriate and individualized approach to treatment.

Heart failure present immediately at birth is rare and is generally attributed to heart muscle dysfunction caused by birth asphyxia with myocardial ischemia, neonatal sepsis, hypoglycemia, or severe anemia or polycythemia. Overall, fetal and neonatal arrhythmias (either sustained tachycardia or bradycardia) are much less common causes of heart failure at birth. Least common are congenital cardiovascular defects that may present with heart failure at birth (Ebstein anomaly with severe tricuspid regurgitation, absent pulmonary valve syndrome, and large systemic arteriovenous malformations).

Heart failure beginning in the first week of life is most likely associated with a structural defect involving the left heart (critical aortic stenosis, severe coarctation or interrupted aortic arch, hypoplastic left heart syndrome). Less common are other forms of congenital structural defects and heart muscle dysfunction. Renal disorders that cause profound renal failure or neonatal systemic hypertension may present in the first week of life with signs of heart failure. Similarly, certain endocrine abnormalities may cause heart failure in neonates during the first week or two after birth.

Previously well newborns who develop heart failure in the first 2 to 8 weeks of life are most likely to have a structural defect that results in a left-to-right shunt. These infants are generally asymptomatic until pulmonary vascular resistance and blood hemoglobin concentration fall postnatally and the magnitude of pulmonary blood flow becomes sufficiently large to cause signs and symptoms of heart failure due to maldistribution of blood flow (pulmonary overcirculation with or without inadequate systemic blood flow). Other forms of congenital cardiovascular malformations can present in the first 2 weeks to 2 months of life, including complex defects such as various forms of single ventricle, obstructive lesions that are not critical at birth but gradually produce symptoms, cardiomyopathies, and rarely, heart failure due to severe pulmonary problems.

Therapeutic Guidelines

Table 11-2 lists the major objectives of the treatment of chronic heart failure in infants. Normalization of altered hemodynamics remains the primary objective during the acutely decompensated phase of heart failure. The effective long-term treatment of the heart failure syndrome requires attention to the neurohormonal derangements involved in the pathophysiology of heart failure.

The treatment objectives for a neonate with heart failure may be somewhat different than those for an adult patient. Often, heart failure in infants with structural heart disease is managed for a relatively short period of time until surgical or catheter-based intervention is undertaken. For example, an infant with left ventricular failure as a result of severe aortic stenosis will be treated medically until stabilized and then referred for definitive therapy. However, heart failure may persist in some of these infants because of preexisting myocardial injury or incomplete relief of structural abnormalities (eg, residual aortic stenosis and aortic insufficiency after aortic valvuloplasty).

This chapter presents a general approach to management of heart failure in newborn and young infants. Additional details of the basic and clinical pharmacology of the various drugs and drug classes are presented in Chapter 12.

Shock and Acute Heart Failure (Decompensated State)

The management of shock and acutely decompensated heart failure requires immediate "normalization" of the altered hemodynamics. The therapeutic approach consists primarily of intravenous administration of diuretics, inotropic agents, and vasodilators. In addition, the therapeutic and deleterious effects of other factors such as oxygen, ventilation (spontaneous vs assisted) and the need to maintain patency of the ductus arteriosus patency must be considered on an individual basis, depending on the specific anatomy and pathophysiology. Additional details

■ **TABLE 11-1.** Differential Diagnosis of Heart Failure in Newborn and Young Infants Depending on the Age at Onset

Heart failure present or starting at birth

1. Neonatal heart muscle dysfunction
   - Birth asphyxia; transient myocardial ischemia
   - Sepsis
   - Myocarditis
   - Hypoglycemia
   - Hypocalcemia
2. Neonatal hematological abnormalities
   - Severe anemia
   - Hyperviscosity syndrome
3. Neonatal heart rate abnormalities
   - Sustained supraventricular tachycardia
   - Congenital complete (3°) atrioventricular block
4. Structural abnormalities
   - Tricuspid regurgitation (eg, Ebstein anomaly)
   - Pulmonary regurgitation (eg, absent pulmonary valve syndrome)
   - Systemic arteriovenous malformation

Heart failure onset in the first 1-2 weeks of age

1. Structural abnormalities
   - Critical aortic stenosis
   - Coarctation of the aorta or interrupted aortic arch
   - Hypoplastic left heart syndrome
   - Total anomalous pulmonary venous connection (with obstruction)
   - Patent ductus arteriosus (preterm infants)
2. Heart muscle dysfunction or arrhythmias (listed above in onset at birth)
3. Renal abnormalities
   - Renal failure
   - Severe systemic hypertension
4. Endocrine diseases
   - Hyperthyroidism
   - Adrenal insufficiency

Heart failure onset in the first 2 months of age

1. Structural abnormalities
   - Ventricular shunt (ventricular septal defect, single ventricle, atrioventricular septal defect)
   - Aortic to pulmonary shunt (patent ductus arteriosus, truncus arteriosus, aorticopulmonary window)
   - Left heart obstructive lesions (aortic stenosis, coarctation, mitral stenosis)
   - Atrial shunt (atrial septal defect, non-obstructed total anomalous pulmonary venous connection; usually with associated lung disease such as bronchopulmonary dysplasia if heart failure is present)
2. Heart muscle dysfunction
   - Myocarditis
   - Cardiomyopathy
   - Anomalous left coronary artery from the pulmonary artery
   - Metabolic diseases (eg, Pompe disease)
   - Tachycardia-associated cardiomyopathy
3. Pulmonary abnormalities
   - Hypoventilation (airway obstruction, skeletal muscle myopathies, central hypoventilation syndromes)
   - Bronchopulmonary dysplasia
4. Renal and endocrine diseases
   - Renal failure
   - Hyper- or hypothyroidism
   - Adrenal insufficiency

■ **TABLE 11-2.** Objectives of Chronic Heart Failure Treatment

Improve survival
Reduce morbidity associated with heart failure
Maintain normal growth
Reduce heart failure symptoms
Halt or delay progression of heart failure
Decrease neurohormonal activation that occurs in heart failure

regarding the initial treatment of symptomatic newborns with congenital heart defects are presented in Chapter 5.

Chronic Heart Failure Syndrome
(Compensated State)

Treatment of adult patients with compensated congestive heart failure is directed at modifying or interrupting the excessive neurohormonal activity. Treatment objectives in adults include reduction of morbidity and hospitalization, increased long-term survival and improved quality of life (enhanced exercise capacity and reduction in symptoms). Drugs such as angiotensin-converting enzyme inhibitors, angiotensin receptor blockers, aldosterone antagonists, and β-adrenergic receptor blockers have all emerged as important agents in the treatment of adult patients with heart failure. Whether and to what extent these processes play a role in newborn and young infants with inadequate systemic output remain to be determined. However, based upon studies in adults and animals, it is reasonable to predict that similar mechanisms are operative in human neonates with heart failure, although there may be both qualitative and quantitative age-related differences. A great deal of additional research is needed to characterize the neurohormonal responses to heart failure and to heart failure therapy in preterm and term infants. The major classes of drugs used to treat chronic heart failure include diuretics, inotropes, vasodilators, and neurohormonal modulators.

Diuretics. Diuretics produce symptomatic improvement in neonates with pulmonary congestion. By reducing preload diuretics also decrease wall stress, a potent stimulus for myocardial remodeling. However, diuretics should not be used in the management of patients without signs or symptoms related to pulmonary congestion. Furthermore, when used alone, diuretics may have deleterious effects because of neurohormonal activation (stimulation of the sympathetic nervous system and activation of the renin-angiotensin-aldosterone system) caused by intravascular volume depletion.

Three classes of diuretics are commonly used for the treatment of congestion related to heart failure in infants. Loop diuretics, mainly furosemide, are potent drugs that retain their effectiveness even at very low glomerular filtration rates. The neonatal response to these loop diuretics is reduced because of immaturity of renal secretory mechanisms. Thiazide diuretics (eg, hydrochlorothiazide, chlorothiazide) act in the distal tubules. They are less potent than loop diuretics and are more affected by low cardiac output and thus low glomerular filtration rate. Potassium sparing diuretics (eg, spironolactone) also act in the distal tubules. Spironolactone diminishes myocardial fibrosis by blocking aldosterone receptors in the myocardium. Potassium sparing diuretics should be used with caution in infants being treated concomitantly with an angiotensin-converting enzyme inhibitor because of the potential for hyperkalemia.

Diuretic therapy is commonly initiated with a loop diuretic. However, in resistant cases, a thiazide diuretic is added. This combination impairs post-diuretic sodium retention and blocks the adaptive processes that develop during chronic loop diuretic therapy. When a thiazide is combined with a loop diuretic, the thiazide should be given approximately 30 to 60 minutes before the loop diuretic to permit transport in the downstream segment to be blocked fully before it is flooded with solute from the thick ascending limb. This strategy will optimize the natriuretic response.

Inotropic agents. For the long-term management of impaired contractility the most commonly used drug is digoxin. Drugs that act via cyclic AMP-dependent mechanisms (eg, β-adrenergic agonists and phosphodiesterase inhibitors) may acutely improve hemodynamics. However, in clinical trials conducted in adult patients, chronic administration of β-agonists or phosphodiesterase inhibitors does not improve symptoms or exercise tolerance. Furthermore, treatment with these drugs increases mortality and morbidity in the long term in adult patients with ischemic heart disease. In contrast, milrinone (a phosphodiesterase inhibitor) is commonly used to treat cardiac dysfunction and decompensation in children. The long-term effects of β-agonists or phosphodiesterase inhibitors in infants and young children have not been studied.

Although digoxin is often thought of as a positive inotropic agent in infants, the effect on contractility is modest, at best. In addition, digoxin may improve symptoms even in the absence of a measurable change in cardiac contractile function. For these reasons, the major beneficial effects of digoxin therapy in chronic heart failure are likely attributable largely to neurohormonal modulation (see following text and Chapter 12).

Vasodilators. Vasodilators are used in the treatment of heart failure in children with impaired ventricular function, semilunar valve regurgitation, or left-to-right shunts. In situations of depressed cardiac contractile function, the administration of a vasodilator may reduce impedance to ejection and improve cardiac output. In an infant with a large left-to-right shunt at the ventricular or arterial level, the magnitude of the shunt is dependent on the relative ratio of systemic to pulmonary vascular resistance. Cardiac contractile function is generally normal or only mildly depressed. An arteriolar dilator may improve systemic output by decreasing systemic vascular resistance, thereby increasing left ventricular output into the aorta and diminishing the magnitude of left-to-right shunt. However, it is important to note that systemic vascular resistance is low in the normal newborn and in newborns with large left-to-right shunts who have warm and well-perfused extremities. The benefit of vasodilators in these infants is questionable. Moreover, the reduction in left-to-right shunt volume depends on the reactivity of the pulmonary vascular bed as well. If the pulmonary vascular resistance is normal or only mildly elevated (which is commonly the case), then a reduction in systemic vascular resistance by arteriolar dilatation results in increased systemic output and reduction of left-to-right shunt. However, if the pulmonary vascular resistance is elevated and also decreases in response to drug therapy (a less common scenario), there may not be any overall change in the magnitude of the left-to-right shunt. Surgical repair of the defect should be considered the first line of therapy for infants with heart failure due to a large left-to-right shunt. Medical management is indicated only to prepare the infant for surgery or in the case wherein extenuating circumstances preclude surgical intervention.

Angiotensin-converting enzyme inhibitors are widely used for treating chronic heart failure in adults. The preference of angiotensin-converting enzyme inhibitors over older classes of vasodilators is related to the effects of different classes of vasodilators on neurohormonal activation. Arteriolar dilators (eg, hydralazine, nifedipine) promote activation of the renin-angiotensin-aldosterone system and the sympathetic nervous system, resulting in reflex tachycardia, and sodium and water retention; these responses are deleterious in the long-term treatment of adults with the heart failure syndrome. In contrast, treatment with an angiotensin-converting enzyme inhibitor avoids the deleterious effects of activation of the renin-angiotensin-aldosterone system. Their use has been shown to significantly improve long-term survival in adult patients with chronic congestive heart failure. It is advisable to begin patients on relatively low doses and then increase the dose to target levels as tolerated. Reduction of diuretic doses to increase circulating blood volume may be necessary if the patient becomes hypotensive after administration of angiotensin-converting enzyme inhibitors. Because of the favorable effects on neurohormonal modulation (see following text and Chapter 12), treatment with an angiotensin-converting enzyme inhibitor is recommended even for asymptomatic adults with objective evidence of depressed cardiac function. Presently, it is not known whether such therapy will have the same long-term beneficial effects in infants as has been shown in adults. Furthermore, safety, efficacy, impact of maturational changes in

the renin-angiotensin-aldosterone system on drug responses, and pharmacokinetics of various drugs in this class remain to be defined in infants.

Neurohormonal modulation. As described in the preceding discussion, the heart failure syndrome is characterized by generalized and organ-specific increases in sympathetic efferent discharge, activation of the renin-angiotensin-aldosterone system, and stimulation of mediators of myocardial remodeling. The current treatment of chronic heart failure is directed at "resetting" this neurohormonal imbalance. Drugs currently used for this purpose in adults include digoxin, angiotensin-converting enzyme inhibitors, β-adrenergic receptor blockers, aldosterone antagonists, and angiotensin receptor blockers.

Many of these drugs have not been studied in neonates with heart failure. Even old drugs such as digoxin have not been studied in appropriately designed prospective clinical trials of heart failure in infants and children. Although the neurohormonal responses to digoxin have not been defined in infants, the beneficial effects of digoxin in infants with heart failure due to a left-to-right shunt and apparently normal cardiac contractility suggests that neurohormonal modulation by digoxin may play a role in this population, as well. Similarly, no prospective randomized controlled trials of angiotensin-converting enzyme inhibitor therapy for heart failure have been conducted in infants. However, published reports of infants and children with left-to-right shunts or dilated cardiomyopathy describe beneficial hemodynamic and clinical responses to angiotensin-converting enzyme inhibitors (mainly captopril or enalapril).

For many years, the use of β-blockers was contraindicated in patients in heart failure based on the premise that the high sympathetic tone present in compensated heart failure provided the needed hemodynamic support. As understanding of pathophysiology of heart failure has expanded, attempts to modulate neurohormonal responses in heart failure have lead to the incorporation of β-blockers in the treatment of the heart failure syndrome with markedly beneficial long-term results. Third-generation β-blockers such as bucindolol and carvedilol have added vasodilator properties that appear to provide a more favorable hemodynamic profile. Carvedilol also has antioxidant properties that are though to provide an added cardioprotective benefit against the deleterious effects of oxygen-free radicals.

Clinical studies have confirmed increased sympathetic nervous system activity in infants and children with heart failure due to both congenital and acquired causes. There have been several reports of beneficial responses to β-blockers in children, but these studies are uncontrolled or retrospective. Results from the only randomized controlled trial of β-blocker therapy (carvedilol) in children with heart failure were reported in 2007. This study failed to show a beneficial effect of carvedilol on a composite measure of heart failure outcomes. However, event rates were lower than expected, the study population was heterogeneous, and the trial may have been underpowered. Furthermore, the improvement rate among placebo-treated patients was higher than predicted and trough carvedilol concentrations in the blood were lower than expected (based on adult studies). Additionally, the high proportion of infants and toddlers may have impacted the overall results as this age group tends to have high spontaneous improvement rates. At this time, the role of β-blocker therapy in neonates and infants remains uncertain and further studies are necessary.

Spironolactone, an aldosterone receptor antagonist, decreases ventricular fibrosis that occurs as part of cardiac remodeling in heart failure in adult patients. However, these responses to heart failure and to therapeutic interventions have not been formally studied in infants and children. Although spironolactone has been used routinely as a potassium sparing diuretic in infants with heart failure, it is not known whether these additional beneficial effects occur in this population.

Angiotensin receptor blockers are a newer class of drugs (eg, losartan, valsartan, and candesartan) that have been tested in adult patients with heart failure. Theoretically, these drugs may provide incremental benefits over angiotensin-converting enzyme inhibitors, but these drugs have not been studied in neonates and young infants with heart failure.

In summary, despite an enlarging body of evidence in adult patients related to the favorable effects of drugs

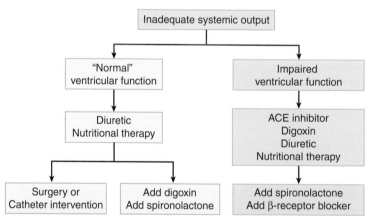

FIGURE 11-3. General therapeutic approach to newborn and young infants with chronic compensated heart failure syndrome. Systemic output may be inadequate due to abnormal distribution of blood flow (eg, large left-to-right shunt) or to impaired ventricular contractile function. Infants with heart failure due to a large left-to-right shunt generally exhibit normal or near normal ventricular contractile function. In that situation, drug therapy is generally initiated with a diuretic (eg, furosemide). If the infant fails to respond satisfactorily and extenuating circumstances preclude surgical repair, then digoxin and/or spironolactone may be added. Surgical or catheter-based intervention is indicated if heart failure cannot be managed with maximal medical and nutritional therapy. If heart failure is due primarily to depressed ventricular function, therapy is generally initiated with an ACE inhibitor, digoxin, and a diuretic. In mild cases, digoxin and a diuretic may be used in combination. Administration of a diuretic alone should be avoided because of potential neurohormonal activation. Although unproven in infants, ACE inhibitor therapy is helpful in the management of heart failure in adults. If a patient fails to respond satisfactorily to the combination of an ACE inhibitor, digoxin, and a diuretic, then a β-adrenergic receptor blocker and/or spironolactone should be added. Clinical status and electrolytes should be monitored (spironolactone may promote hyperkalemia, especially if administered concomitantly with an ACE inhibitor). Optimization of nutritional status and caloric intake is an essential component of heart failure therapy in newborn and young infants regardless of the etiology and pathophysiology.

targeted at the neurohormonal derangements observed in heart failure, little or no information is available to support the use of these drugs in infants. Extrapolating from adult studies can be misleading and inappropriate due to important developmental differences in receptor-effector systems and circulatory physiology. However, it is important to recognize that neurohormonal activation and its pharmacological modulation may be important in the chronic heart failure syndrome in newborn and young infants. Based upon our current understanding of pathophysiology, a general approach to medical therapy for the chronic heart failure syndrome in infants is presented in Figure 11-3. Infants with refractory heart failure and failure to thrive despite medical management should undergo surgical repair or palliation (if a surgical approach is possible) without further delay.

Device Therapy

Use of extracorporeal membrane oxygenation and ventricular assist devices is discussed in Chapter 13.

■ NUTRITIONAL THERAPY

Overview

Nutritional therapy is perhaps one of the most important (and often overlooked) aspects in the comprehensive management of infants with heart disease. Acute and chronic malnutrition is common in infants with congenital and acquired heart disease and may be related to the complexity of the medical condition. For example, 80% of infants with complex single ventricle exhibit chronic malnutrition. When faced with a newborn with significant structural heart disease, caretakers may focus on the acute medical and surgical aspects of the condition and not give the nutritional aspects of neonatal care sufficient priority. Early attention to nutritional needs may ultimately have important positive influences on overall growth, well-being and long-term outcome. Failure to establish adequate growth in an infant awaiting surgical repair or palliation should be considered a failure of medical therapy, and constitutes an indication for surgical intervention including heart transplantation if other operative intervention is not available.

Etiology of Failure to Thrive

Inadequate growth may result from a variety of factors. Infants born with congenital heart defects have a higher incidence of chromosomal abnormalities. Patients with trisomy 21, deletion 22q11 (DiGeorge) syndrome or Turner syndrome do not have normal linear growth. Many infants born with congenital heart disease are appropriately grown for gestational age, but the incidence of intrauterine growth retardation in infants with congenital heart disease is around 5% to 15%. The role of intrauterine growth retardation in long-term growth failure is not always clear, however. In addition, other factors such as maternal alcohol and drug consumption and cigarette smoking may play a role in intrauterine growth retardation. Extracardiac congenital anomalies that may contribute to postnatal failure to thrive include gastroschisis, malrotation, and other intestinal abnormalities. Intestinal malabsorption does not commonly play an important role in poor weight gain in patients with cardiac disease. However, mild malabsorption may occur as a result of impaired intestinal perfusion and/or bowel wall edema and may contribute to poor weight gain when combined with other factors.

In general, the most common cause for failure to thrive in infants with heart failure is a combination of decreased caloric intake and increased energy expenditure. Infants with heart failure simply do not feed well. Newborn and young infants with heart failure tire easily and may be unable to suckle effectively. Fatigue may also result from chronic hypoxia and diminished energy reserves. In addition, pronounced tachypnea may interfere with feeding in young infants, as they are unable to coordinate sucking, swallowing, and breathing. The increased work of breathing causes increased intra-abdominal pressure, which may explain the higher frequency of vomiting in these infants, another cause of decreased caloric intake. Discoordination of sucking and swallowing, delayed gastric emptying, vomiting, and increased total energy expenditure all contribute to growth failure in neonates with heart disease. Although resting energy expenditure may be normal or only slightly elevated, total energy expenditure is significantly increased in infants with heart failure due to increased energy requirements associated with the work of breathing and feeding.

Diagnosis

Failure to thrive is the chief sign among infants with many types of heart disease, especially chronic heart failure. Diminished growth velocity is obvious from plotting the infant's length, weight, and head circumference on a growth chart. Weight is affected earliest and most severely, then length is suppressed, and only with severe failure to thrive is head growth impaired. A number of biochemical markers have been used to assess nutritional status. Serum albumin is widely used and hypoalbuminemia has been associated with increased length of hospital stay and risk of death. However, because of its long half-life and high rate of intravascular/extravascular exchange, serum albumin seems to be a better measure of disease severity than nutritional status. Prealbumin has a half-life of 2 days and serum concentrations correlate better with positive nitrogen balance than do albumin or transferrin levels. Additional testing for other etiologies of failure to thrive is not necessary in these infants, unless there is a marked discrepancy between the apparent clinical severity of heart failure and the severity of growth failure.

Treatment

Calorie and protein requirements of infants with heart disease are generally greater than that of normal infants. Normal infants require 100 to 120 kcal/kg/d for optimal growth. Infants with heart disease may require 120 to 160 kcal/kg/d to maintain appropriate weight gain (approximately 30 g/d in term neonates). Standard infant formulas and breast milk contain 20 kcal/oz. Infants with significant heart failure may not be able to tolerate the fluid load necessary to provide sufficient calories. In this setting, formula (or fortified breast milk) with a higher caloric density should be employed. Fluid requirements must be individualized and may change, depending on the course of the disease and changes in diuretic therapy. In general, sodium restriction is not recommended for neonates with heart failure since provision of less than 2 mEq/kg/d may result in hyponatremia and growth impairment.

The caloric density of standard infant formula or breast milk may be increased to 24 to 30 kcal/oz using either of two general methods (formula greater than 30 kcal/oz can be used, but this often produces an osmotic diarrhea). One method is to prepare concentrated or powdered formula with less water. This has the advantage of being relatively simple, but carries the disadvantage of high solute (and sodium) load. In a similar fashion, breast milk can be supplemented with powdered formula. Generally infants will tolerate formula or breast milk concentrated to 24 to 27 kcal/oz. If the caloric density required exceeds 27 kcal/oz, then the concentration method should not be used to further increase caloric density. Instead, the alternative method of adding supplements to formula or breast milk should be employed to increase the caloric density. Several commercial breast milk fortifiers are available that

have been developed for preterm infants. Caloric density should not be increased abruptly as that is likely to produce emesis and/or diarrhea. Instead, caloric density should be increased by 3 kcal/oz every 24 hours as tolerated (defined as minimal emesis and no diarrhea). Thus, it will take about 3 days to incrementally advance an infant from 20 to 30 kcal/oz.

Increasing the caloric content of infant formula or breast milk may increase the respiratory quotient if all of the added calories are in the form of a glucose polymer. Infants with chronic heart failure are prone to contraction alkalosis (secondary to diuretic therapy) which, if combined with an increased carbohydrate load, may lead to either inadequate ventilation or to even greater caloric expenditure from excessive use of respiratory muscles.

Comprehensive nutritional therapy includes not only provision of sufficient calories and nutrients, but also involves attention to specific feeding problems and educational efforts to ensure the family's ability to provide specialized care at home. It is often helpful to enlist the assistance of nutritionists and social workers for infants with especially difficult or demanding nutritional needs. In addition, occupational and physical therapists with special expertise in infant oral-motor feeding techniques may provide invaluable advice and practical assistance.

If an infant is failing to thrive despite attention to feeding issues and increased caloric density, it may be necessary to intensify nutritional support by providing nasogastric or orogastric feeds, or feeding via a gastrostomy tube. Occasionally, a fundoplication is necessary when a gastrostomy tube is placed if the infant has persistent emesis despite maximal gastroesophageal reflux therapy. The most effective method of improving nutritional status is by 24-hour continuous enteral feeding. If the infant is at home, it is easier for the family if the feeding is for a total of 18 to 20 hours per day to allow time for bathing, formula preparation, travel, etc. The disadvantage to strict tube feeding and completely avoiding oral feeding is that this approach may contribute to poor oral-motor function and delay progression of adequate oral intake. It is therefore recommended that tube feeding be combined with strategies to maintain oral-motor feeding skills.

For long-term combined oral and tube feeding, the tip of a small and very soft feeding tube is placed in the stomach via a nostril and taped it in place. The nasogastric tube can be used for up to 6 weeks before removing and changing. Several approaches can be used to combine oral feeding with tube feeding to provide adequate caloric intake and maintain oral-motor feeding skills. One approach is to allow the infant to feed by nipple for a restricted period of time (generally 10, 15, or 20 min) and then administer the remainder of the prescribed volume via the nasogastric tube. It is very important that the parents and the nursing staff observe the strict limit on nippling time. Another commonly used approach is to encourage ad-libitum oral feeding of calorically enriched formula (or breast milk) throughout the day (8-12 h) and then provide the balance of the daily nutritional needs by continuous feeding at night.

Variations on these regimens are possible and there is no one single approach that will be suitable for all infants and families. However, regardless of which specific regimen is used, it is of utmost importance that infants receive all of their prescribed feedings each day or they will not gain weight well. This must be emphasized to parents and to nursing staff. In addition, parents should be informed that solid foods provide fewer calories per volume as compared to 24 to 30 kcal/oz formula. As such, it is often recommended that the introduction of solid foods be delayed in infants with moderate to severe growth failure.

■ MISCELLANEOUS MEDICAL PROBLEMS

Infective Endocarditis

Neonates with cardiac structural defects are at risk for infective endocarditis, although the incidence is low. The most common presentation is that of unexplained fever, often in the setting of indwelling intravascular catheters. Newborns without structural heart disease may also acquire infective endocarditis related to the presence of intravascular catheters. The organisms most frequently recovered in cases of neonatal infective endocarditis include coagulase-positive and coagulase-negative staphylococci, fungi (*Candida* species), and gram-negative organisms. This pattern is different from that observed in older children and adults with infective endocarditis.

Diagnosis

The diagnosis of infective endocarditis in newborns can be difficult and requires thoughtful and comprehensive assessment. Unexplained fever requires a thorough evaluation for sources of fever. Blood cultures are an essential part of the diagnostic workup. Studies in adult patients demonstrate that the bacteremia of endocarditis is continuous, so cultures can be taken anytime (it is not necessary to wait for a "fever spike"). Because the number of viable organisms in the blood may be relatively low, it is helpful to obtain two or three separate sets of blood cultures drawn several hours apart. Since staphylococci are common causes of both neonatal endocarditis and false-positive contamination of culture specimens, it is imperative that strict attention be paid to maintain sterile techniques during procurement of the specimens. Laboratory findings include leukocytosis and elevated acute-phase reactants (C-reactive protein and erythrocyte sedimentation rate). Urinalysis and culture should be performed as bacteria or fungi may be isolated from the urine. In addition, there may be proteinuria or hematuria, consistent with an inflammatory process.

Echocardiography plays an important role in determining the presence or absence of structural cardiac defects. Furthermore, ultrasound can be used to image the tips of intravascular catheters in an effort to determine whether there is evidence of a vegetation or thrombus on the catheter or adjacent tissue. However, it is important to stress that echocardiography is not diagnostic of either the presence or absence of infective endocarditis. In other words, even in the setting of a completely normal echocardiogram, endocarditis may be present. Conversely, a "positive echocardiogram" does not necessarily indicate the presence of infection. Thus, the echocardiogram cannot "rule out" endocarditis. Echocardiography is very helpful in the setting of positive blood cultures and a definite intracardiac or intravascular mass (vegetation) observed echocardiographically. Serial echocardiograms can be used to monitor progress and resolution of the vegetation.

A common clinical problem arises when an infant with congenital heart disease who has an intravascular catheter develops signs and symptoms of infection. The question arises as to whether this represents an infected catheter or true endocarditis. It is helpful to obtain cultures drawn through the catheter and from a separate site. If the culture from the catheter is positive in the absence of a positive peripheral culture, then an infected catheter (and not endocarditis) is most likely. If the culture drawn through the catheter and the peripheral culture are both positive, the situation is less clear and the source of bacteremia could be the catheter, endocarditis, or some other source. In this case, some centers compare the time it takes for the cultures from the catheter and a peripheral site to become positive. If the two cultures are positive simultaneously, then bacteremia is less likely to be from the catheter; if the culture from the catheter becomes positive more quickly than the peripheral culture, then the catheter is considered as the source of the infection and removal is advised. If evidence of ongoing infection persists even after the infected catheter is removed, then a reassessment for the possibility of endocarditis is warranted. In some cases, removal of the catheter is not feasible. There have been reports of successful treatment without removing the catheter, but this often requires prolonged therapy and is not recommended as the first choice if the catheter is thought to be the source of the infection.

Therapy

Appropriate targeted treatment of infective endocarditis requires identification of the responsible organism. The importance of obtaining proper cultures prior to initiating antimicrobial therapy cannot be underestimated. Culture-negative endocarditis in neonates is exceedingly rare, so a broad-spectrum approach to therapy is generally not necessary. When there is a high index of suspicion and culture results are pending, it is reasonable to initiate therapy directed at the most likely organism (eg, staphylococci). Therapy should be modified once culture and sensitivity results are available.

Treatment of fungal endocarditis in neonates can be an extremely challenging clinical problem. These infants often have multiple sites of infection and require a prolonged course of antifungal therapy. If there is evidence of an infected intracardiac or intravascular thrombus, then surgical intervention may be necessary. This is especially important in the setting of an infected prosthetic material (such as a shunt or intracardiac patch). It is difficult to resolve a fungal infection of a prosthetic material without removal of the infected prosthesis.

Endocarditis Prophylaxis

Prophylaxis of infective endocarditis should follow specific guidelines recommended by the American Heart Association (see *Suggested Readings*). Infants with congenital heart disease undergoing cardiac surgery should receive antibiotic prophylaxis directed toward staphylococci (a cephalosporin or vancomycin) but treatment should be restricted to the perioperative period (no longer than 48 h postoperatively). There is no evidence that a longer course of antibiotic "prophylaxis" for cardiac surgical patients is beneficial and indeed, there may be an increased incidence of acquired infections with other organisms (especially in neonates).

Routine circumcision does not require endocarditis prophylaxis. Similarly, prophylaxis is not indicated for infants with a patent foramen ovale who are undergoing unrelated surgical procedures. Current American Heart Association guidelines should be followed for infants with structural cardiac defects who require invasive diagnostic or surgical procedures.

Intracardiac and Intravascular Thrombi

Formation of a clot at the tip of an indwelling catheter is an extremely common phenomenon. Similarly, a thrombus may form on the wall of the atrium at the site where a catheter tip is located. These situations can present a challenge as to the proper course of therapy. Ultrasound can be very helpful in defining the location, extent, and size of such thrombi. In many cases, there is no need for any specific intervention. If a large mobile mass is observed, then it may be appropriate to administer heparin in an attempt to prevent extension of the clot. Heparin is not thrombolytic, but it may prevent enlargement and allow normal thrombolytic processes to resolve the clot. Removal of the indwelling catheter may be necessary for complete resolution. There is a risk of embolization when there is a large mobile thrombus. Most infants will have a patent foramen ovale, so the risk of systemic embolization exists. However, significant embolic complications appear to be quite rare, although relatively little data are available. Risks of heparin therapy must be considered, especially in critically ill neonates and preterm infants.

If a catheter becomes occluded, it is generally recommended that the catheter be removed and replaced. It is important not to forcibly flush a clotted catheter, as this can promote embolization. If replacement of the catheter is not feasible, then dissolution of the clot can be attempted by filling the catheter with a small volume (equal to the catheter volume) of either 25,000 units of streptokinase or tissue plasminogen activator at a concentration of 1 mg/mL. The catheter is clamped for a period of time (1-4 h with streptokinase and 5-15 min with tissue plasminogen activator) and then the contents are aspirated.

SUGGESTED READINGS

Pathophysiology and Overview of Heart Failure

Anker SD, von Haehling S. Inflammatory mediators in chronic heart failure: an overview. *Heart.* 2004;90:464-470.

Braunwald E. Biomarkers in heart failure. *N Engl J Med.* 2008;358:2148-2159.

Shaddy RE, Tani LY. Chronic congestive heart failure. In: Allen HD, Driscoll DJ, Shaddy RE, Feltes TF, eds. *Moss and*

Adams' Heart Disease in Infants, Children, and Adolescents, Including the Fetus and Young Adult. 7th ed. Philadelphia, PA: Lippincott Williams & Wilkins; 2008:1495.

Shaddy RE, Wernovsky G, eds. *Pediatric Heart Failure.* Boca Raton, FL: Taylor & Francis Group; 2005.

Treatment of Heart Failure

Balaguru D, Artman M, Auslender MA. Management of heart failure in children. *Curr Prob Pediatr.* 2000;30(1):1-35.

Balaguru D, Auslender M. Vasodilators in the treatment of pediatric heart failure. *Prog Pediatr Cardiol.* 2000;12(1):81-90.

Grenier MA, Fioravanti J, Truesdell SC, et al. Angiotensin-converting enzyme inhibitor therapy for ventricular dysfunction in infants, children and adolescents: a review. *Prog Pediatr Cardiol.* 2000;12(1):91-111.

Leitch CA. Nutritional aspects of pediatric heart failure. In: Shaddy RE, Wernovsky G, eds. *Pediatric Heart Failure.* Boca Raton, FL: Taylor & Francis Group; 2005:621.

Lowrie L. Diuretic therapy of heart failure in infants and children. *Prog Pediatr Cardiol.* 2000;12(1):45-55.

Rosenthal D, Chrisant MRK, Edens E, et al. International Society for Heart and Lung Transplantation: practice guidelines for management of heart failure in children. *J Heart Lung Transplant.* 2004;23(12):1313-1333.

Shaddy RE, Boucek MM, Hsu DT, et al. Carvedilol for children and adolescents with heart failure: a randomized controlled trial. *JAMA.* 2007;298(10):1171-1179.

Clinical Assessment of Heart Failure Severity

Connolly D, Rutkowski M, Auslender M, Artman M. The New York University pediatric heart failure index: a new method of quantifying chronic heart failure severity in children. *J Pediatr.* 2001;138(5):644-648.

Ross RD, Bollinger RO, Pinsky WW. Grading severity of congestive heart failure in infants. *Pediatr Cardiol.* 1992; 13(2):72-75.

Tissieres P, Aggoun Y, Da Cruz E, et al. Comparison of classifications for heart failure in children undergoing valvular surgery. *J Pediatr.* 2006;149:210-215.

Endocarditis

Milazzo AS, Li J. Bacterial endocarditis in infants and children. *Pediatr Infect Dis J.* 2001;20(8):799-801.

Millar BC, Jugo J, Moore JE. Fungal endocarditis in neonates and children. *Pediatr Cardiol.* 2005;26:517-536.

Taubert KA, Gewitz M. Infective endocarditis. In: Allen HD, Driscoll DJ, Shaddy RE, Feltes TF, eds. *Moss and Adams' Heart Disease in Infants, Children, and Adolescents, Including the Fetus and Young Adult.* 7th ed. Philadelphia, PA: Lippincott Williams & Wilkins; 2008:1299.

Wilson W, Taubert KA, Gewitz M, et al. Prevention of infective endocarditis: guidelines from the American Heart Association. *Circulation.* 2007;116:1736-1754.

Cardiovascular Drug Therapy

■ GENERAL PRINCIPLES OF PHARMACOLOGICAL THERAPY

Although a large number of specific therapeutic agents are available for treatment of patients with cardiovascular disease, most of these drugs have never been tested in clinical trials conducted in infants and children with heart disease. Testing in the pediatric population has been included only recently as a requirement for gaining Food and Drug Administration approval for a new drug. Even so, most drugs currently used to treat infants with cardiac conditions have not undergone appropriate randomized prospective clinical trials in this population.

The number of drugs available to treat cardiovascular disorders is enormous. Rather than attempting to maintain extensive knowledge about each specific drug, it is much more practical to understand principles and mechanisms of action according to drug classification. Practical differences among drugs within a given class are often of minimal clinical significance. A useful approach is to understand general mechanisms of action and to become familiar with one or two specific agents within a given class. In this manner, a small "personal" formulary can be developed which greatly simplifies the amount of information necessary to provide appropriate therapy. It is important to stay current, be alert to new drug developments, and be willing to modify the approach to drug therapy as new information becomes available.

As mentioned in the preceding discussion, relatively few drugs have been tested in neonates with heart disease. Thus, any drug therapy in infants should be founded on sound principles of clinical pharmacology. Ideally, drug administration is justified only if sufficient data exist to indicate that the overall morbidity or mortality of the disease is reduced by therapy *and* the beneficial effects outweigh the adverse drug effects. However, information regarding basic and clinical pharmacology of many drugs is simply not available in the neonatal population. Drug therapy for infants with cardiovascular disease is therefore usually extrapolated from studies performed in adult patients or older children and is often guided by personal experience, anecdotal reports, tradition, or uncritical acceptance of drug advertising. Medications are often administered on the basis of personal belief that a drug is effective, sometimes even in the face of scientific evidence to the contrary.

The general concept of rational drug therapy (Table 12-1) is to prescribe drugs in an attempt to maximize efficacy and to minimize adverse drug effects. This implies that therapy is tailored to the needs of a particular patient and clinical situation. Nowhere is this more important than in the newborn population. In many instances, the adverse or toxic effects of a drug in neonates do not become clear until the drug has been marketed for many years. Even though a drug is commercially available and has been used in adults, it may not be equally safe and effective in a newborn with heart disease.

Adherence to the general features of rational drug therapy described in Table 12-1, which avoids prescribing on

■ **TABLE 12-1.** Guidelines for Rational Drug Therapy

- Reasonable certainty of the diagnosis
- Understanding of the disease pathophysiology
- Knowledge of the clinical pharmacology of the available drugs for the condition
- Individualizing the specific drug and dose for the particular patient
- Defining endpoints of efficacy and toxicity
- Appropriate monitoring for therapeutic and toxic endpoints
- Willingness to change therapy if drug efficacy is not apparent or if unacceptable toxicity occurs

the basis of personal beliefs, will most certainly improve use of medications and promote a rational approach to drug therapy. A firm understanding of the pathophysiology of the disease being treated is also necessary to provide effective drug therapy so it is important to make every attempt to establish a diagnosis with certainty.

Application of drug therapy to a specific neonatal patient should be considered a "therapeutic experiment." Even in the rare case that specific information regarding the pharmacology, pharmacodynamics, and pharmacokinetics of a particular drug is available for neonates, an individual patient may not have been exposed to the specific chemical entity to be administered. Furthermore, although the drug may have been tested in neonates with other conditions, the underlying pathophysiology and genetic makeup of a specific patient may affect the response to the medication. If drug administration is approached as a therapeutic experiment in every patient, a heightened awareness of drug efficacy and toxicity will result. It is imperative to set endpoints of therapy, to monitor appropriately for such endpoints, and to observe carefully for adverse drug effects. The approach to rational and age-appropriate drug therapy must be based on a firm understanding of drug metabolism, distribution, receptor/effector ontogeny, and knowledge of the molecular and cellular processes involved in regulation of cardiovascular function in preterm and term neonates.

■ PHARMACOKINETIC PRINCIPLES

Pharmacokinetics defines drug concentrations in mathematical and kinetic terms. Absorption, distribution, metabolism, and excretion all affect the pharmacokinetic profile of a particular drug. Each of these processes can be described in quantitative terms. These principles are especially useful if the pharmacodynamic effects of a particular drug can be related to the concentration of the drug. Fortunately, for most drugs, a close relationship exists between the pharmacodynamic action of the drug and the concentration of the drug at the receptor site of action. Thus, understanding the various factors that influence the overall pharmacokinetic profile of a given drug is important.

Absorption

The most direct route for delivery of most medications is by injection into the bloodstream. However, drugs can be administered by intravenous or intra-arterial infusion or by extravascular routes (orally, sublingually, intramuscularly, subcutaneously, rectally, or by inhalation). For extravascular routes of administration, the drug must be absorbed across cell membranes to reach the bloodstream, where distribution subsequently occurs. In selected cases, inhalational therapy provides a high concentration of the drug at the site of action in the lungs (eg, nitric oxide therapy). Most drugs move through membranes by passive diffusion and therefore drug movement is regulated by the physicochemical properties of the drug, membrane characteristics, pH, and local blood flow.

Drug absorption following intramuscular injection is generally erratic and less reliable than other routes. Perfusion and blood flow to muscle beds is variable and may change rapidly, especially in critically ill newborns. Neonates and preterm infants may have relatively little muscle mass, which makes injection technically difficult. Furthermore, many drugs are insufficiently soluble and are not amenable to intramuscular administration. Thus, intramuscular injections in neonates should be avoided.

Gastrointestinal Absorption

Diffusion largely drives drug absorption from the gastrointestinal tract. The rate and extent of drug absorption are therefore influenced by gastrointestinal motility, absorptive surface area, pH (which affects ionization of the drug), and gastrointestinal contents. Developmental changes in gastrointestinal characteristics include a relatively greater gastrointestinal surface area (relative to body size), higher gastric pH, delayed gastrointestinal transit time, and the presence of β-glucuronidase in the intestinal lumen. Despite important differences in gastrointestinal function, very few controlled studies of oral drug bioavailability in neonates are available. A relatively higher gastric

pH will reduce the absorption of enterally administered drugs that are poorly ionized. In contrast, the relatively larger surface area of the newborn gastrointestinal tract may potentially increase absorption of many drugs. Gastric emptying and intestinal transit times are often reduced in newborns, but these may fluctuate considerably. For these reasons, drug absorption varies considerably not only among different patients, but even within the same patient at different times.

Drug Distribution

Distribution refers to the processes involved in partitioning of a drug among the various body tissues and organs. In general, the movements of drugs throughout tissues are reversible from one location to another and are affected by relative concentrations of the drug at various sites. Drug concentrations in various compartments are in turn determined by many factors, including blood flow, physicochemical properties of the drug, pH, composition of body fluids and tissues, drug binding in the plasma, and drug binding to other tissue proteins. The route of administration is an important determinant of drug distribution, especially in the early phases after administration. Following oral administration, the liver is the first major organ to encounter a drug, whereas the heart and lungs will receive the greatest initial concentration of a drug administered intravenously. The free drug concentration is generally the most reliable determinant of the concentration of the drug at the receptor sites. Therefore, binding to plasma proteins can be an important factor in modulating drug distribution, dose response relationships, and drug clearance. In general, fundamental age-related differences in the composition of the proteins involved in drug binding diminish binding of drugs to plasma proteins in newborns compared with adults.

Body Composition

Important changes in body composition occur during development that may have profound effects on drug distribution. In a normal full-term infant, total body water makes up approximately 75% to 80% of body weight. After birth, there is a rapid fall in total body water and a relative increase in intracellular fluid. By 1 year of age, total body water makes up approximately 60% of body weight. Fat tissue represents only approximately 3% of total body weight in a 28-week-gestation premature infant, in contrast to 15% to 28% of the body weight as fat in a term newborn. In newborns, especially premature newborns, the relatively greater proportion of total body water and the relatively lower total body fat content undoubtedly affect the apparent volume of distribution of many drugs. Apparent volume of distribution is the theoretical volume of fluid into which the total amount of drug administered would have to be diluted to produce the resulting concentration in the plasma. Apparent volume of distribution is influenced by a number of patient variables (including regional perfusion, distribution of fat, muscle and body water, and cell permeability) and drug variables (including protein binding, lipid, and water solubility). Many commonly used drugs have a larger apparent volume of distribution in premature and newborn infants (eg, furosemide, theophylline, and aminoglycosides). This becomes especially important when a loading dose is administered, since the volume of distribution is a major determinant of an appropriate loading dose.

Metabolism

The two major categories of metabolic or biotransformation reactions are the nonsynthetic (phase I) reactions, such as oxidation, reduction, or hydrolysis, and the synthetic (phase II) reactions, such as sulfation or glucuronidation. Phase I reactions often are followed by a phase II reaction. These processes enhance water solubility of a drug and promote clearance. Most drug metabolism occurs in the liver, but other organs and tissues can contribute significantly to drug metabolism (blood, lungs, gastrointestinal tract, and kidneys). In addition to facilitating more rapid drug clearance, biotransformation may result in either toxic or therapeutically active metabolites. Hepatic metabolism is generally reduced in newborns compared with adults, but this does not necessarily apply to all drugs. In the neonatal period, most phase I and phase II reaction rates are diminished and are more readily saturated. As a result, neonates generally exhibit reduced clearance rates and longer half-lives for drugs that are eliminated by biotransformation. However, drug metabolism may change rapidly in the first few months after birth, necessitating appropriate dosage adjustments. Table 12-2 highlights selected aspects of neonatal drug metabolism.

Some drugs, such as angiotensin-converting enzyme inhibitors, are administered in the form of a prodrug. Prodrugs are inactive dosage forms (usually salts or esters) that must be hydrolyzed to release the active form of the drug. Hydrolysis and esterase activity may be quite variable in newborns. Relatively little information is currently available regarding the potential impact of age-related differences in de-esterification.

■ **TABLE 12-2.** General Features of Drug Metabolism in Neonates

- Drug metabolism and clearance vary according to gestational age and are often variable even among patients of comparable gestation
- Biotransformation processes are slower than in adults
- Elimination is slower compared with adults
- Novel biotransformation pathways may exist in neonates
- Esterase activity is reduced compared with adults

Excretion

Renal excretion is the major pathway for the elimination of most drugs and drug metabolites. Maturation of renal function is well characterized and newborn renal function clearly differs considerably from that in adults. Changes in renal function that occur with gestational age, chronological age, and with underlying disease state must be considered for every drug that is eliminated principally via the kidneys. Since congenital heart disease may be associated with reduced renal perfusion, renal function must be monitored in these patients.

■ THERAPEUTIC DRUG MONITORING

All of the aforementioned changes in body composition, drug metabolism, and renal elimination combine to make precise drug dosing complicated in neonates. Rational use of therapeutic drug monitoring can be very helpful, especially in critically ill newborns. The capability to measure the plasma concentration of the most commonly used drugs is widely available. However, a clear relationship between the plasma drug concentration and the pharmacodynamic or toxic effects must be present to provide maximal benefit.

Although guidelines are available for "therapeutic" drug concentrations for many cardiovascular drugs, these values are derived largely from adult population studies. An individual infant may be more or less sensitive to the therapeutic and toxic effects of a specific drug. Some patients will obtain a beneficial effect at steady-state plasma concentrations lower than the therapeutic threshold listed by the laboratory. In these cases, increasing the dosage simply to achieve a laboratory value within the therapeutic range is not necessary and could be harmful. Conversely, maintaining a higher than usual steady-state plasma concentration to achieve efficacy is acceptable if toxicity is absent. Therapeutic drug monitoring is especially useful for antiarrhythmic drugs in complex patients, critically ill patients receiving multiple drugs, or infants with impaired renal and/or hepatic function.

■ DRUG INTERACTIONS

Drug interactions represent an often-neglected source of potential morbidity. In contrast to adult patients with multiorgan system diseases and multiple drug therapies, neonates are generally managed with a limited number of medications. However, potential adverse drug interactions may exist among the most commonly used cardiovascular drugs in newborns. Thus, it is important to keep in mind the potential for adverse events caused by interactions among the various drugs administered to an infant with heart disease. Table 12-3 lists some of the most commonly used cardiovascular drugs in the neonatal period and the clinically relevant drug-drug interactions that might occur with their use. This is a selected and limited listing. Additional references should be consulted when using other drug combinations. Many hospital pharmacies automatically survey for potential drug interactions, but even if they do not, hospital pharmacists are generally an excellent source of information regarding drug interactions.

■ CARDIOVASCULAR PHARMACOLOGY

As understanding of the cellular and molecular aspects of cardiovascular diseases in adult patients has increased, cardiovascular drug therapy has expanded considerably in the past few decades. Many drugs are marketed for the treatment of heart failure and hypertension. In contrast, far less

attention has been directed toward the immature heart and cardiovascular system. Although there are relatively few developmental studies, in almost every study published to date, drugs developed for adults affect contractile function in a qualitatively and/or quantitatively different fashion in immature myocardium. As described in Chapter 2, the fundamental processes involved in contraction, relaxation, and calcium regulation undergo maturational changes in the perinatal period. Important age-related differences exist in virtually all of the cellular components and signaling pathways that are involved in the mechanism(s) of action of conventional pharmacological agents. As a result, the responses to these drugs in the immature cardiovascular system are often poorly understood and may be unpredictable and suboptimal.

This chapter provides an overview of drugs that are most commonly used for cardiovascular diseases in neonates. The emphasis is on the management of heart failure, since heart failure (acute and compensated) is a relatively common problem in this patient population. Dosage guidelines for commonly used cardiovascular drugs are presented in Table 12-4. Antiarrhythmic agents are discussed in Chapter 10.

■ POSITIVE INOTROPIC AGENTS

The three major classes of inotropic agents presently used in infants include cardiac glycosides, β-adrenergic agonists, and phosphodiesterase inhibitors. In every case, important developmental differences influence the responses to drugs from among these classes. For example, age-related changes occur in β-adrenergic receptor/effector coupling, G protein distribution, adenylyl cyclase activity/isoform expression, cAMP-dependent protein kinase activity, and expression

---

■ TABLE 12-3. Common Cardiovascular Drug Interactions in Neonates

Drug	Interaction	Effect
Digoxin	Amiodarone	Reduced digoxin clearance (decrease digoxin dose)
	Amphotericin B	Hypokalemia (digoxin toxicity; monitor serum K^+)
	Diuretics	Hypokalemia (digoxin toxicity; monitor serum K^+)
	Flecainide	Reduced digoxin clearance (decrease digoxin dose)
	Spironolactone	Possible reduced digoxin clearance (monitor digoxin level)
Furosemide	Aminoglycosides	Increased nephro- and ototoxicity
Adenosine	Theophylline; caffeine	Diminished adenosine effect (increase adenosine dose)
ACE inhibitors	Furosemide	Potential for renal dysfunction
	Spironolactone	Hyperkalemia

■ **TABLE 12-4.** Dosage Guidelines for Cardiovascular Drugs in Neonates

Drug	Dose	Comments
DIURETICS		
Bumetanide	0.01-0.05 mg/kg/dose IV or PO (qd or qod) (maximum 0.1 mg/kg/d)	
Chlorothiazide	20-40 mg/kg/d PO bid 1-4 mg/kg/dose IV q6-12h	
Ethacrynic Acid	0.5-1.0 mg/kg IV	May repeat in 12-24 h
Furosemide	1-2 mg/kg IV or PO q6-12h; continuous IV infusion: 0.01-0.05 mg/kg/h, titrate up as necessary	Dose interval may be shortened to 4 h. May produce hypokalemia
Hydrochlorothiazide	2-3 mg/kg/d PO in 2 divided doses	
Mannitol	0.5-1 g/kg IV	After urine flow is established, lower doses (0.25-0.5 g/kg) are recommended. Repeat every 6 h as clinically indicated. Use caution in newborn infants
Metolazone	0.2-0.4 mg/kg PO qd	
Spironolactone	1-3.5 mg/kg/d PO	Potassium-sparing diuretic. May administer in 1 or 2 daily doses. Caution in combination with ACE inhibitors (may produce hyperkalemia)
VASODILATORS AND ANTIHYPERTENSIVES		
Atenolol	0.5-2 mg/kg/d PO	May be given once per day
Captopril	0.1-0.5 mg/kg/dose PO q8h	Maximum pediatric dose = 4-6 mg/kg/24 h (divided tid)
Carvedilol	0.1-0.4 mg/kg/dose PO bid	Monitor blood pressure and signs of fluid retention
Enalapril	0.1-0.4 mg/kg/d PO	Administer once daily or divide bid
Enalaprilat	5-10 µg/kg/dose IV q8-24h	
Esmolol	Loading dose = 500 µg/kg IV over 2-4 min; initial maintenance = 50-200 µg/kg/min continuous IV infusion	May increase in 50-100 µg/kg/min increments up to maximum of 1000 µg/kg/min. Mean effective dose = 500-600 µg/kg/min
Fenoldopam	0.1-0.3 µg/kg/min continuous IV infusion	Monitor blood pressure
Nifedipine	0.1-0.5 mg/kg PO q8h	May depress cardiac contractility in infants
Nesiritide	0.01-0.03 µg/kg/min continuous IV infusion	Monitor urine output and serum electrolytes
Nitric oxide	1-40 ppm via inhalation	Pulmonary vasodilator
Nitroglycerin	0.5-3 µg/kg/min continuous IV infusion	Maximum = 10 µg/kg/min
Nitroprusside	0.5-3.0 µg/kg/min continuous IV infusion	Maximum = 10 µg/kg/min
Phentolamine	0.05-0.1 mg/kg/dose IV; maximum single dose = 5 mg 2.5-15 µg/kg/min continuous IV infusion	Treatment of extravasation (due to dopamine, dobutamine, norepinephrine, epinephrine, or phenylephrine); dilute 5-10 mg in 10 mL normal saline and infiltrate area subcutaneously. Do not exceed 0.1-0.2 mg/kg or 5 mg total
Propranolol	0.5-1 mg/kg/d PO (divided tid or qid)	May increase to maximum of 8-10 mg/kg/d PO

(Continued)

■ **TABLE 12-4.** Dosage Guidelines for Cardiovascular Drugs in Neonates (*Continued*)

Drug	Dose	Comments
Prostaglandin E_1	Initial dose 0.05 µg/kg/min continuous IV infusion May increase to 0.1-0.15 µg/kg/min	Lower doses (as low as 0.01 µg/kg/min) may be effective Tapering to lowest effective dose is recommended. May cause apnea and/or hypotension, especially if a bolus is given
Sildenafil	Orally: 0.5-3.0 mg/kg/dose, given q6h Intravenously: loading dose 0.4 mg/kg over 3 h; followed by continuous infusion at 1.6 mg/kg/d	Limited experience with intravenous administration in neonates
INOTROPIC AGENTS AND VASOPRESSORS		

Digoxin	Total digitalizing dose:
	  Preterm infant 10 µg/kg PO
	  Term infant 10-20 µg/kg PO
	  Maintenance dose: 5-10 µg/kg/d PO
		IV dose is approximately 80% of PO dose. Reduce dose in renal dysfunction. Narrow therapeutic index

Dobutamine	2-20 µg/kg/min continuous IV infusion	
Dopamine	2-20 µg/kg/min continuous IV infusion	
Epinephrine	Acute: 0.1 mL/kg of 1:10,000 (0.01 mg/kg) Continuous IV infusion: 0.1-1 µg/kg/min	
Isoproterenol	0.05-1 µg/kg/min continuous IV infusion	Rarely require > 0.5 µg/kg/min
Milrinone	Loading dose = 0.1 mg/kg IV over 15-30 min Continuous IV infusion = 0.5-0.75 µg/kg/min	Loading dose may promote hypotension
Norepinephrine	0.05-1 µg/kg/min continuous IV infusion	Rarely require > 0.5 µg/kg/min
Phenylephrine	0.5-5 µg/kg/min continuous IV infusion	
Vasopressin	0.0001-0.0005 units/kg/min continuous IV infusion	Maximum dose 0.001 units/kg/min. Monitor blood pressure, urine output, and cardiac function

and distribution of cyclic nucleotide phosphodiesterases. Little is known regarding the determinants of the maturational changes in responses to cardiac glycosides (such as digoxin). Nonetheless, these drugs are widely used in the neonatal population, even though documentation of their efficacy and safety may be inadequate in many cases.

Digoxin

Digoxin is the cardiac glycoside recommended for use in neonates. The primary mechanism of action of digoxin related to inhibition of sarcolemmal Na^+-K^+ ATPase activity (Figure 12-1). This inhibition produces a slight increase in intracellular sodium concentration. This change in the transsarcolemmal sodium gradient affects sodium-calcium exchange activity, which causes an increase in intracellular calcium concentration. As a result, more calcium is available for delivery to and from the contractile proteins and contractility increases. In addition to direct myocardial effects, digoxin slows cardiac conduction and heart rate.

Digoxin is readily absorbed from the gastrointestinal tract. In general, this is the preferred route of administration, but digoxin may be administered intravenously if necessary. Peak serum levels occur approximately 30 to 90 minutes after an oral dose. During the initial phase of distribution, the drug is distributed to tissue binding sites. Following distribution and tissue binding, digoxin is excreted by the kidneys with a half-life of approximately 20 hours in infants (compared with 40 h in older children). The half-life is increased in premature infants due to slower renal elimination. The clearance of digoxin is

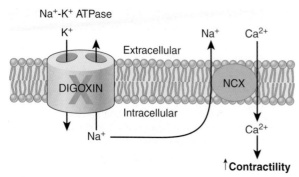

FIGURE 12-1. Cellular mechanism of action of digoxin. Digoxin inhibits the plasma membrane sodium pump (Na^+-K^+ ATPase). This results in a slight increase in intracellular sodium concentration, which then influences the activity of the sodium-calcium exchanger (NCX). The net effect within the myocyte is an increase in intracellular calcium with more calcium delivered to the contractile protein complex. This provides a positive inotropic effect. However, digoxin binds to sodium pumps ubiquitously distributed throughout the body. The overall response to digoxin therapy in heart failure involves changes in neurohormonal activity mediated by the actions of digoxin in other organs besides the heart (see text for more details).

directly related to renal function, and the dosage must be adjusted in patients with impaired or immature renal function.

Because digoxin has a large volume of distribution, therapy may be started with administration of a loading dose. The loading dose (digitalization dose) is generally divided over 12 to 24 hours (half total loading dose initially; one-fourth 6-12 h later; one-fourth 12-24 h after the initial dose). It should be recognized, however, that administration of a loading dose is associated with a higher incidence of toxic effects in newborns. Rarely is digoxin required as an emergency and other drugs are available that can be given intravenously until digoxin reaches steady-state levels (approximately 5 days after starting maintenance therapy). Thus, it is reasonable in most cases to begin maintenance dose therapy without a loading dose. Digoxin may be given once daily based on pharmacokinetic studies in infants. This may simplify the medical regimen and in general, once a day dosing improves compliance. However, many pediatric cardiologists prescribe twice a day dosing of digoxin.

Although digoxin concentration in the blood can be readily measured, routine monitoring of serum digoxin levels is not necessary. In addition, the presence of endogenous digoxin-like immunoreactive substances in infants

may confound interpretation of serum digoxin concentrations in newborns. The concentration of endogenous digoxin-like immunoreactive substances may change postnatally, which confounds the interpretation of serum digoxin levels even more. If drug concentration monitoring is performed, trough serum concentrations (as opposed to peak levels) should be used to guide adjustments in therapy. Because of the lack of relationship between higher serum levels and a greater therapeutic effect, the target serum digoxin levels should range between 1 to 2 ng/mL in neonates (similar to infants and older children). The major indication for obtaining a serum digoxin concentration is in cases of known or suspected digoxin toxicity. This occurs most commonly in cases of accidental overdose and in complicated patients with renal failure and/or those on medications that may interfere with digoxin clearance. Newborns and infants are less prone to arrhythmias induced by digoxin than are adults with ischemic heart disease.

The major indication for digoxin is heart failure with impaired myocardial contractile function. Numerous studies in adult patients have confirmed the beneficial effects of digoxin for congestive heart failure. However, controversy exists regarding the magnitude of the positive inotropic effect of digoxin in newborns with heart disease. No randomized, prospective, controlled clinical trials of digoxin have been performed in this population. Thus, recommendations are based largely on inferences drawn from adult studies and animal experiments. Digoxin is commonly used as first-line therapy for infants and children with heart failure due to systemic ventricular dysfunction.

The efficacy of digoxin for infants with heart failure due to a large left-to-right shunt is controversial. Most infants with intracardiac left-to-right shunts have apparently normal systolic ventricular function and likely do not benefit from a positive inotropic agent. Manipulation of loading conditions with diuretics is a more rational approach and should be used initially. However, some patients who are very tachycardic because of sympathetic nervous system stimulation may benefit from the decreased sinoatrial node rate mediated by digoxin. Consistent with this approach, digoxin has been shown to exert important neurohormonal modulating effects in adult patients with congestive heart failure (Table 12-5). These effects may provide substantial benefits, even in the absence of measurable objective changes in cardiac function. However, the neurohormonal effects of digoxin remain to be studied in neonates with heart disease.

■ **TABLE 12-5.** Neurohormonal Effects of Digoxin

- Restores baroreceptor sensitivity
- Increases vagal tone
- Decreases central sympathetic outflow
- Decreases myocardial response to β-adrenergic receptor stimulation
- Decreases plasma norepinephrine
- Decreases activation of the renin-angiotensin-aldosterone system

Digoxin has a narrow therapeutic window and one must always be alert to the potential for digoxin toxicity. Common signs and symptoms of systemic toxicity in adults (anorexia, vomiting, visual disturbances, and central nervous system disturbances) may be especially difficult to recognize in infants. Digoxin toxicity should be suspected in any neonate receiving digoxin who manifests apathy toward feeding or feeding intolerance. Cardiac toxicity in infants often manifests as high-degree atrioventricular block (second or third degree) with resulting bradycardia. Prolongation of the PR interval is an expected consequence of digoxin effect and is not a sign of toxicity. In addition to atrioventricular block, virtually any type of arrhythmia can be produced by digoxin toxicity. Unless toxicity is suspected, it is not necessary to routinely obtain an electrocardiogram (ECG) or measure the heart rate prior to administration of digoxin. Drugs that may predispose to digoxin toxicity include diuretics (hypokalemia) and amiodarone (reduced elimination of digoxin). Treatment of acute digoxin toxicity requires hemodynamic and ECG monitoring, temporary cardiac pacing if necessary, normalization of serum potassium levels, and antiarrhythmic drug therapy. In cases of life-threatening arrhythmias, specific Fab antibody fragments should be administered intravenously.

■ ADRENERGIC AGONISTS

The responses to adrenergic agonists are mediated by specific receptors. Although grossly oversimplified, a convenient scheme for understanding the predominate actions of adrenergic agonists is to consider that the heart contains mainly β_1-, the lungs contain β_2-, and the vasculature contains β_2- and α-adrenergic receptors. Stimulation of β_1-adrenergic receptors in the mature heart increases rate, contractility, relaxation, and conduction. These events are

mediated by G-protein coupled stimulation of adenylyl cyclase, generation of cAMP, activation of cAMP-dependent protein kinase, and phosphorylation of key regulatory proteins involved in calcium regulation (Chapter 2). Stimulation of β_2-adrenergic receptors in the lungs produces bronchodilation and modest pulmonary vasodilation. Systemic vasoconstriction results from activation of α-adrenergic receptors. In contrast to most of the vascular bed, skeletal muscle vasculature contains β_2-adrenergic receptors, which promote vasodilation when activated. Dopaminergic receptors in the splanchnic and renal vascular beds produce vasodilation in response to dopaminergic agonists (eg, dopamine).

Age-dependent changes in receptor expression, receptor-effector coupling, kinase activities, substrate availability, phosphatase activities, and cAMP hydrolysis by phosphodiesterases all contribute to age-related variability in responsiveness to adrenergic agonists. Loading conditions, volume status, and responsiveness of the peripheral vasculature can also influence the responses to these agents, especially in critically ill infants. Therefore, adrenergic agonists must be carefully titrated and appropriate hemodynamic monitoring is required. Drugs in this class undergo rapid metabolism and are administered by continuous intravenous infusion. Comparison of the relative effects on β, α, and dopaminergic receptor subtypes for various drugs is presented in Table 12-6.

Dopamine

Dopamine is an endogenous catecholamine precursor of norepinephrine with direct cardiac β_1-adrenergic agonist effects. In addition, dopamine indirectly stimulates β_1 receptors by promoting the release of norepinephrine from presynaptic sympathetic nerve terminals within the

■ **TABLE 12-6.** Effects of Agonists on Adrenergic Receptor Subtypes

Drug	Predominant agonistic effects
Dopamine	$\beta_1 = DA_1 > \alpha$
Dobutamine	β_1
Epinephrine	$\beta_1 = \beta_2 = \alpha$
Fenoldopam	DA_1
Phenylephrine	α
Norepinephrine	$\beta_1 = \alpha$
Isoproterenol	$\beta_1 = \beta_2$

myocardium. Unlike the other related catecholamines, dopamine exhibits specific dopaminergic receptor agonism (dopamine DA_1 receptor agonist). Dopamine has little or no effect on β_2-adrenergic receptors, but at higher concentrations it stimulates α_1-adrenergic receptors.

At low to moderate doses, the major action of dopamine is to increase contractility (β_1 effect) and to dilate the renal vascular bed (DA_1 effect). At higher rates of infusion, α_1 receptor stimulation becomes more pronounced and vasoconstriction occurs. In addition, the renal vasodilating effect is overcome at higher concentrations.

Dopamine has gained considerable popularity for use in newborns. Dopamine is indicated in neonates with depressed cardiac output related to impaired contractile function. Low to moderate doses are thought to incur an additional advantage by increasing renal blood flow and maintaining urine output, although this has not been proven rigorously. At conventional doses, dopamine has little effect on pulmonary vascular resistance. High rates of infusion may increase systemic vascular resistance because of α_1-mediated vasoconstriction. Extreme vasoconstriction with peripheral gangrene is associated with use of moderate or high doses in critically ill patients with circulatory insufficiency. Dopamine has minimal effect on heart rate, but high concentrations may induce sinus tachycardia and provoke arrhythmias. Dopamine clearance is slowed in the presence of hepatic or renal dysfunction. Dopamine should ideally be infused through a central catheter, but if the drug must be administered in a peripheral vein, care should be employed to avoid extravasation. Careful hemodynamic monitoring is imperative to titrate the dosage to the desired hemodynamic responses. Dopamine should not be mixed with sodium bicarbonate because alkaline solutions inactivate the drug.

Fenoldopam

Like dopamine, fenoldopam is a selective DA_1 agonist, but in contrast, fenoldopam is more potent than dopamine and does not stimulate α- or β-adrenergic receptors at conventional dosages. This pharmacologic profile results in dilation of the renal and splanchnic beds, increased renal blood flow and glomerular filtration rate, and diuresis. Fenoldopam is used primarily for treating hypertension in adults, but some centers have used intravenous fenoldopam in neonates in an effort to promote diuresis. Potential advantages of fenoldopam include rapid titration and few side effects beyond excessive hypotension. However, the limited published results in oliguric neonates

and in newborns immediately after cardiac surgery do not provide compelling evidence for a dramatic benefit from fenoldopam infusion. Additional prospective studies will be needed to determine if fenoldopam should play a role in the management of neonates with heart disease.

Dobutamine

Dobutamine is a racemic mixture with complex actions involving α- and β-adrenergic receptors. The net response to conventional dosages in adult patients is that of β_1 agonism with relatively little effect on β_2 receptors, α receptors, or DA_1 receptors. The usual pharmacodynamic response to dobutamine in children is an increase in contractility and cardiac output with minimal effects on pulmonary vascular resistance or heart rate. Systemic vascular resistance may decline because of improved cardiac output. In contrast to dopamine, dobutamine does not dilate the renal vascular bed. Dobutamine is often selected in situations for which the primary goal of therapy is to improve ventricular contractility.

Dobutamine may be administered as a single drug or as an adjunct to the infusion of other agents. Wide variability in drug clearance and in hemodynamic responses requires individual titration of dobutamine therapy in infants. As with the other sympathomimetic drugs, central venous administration with careful hemodynamic monitoring is recommended. At conventional doses, dobutamine appears to be well tolerated in neonates. As the dosage increases, dobutamine may adversely increase heart rate and myocardial oxygen demand. Dobutamine is reported to be less arrhythmogenic than the other sympathomimetic amines in adults, but comparative data in neonates are not available.

Epinephrine

Epinephrine is an endogenous catecholamine produced by the adrenal medulla that has extremely potent effects on α- and β-adrenergic receptors. Hemodynamic responses are dose-dependent. At low concentrations, the predominant effects are increased heart rate, contractility, and systolic blood pressure due to β_1-adrenergic stimulation. As the dose increases, diastolic blood pressure may decline slightly due to β_2-adrenergic effects in the peripheral vascular beds. At higher doses, α-adrenergic effects become prominent and pronounced vasoconstriction occurs.

The major indication for epinephrine is for patients with cardiovascular collapse associated with low cardiac output who have failed to respond adequately to dopamine and/or dobutamine. Epinephrine must be infused cautiously with careful hemodynamic monitoring. The initial infusion rate should be at the lower end of the recommended dosage and then gradually increased as needed. The major life-threatening toxic effect of epinephrine is the induction of ventricular arrhythmias, but this is relatively uncommon in neonates. Epinephrine increases myocardial oxygen requirements because of its prominent inotropic and chronotropic effects. High doses may produce myocardial ischemia, especially in cases involving either coronary artery anomalies or significant ventricular hypertrophy. Tissue ischemia can occur because of peripheral vasoconstriction, especially with high rates of infusion. Urine output should be monitored carefully. Because subcutaneous infiltration at peripheral infusion sites may result in cutaneous necrosis, epinephrine should be administered via a central catheter.

Phenylephrine

Phenylephrine is an α_1-adrenergic receptor agonist with relatively little effect on other adrenergic receptors. The hemodynamic effects of phenylephrine are related primarily to vasoconstriction and increased systemic vascular resistance. There may be a reflex decrease in heart rate. Phenylephrine is administered by continuous intravenous infusion. Administration of phenylephrine in neonates is indicated in conditions such as septic shock where the primary goal of therapy is to promote vasoconstriction. Phenylephrine is also used acutely during hypercyanotic episodes in congenital heart defects such as tetralogy of Fallot to increase systemic resistance, reduce the right-to-left shunt, promote an increase in pulmonary blood flow, and thereby improve systemic oxygenation.

Norepinephrine

Norepinephrine is an endogenous catecholamine that has β_1- and α-adrenergic agonist effects, but in contrast to epinephrine and isoproterenol, norepinephrine does not stimulate β_2 receptors (at conventional concentrations). Infusion of norepinephrine increases systolic and diastolic blood pressure, systemic vascular resistance, and contractility. Heart rate may remain unchanged or even decrease by virtue of opposing effects of norepinephrine on myocardial β_1 receptors and reflex baroreceptor activation with vasodilation. The prominent α-adrenergic effects of norepinephrine result in systemic vasoconstriction and may reduce renal perfusion and urine output.

Norepinephrine is rarely used as a positive inotropic agent because of significant elevation of systemic vascular resistance, reduction in renal blood flow, and increased myocardial oxygen demand. Norepinephrine may be useful in gravely ill patients with cardiovascular collapse associated with profound peripheral vasodilation, such as hyperdynamic septic shock. Some infants exhibit little vascular tone following cardiopulmonary bypass surgery and norepinephrine may be helpful temporarily in supporting the systemic blood pressure. Adverse effects of norepinephrine include arrhythmias, tissue ischemia secondary to extreme vasoconstriction, and skin necrosis if cutaneous infiltration occurs. Norepinephrine should be administered through a central venous catheter.

Isoproterenol

Isoproterenol is a synthetic catecholamine with potent nonselective β-adrenergic agonism and no significant effect on α-adrenergic receptors. Isoproterenol increases cardiac contractility and heart rate (β_1 effect), and reduces systemic vascular resistance due to dilation of skeletal muscle, renal, and splanchnic beds (β_2 effect). Isoproterenol is a potent bronchodilator and may be particularly beneficial in patients with pulmonary disease and bronchoconstriction.

Bradycardia caused by atrioventricular block or sinus node dysfunction is probably the most common indication for isoproterenol in young infants. These patients may be managed temporarily by infusing isoproterenol until pacing can be instituted (either a temporary pacing catheter or a permanent pacemaker). Although isoproterenol increases myocardial contractility and therefore increases cardiac output, this agent causes a much greater increase in heart rate than milrinone, dobutamine, or dopamine. Since many infants with low cardiac output are already tachycardic, isoproterenol is used rarely. The major adverse effects of isoproterenol include sinus tachycardia, atrial and ventricular arrhythmias. The increase in contractility and heart rate may produce excessive myocardial oxygen requirements or impaired time for diastolic filling, thereby limiting the utility of isoproterenol in some patients.

■ PHOSPHODIESTERASE INHIBITORS

A family of phosphodiesterase enzymes with distinct properties and subcellular distributions controls the degradation of intracellular cAMP and cGMP. Drugs that selectively inhibit cAMP phosphodiesterase activity exert a positive inotropic effect in mature myocardium that is mediated by elevated cAMP and activation of protein kinase A (Chapter 2). Experimental studies in immature animals indicate significant age-related changes in expression of various phosphodiesterase isoenzymes. For example, newborn rabbit myocardium is insensitive to the effects of selective inhibitors of phosphodiesterase type 3 (eg, milrinone), because of a relative lack of this enzyme. Development of the phosphodiesterase system in human myocardium has not been characterized, but virtually every immature mammalian species studied to date exhibits little or no positive inotropic response to milrinone. Despite these observations, milrinone has gained widespread usage in the preoperative and postoperative management of infants with ventricular dysfunction. However, whether the apparently beneficial hemodynamic responses are primarily due to increased contractility or to pulmonary and systemic vasodilation is unclear.

Milrinone

Milrinone is a second-generation phosphodiesterase inhibitor that is used in infants and children with heart disease. The clinical benefits of milrinone in infants with low cardiac output after cardiac surgery may be due to systemic and pulmonary vasodilation. Additionally, species differences between humans and animals and the relative maturity of the human myocardium at birth may result in milrinone-induced increases in ventricular contractility. Milrinone has lower clearance in infants than in older children and is associated with the development of thrombocytopenia in newborns and older infants. The use of milrinone is restricted to intravenous administration. Published experience with milrinone in neonates is relatively limited, but it seems to be effective and well tolerated. In particular, milrinone is not arrhythmogenic.

■ DIURETICS

Diuretics remain a mainstay of anticongestive therapy in adults and are used mainly to improve symptoms associated with a congested circulatory state. However, diuretics do not improve the neurohormonal alterations that contribute to the heart failure syndrome. Aggressive diuresis can actually promote activation of the sympathetic nervous system and the renin-angiotensin-aldosterone system (Chapter 11). The clinical response to a diuretic depends on effective delivery of salt and water to the renal tubule. Hypovolemia, decreased renal blood flow, reduced glomerular filtration rate, or sodium depletion may reduce diuretic efficacy. Diuretics can be classified according to their pharmacological effects at various sites within the nephron (see following text). Relative potency and adverse effects vary among the different classes.

Loop Diuretics

These agents are potent diuretics and have been widely used in neonatal nurseries for a variety of indications, including heart disease. The most commonly used drug is furosemide, but ethacrynic acid and bumetanide are also available. Loop diuretics inhibit chloride-sodium-potassium cotransport in the thick ascending limb of the loop of Henle. This reduces reabsorption of chloride, sodium, and potassium, and increases net excretion of free water.

Furosemide

Furosemide exerts many effects, some of which are mediated through stimulation of renal prostaglandins. Furosemide increases renal blood flow, enhances renin release, and reduces renal vascular resistance. It has diuretic and nondiuretic pulmonary effects and appears to reduce pulmonary transvascular fluid filtration.

Major clinical indications for furosemide in newborns with heart disease include acute and chronic management of congestive circulatory states and diuresis following cardiac surgery. Furosemide may be administered orally or intravenously. The drug is primarily excreted unchanged by the kidneys and the dosage must be adjusted in renal failure or in infants with immature renal function. In preterm infants, the plasma half-life is approximately 20 hours, compared with 8 hours in term infants and 1 hour in adults.

Adverse effects of furosemide include excessive contraction of extracellular volume, electrolyte imbalances, and ototoxicity. Hyponatremia in older patients with congestive heart failure is generally due to excess total body water. However, in newborn infants with limited sodium intake, chronic or excessive use of furosemide may promote excessive sodium excretion and contribute to hyponatremia. Hypokalemia is a relatively common side effect of therapy with loop diuretics and serum potassium should be monitored, especially in the acute care setting. Potassium supplementation is often required in the perioperative period for infants with significant congenital heart disease. Hypochloremic metabolic alkalosis is a common occurrence with furosemide therapy and, if severe, chloride supplementation is required. Hypocalcemia and hypomagnesemia are usually not significant clinically, but one must be alert to these potential complications, especially in the immediate postoperative period.

With standard dosage regimens in infants with normal renal function, the risk of ototoxicity is minimal. However, if renal dysfunction is present or if other ototoxic medications are administered concomitantly (such as aminoglycosides), the risk of ototoxicity increases. The dosage of furosemide must be reduced in preterm infants because of immature renal function.

Ethacrynic Acid

Ethacrynic acid is occasionally used acutely in the management of neonates with significant or refractory volume overload. Generally, ethacrynic acid is reserved for use after apparent failure to respond to furosemide. The indications and toxic effects of ethacrynic acid are otherwise comparable to those described for furosemide.

Bumetanide

Bumetanide is a loop diuretic for which fewer data are available in newborns. It is generally reserved for use in infants who have not responded adequately to conventional diuretic regimens. Bumetanide can be administered orally or intravenously. In contrast to furosemide, bumetanide is partially metabolized in the liver with approximately 50% excreted unchanged in the urine. Thus, the dosage should be reduced in cases of hepatic dysfunction. Bumetanide is more potent than furosemide and requires careful attention to dosing. The indications and potential complications are similar to those described for furosemide.

Thiazide Diuretics

Thiazides exert their diuretic effect primarily by inhibiting sodium and chloride transport in the distal convoluted tubule of the nephron. Thiazide diuretics have been available for many years and there is broad experience with these agents. Hydrochlorothiazide and chlorothiazide are the primary thiazide diuretics used in newborn patients with cardiovascular abnormalities. They are generally used chronically for outpatient management of congested circulatory states, but may be useful in the inpatient setting for patients with more advanced heart failure. In this situation, a thiazide diuretic may be used in combination with a loop diuretic and/or a potassium-sparing diuretic.

Hydrochlorothiazide and Chlorothiazide

These two drugs are close structural analogs with similar mechanism of action, diuretic efficacy, and side effects. The main differences relate to dosage, absorption, and

excretion. Following oral administration, a diuretic effect is generally noted within 60 minutes and may persist as long as 12 to 24 hours. Hydrochlorothiazide is more potent than chlorothiazide.

Adverse effects of thiazides include hypokalemia, hyperuricemia, and hypercalcemia. Non-renal effects of thiazide diuretics that have been described in older patients and adults include carbohydrate intolerance and adverse effects on plasma cholesterol and triglycerides. The extent and implications of potential disturbances in cholesterol, lipoproteins, and triglycerides have not been determined in neonates.

Metolazone

Metolazone is an orally available sulfonamide derivative that blocks sodium reabsorption in the distal and proximal convoluted tubule. It exhibits several thiazide properties although it does not have a classic thiazide structure. In general, metolazone is reserved for short-term treatment of edematous states that are resistant to conventional therapy with loop diuretics or thiazides. The combination of metolazone and furosemide can be synergistic and promote marked diuresis. Metolazone is given orally once a day or every other day. The major adverse effects of metolazone include significant volume depletion and severe electrolyte disturbances.

Potassium-Sparing Diuretics

Spironolactone competitively inhibits aldosterone at the distal tubule. By blocking aldosterone effects, spironolactone reduces potassium loss in the urine. The diuretic effect is relatively weak compared with the loop or thiazide diuretics. In most cases, spironolactone is used in combination with either furosemide or hydrochlorothiazide.

The major adverse effect of spironolactone is hyperkalemia. In most patients, this is not a significant problem, but the risk is increased in patients with excessive potassium intake (eg, when coadministered with a potassium supplement), renal dysfunction, or hepatic dysfunction. Care should be exercised if spironolactone is used in combination with an angiotensin-converting enzyme inhibitor because of the propensity for hyperkalemia. Similarly, if coadministration of a potassium supplement is necessary, serum potassium levels must be monitored carefully.

Osmotic Diuretics

The administration of osmotic diuretics is reserved for the acute setting in infants with myoglobinuria or hemoglobinuria associated with rhabdomyolysis or hemolysis.

Therapy includes urinary alkalinization and osmotic diuresis. The most commonly used drug of this class is mannitol. Mannitol produces diuresis by direct osmotic inhibition of water reabsorption in the kidneys. After acute administration, mannitol may temporarily increase intravascular volume before the diuretic response occurs, which may be disadvantageous in patients with severe congestive heart failure. In addition, mannitol may promote brisk diuresis with subsequent volume contraction in some patients. In general, the use of hyperosmotic agents in preterm and term newborns should be avoided if possible because of the potential effects on intracranial hemorrhage.

■ VASODILATORS

The major indications for the use of vasodilators in infants with heart disease are (1) impaired ventricular function; (2) semilunar valve regurgitation; (3) systemic hypertension; and (4) pulmonary hypertension. The selection of a specific drug depends upon the primary goal of therapy, underlying or associated conditions, and whether or not the treatment is acute or chronic in nature. Vasodilators can be categorized in several ways. One classification groups the drug classes according to their major mechanism of action. Table 12-7 presents the major mechanisms of action and a representative drug for each class. Knowledge of the mechanism of action of a given drug provides a framework for understanding the pharmacology and therapeutic applications. As new drugs within a class become available, a great deal regarding the pharmacology of the drug will already be known if one understands the mechanism of action. Another method of classification is to group drugs according to their predominant site of action. As outlined in Table 12-7, vasodilators can be considered as predominately venous, arteriolar, or balanced (comparable effects on arterioles and venules). Depending on the goal of therapy, one may select an agent that has predominant effects on venous capacitance, arteriolar resistance, or both.

Nitrovasodilators

Relaxation of vascular smooth muscle by drugs in this class is mediated by nitric oxide. Nitric oxide activates guanylyl cyclase, resulting in increased formation of cGMP in vascular smooth muscle cells and activation of cGMP-dependent protein kinase. The net effect is relaxation of vascular smooth muscle tone and vasodilation.

Nitroglycerin

Although nitroglycerin affects virtually all smooth muscle in the cardiovascular, respiratory, gastrointestinal systems, the predominant site of action at the usual therapeutic concentrations is the venous vascular bed. Nitroglycerin therefore acts principally to increase venous capacitance, promoting a reduction in atrial and ventricular filling pressures. Nitroglycerin is rarely used in neonates because of the risk of hypotension, but is sometimes administered after cardiac surgery. At low doses there is little effect on systemic vascular resistance, systemic arterial pressure, or heart rate. However, higher doses can produce arteriolar dilation with hypotension and reflex tachycardia.

Nitroglycerin is rapidly metabolized in the liver and is therefore not effective after oral administration. Because of the short plasma half-life, it must be given by continuous infusion. Nitroglycerin is a potent vasodilator that must be used with appropriate hemodynamic monitoring. Patients with decreased intravascular volume (low preload) may respond adversely to nitroglycerin because a further decline in filling pressure may significantly reduce cardiac output. Overdose causes hypotension and tachycardia, which respond quickly to cessation of the infusion or a reduction in dose.

Nitroprusside

Nitroprusside is an extremely potent vasodilator. Hemodynamic responses to nitroprusside result from decreases in venous and arteriolar tone. Nitroprusside reduces systemic vascular resistance, pulmonary vascular resistance, atrial pressures, and may indirectly increase cardiac output. Heart rate may increase slightly in response to nitroprusside.

■ **TABLE 12-7.** Vasodilator Mechanisms and Sites of Action

Predominant mechanism	Drug examples	Predominant site of action
Nitrovasodilator	Nitroglycerin	Venous
Calcium channel antagonist	Nifedipine	Arteriolar
ACE inhibitor	Captopril	Mixed
Angiotensin receptor blocker	Losartan	Mixed
Natriuretic peptide	Nesiritide	Mixed

Nitroprusside is used for treating hypertensive emergencies because it is a potent vasodilator with a rapid onset of action and titratable effects. Nitroprusside is sometimes administered to pediatric cardiac surgical patients in the immediate postoperative period. In addition, it may be effective acutely in children with left ventricular dysfunction or mitral regurgitation. With proper monitoring and dosing, nitroprusside appears to be safe and effective in neonates.

Nitroprusside is rapidly metabolized and must be administered by continuous intravenous infusion. It is subject to photochemical degradation so solutions must be freshly prepared and protected from light during infusion. Because of the rapid onset of action and rapid metabolism, the desired hemodynamic effect can be achieved by careful dose titration. The major adverse effects of nitroprusside are a direct extension of its powerful vasodilator activity. Careful hemodynamic monitoring is imperative in order to avoid significant hypotension.

Nitroprusside is metabolized to thiocyanate and cyanide. Toxic effects in older patients include tachycardia, tachypnea, vomiting, headache, fatigue, anorexia, and disorientation. These signs and symptoms are difficult to detect in newborns. Although red blood cell cyanide and serum thiocyanate concentrations must be monitored in infants receiving long-term or high-dose nitroprusside therapy, the precise relationships between cyanide or thiocyanate concentrations and clinical toxicity are not entirely clear. Chronic thiocyanate toxicity may affect thyroid function and this must be considered in neonates.

Pulmonary Vasodilators

Nitric Oxide

Nitric oxide is an endothelium-derived relaxing factor that is administered as an inhaled gas. This agent causes rapid pulmonary vasodilation but does not affect the systemic vasculature because it is rapidly inactivated by hemoglobin. Therapy with nitric oxide plays a central role in the management of infants with persistent pulmonary hypertension of the newborn. This agent is also beneficial in the perioperative period for neonates with pulmonary arterial hypertension associated with congenital heart disease. Determination of the effectiveness of nitric oxide therapy includes evaluation of oxygenation and pulmonary artery pressure. Echocardiography may be helpful in assessing pulmonary artery pressure noninvasively. Methemoglobin

levels should be monitored regularly in patients receiving high concentrations or prolonged therapy.

Sildenafil

Sildenafil is a potent and selective inhibitor of cyclic nucleotide phosphodiesterase type 5. This isoform is the predominant phosphodiesterase that metabolizes cGMP in the lung vasculature. Inhibition of this phosphodiesterase results in pulmonary vasodilation and increased efficacy of inhaled nitric oxide. Sildenafil can be administered enterally, intravenously, or as an aerosol but most of the published experience in infants to date has been with the oral and intravenous forms. Orally administered sildenafil has been shown to be effective in treating persistent pulmonary hypertension in newborns and is well tolerated. The primary use of sildenafil in neonates with cardiac disease is for those patients with acute or chronic pulmonary hypertension following cardiac surgery. Additional studies are needed in infants with heart disease to define optimal dosing and pharmacokinetics, and to further clarify the role of sildenafil in the immediate postoperative period.

α-Adrenergic Receptor Antagonists

Phentolamine

Phentolamine is a competitive antagonist of α-adrenergic receptors, but it is nonselective and blocks α_1 and α_2 receptors. Blockade of presynaptic α_2-adrenergic receptors may contribute to the tachycardia and arrhythmias that occur at high doses of phentolamine. Administration of phentolamine to patients with low cardiac output produces a decrease in systemic vascular resistance with a resultant increase in cardiac output. Although phentolamine is classified as a mixed vasodilator, the effects on venous capacitance are minimal compared with other mixed vasodilators. Phentolamine reduces pulmonary vascular resistance and pulmonary arterial pressure.

Published experience with phentolamine in children is limited to short-term intravenous administration. In general, phentolamine is effective and well tolerated in infants and children. Adverse effects include significant sinus tachycardia, arrhythmias, and excessive hypotension. The major application of phentolamine in neonates is in the period immediately after cardiac surgery.

Calcium Channel Antagonists

Calcium channel antagonists block the opening of calcium channels in vascular smooth muscle, thereby promoting vasodilation. However, these drugs also block L-type calcium channels in the heart. Newborns are more sensitive to the negative inotropic effects of calcium channel blockers and intravenous administration of calcium channel blockers in infants has been associated with cardiovascular collapse. These drugs must be used cautiously in neonates and infants.

Calcium channel antagonists are categorized into three major chemical classes: phenylalkylamines (eg, verapamil), dihydropyridines (eg, nifedipine), and benzothiazepines (eg, diltiazem). Drugs of the dihydropyridine class exhibit the most pronounced vasodilation and should be selected if that is the primary goal of therapy. Many different dihydropyridine calcium channel antagonists are commercially available in the United States. Most of the published pediatric experience is limited to nifedipine, but the clinically important differences among the various dihydropyridines are slight. In young infants nifedipine is used primarily to treat pulmonary hypertension associated with bronchopulmonary dysplasia. Oral verapamil is used rarely for treatment of older infants with arrhythmias or hypertrophic cardiomyopathy.

Angiotensin-Converting Enzyme Inhibitors

Angiotensin-converting enzyme (ACE) inhibitors play a central role in the management of systemic hypertension and congestive heart failure in adults. However, relatively few rigorous clinical trials have been performed to support the widespread use of ACE inhibitors in infants and children. Despite the relative paucity of data, anecdotal reports and clinical experience support the beneficial effects of these drugs, especially in the short term.

ACE inhibitors block the conversion of angiotensin I to angiotensin II by inhibiting activity of the converting enzyme. In addition, ACE inhibitors reduce the inactivation of vasodilatory bradykinins and diminish production of aldosterone. These concepts are illustrated in Figure 12-2. More recently, it has become apparent that tissue angiotensin-generating systems may be important in local control of cardiac, renal, and vascular function.

Hemodynamic effects of ACE inhibitors include a reduction in systemic vascular resistance and systemic blood pressure. Because patients with congestive heart failure also respond with venodilation, these drugs are classified as balanced vasodilators. Results from studies of the chronic use of ACE inhibitors in adults with heart failure have confirmed significant improvements in survival,

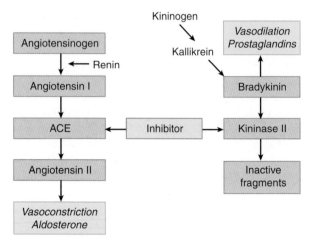

FIGURE 12-2. Effects of angiotensin-converting enzyme inhibitors. ACE inhibitors block the conversion of angiotensin I to angiotensin II, thereby reducing vasoconstriction and aldosterone production mediated by angiotensin II. In addition, the degradation of bradykinin is inhibited by ACE inhibitors. This action promotes vasodilation.

reduction in hospitalizations, and improvements in quality of life. ACE inhibitor therapy does not promote neurohormonal activation. The results of ACE inhibitor therapy for heart failure in adult patients is so compelling that administration of an ACE inhibitor is presently recommended even for patients with asymptomatic left ventricular dysfunction.

Many ACE inhibitors are commercially available in the United States that are similar with regard to their mechanism of action but differ slightly in their pharmacokinetic and metabolic profiles. Most of the published experience in the pediatric population is with captopril and enalapril.

Captopril

Captopril reduces systemic vascular resistance and increases venous capacitance, resulting in increased cardiac output and a reduction in cardiac filling pressures in children with congestive heart failure. Pulmonary vascular resistance generally declines and heart rate is usually minimally affected. Mild to moderate diuresis occurs as a result of increased renal blood flow and a reduction in aldosterone formation.

Captopril is administered orally and peak plasma concentrations occur 1 to 2 hours after a single oral dose. Although the plasma half-life is short (2-3 h), the duration of the clinical effect is usually 6 to 8 hours. Captopril is therefore administered three times a day. Approximately

50% is excreted in the urine unchanged and clearance is reduced in patients with impaired renal function.

Initial pediatric experience with captopril was for the treatment of systemic hypertension in infants and children. Subsequently, captopril was shown to be very effective in the management of congestive heart failure in infants and children related to dilated cardiomyopathy. Captopril is generally well tolerated in most infants, but significant hypotension may occur in volume-depleted patients or in patients with extremely high basal renin activity. When starting captopril therapy for congestive heart failure in infants, the first dose should be low and the blood pressure should be carefully monitored. If the drug is tolerated, then the dosage can be escalated over a few days.

Adverse effects include neutropenia and proteinuria, especially in children with underlying renal disease. Less serious side effects include rash, taste impairment, and minor gastrointestinal disturbances. A dry nonproductive cough is a well-described feature of ACE inhibitor therapy in adults, but this does not seem to be a major problem in neonates. In general, potassium supplements and potassium-sparing diuretics should not be administered concomitantly to patients receiving captopril because of the risk of hyperkalemia.

Enalapril

The mechanism of action, hemodynamics, and clinical indications for enalapril are similar to those described for captopril. Enalapril differs from captopril in that enalapril is a prodrug that must be de-esterified to form the active agent, enalaprilat. Enalaprilat is commercially available for parenteral administration. Enalapril has a slower onset of action and longer half-life than captopril. Generally, enalapril is administered once or twice per day which facilitates compliance compared to captopril. Enalapril has been shown to be effective in the management of infants with congestive heart failure and systemic hypertension. The overall incidence of side effects due to enalapril appears to be lower than that reported for captopril. Because enalapril has a longer duration of action, hypotension may be prolonged if overdose occurs.

Angiotensin Receptor Blockers

Angiotensin receptors exist as distinct subtypes (AT_1, AT_2) that serve to couple angiotensin with specific intracellular responses. Because local tissue production of angiotensin may occur that is not ACE-dependent, more complete local inhibition of the angiotensin pathway can theoretically be achieved by direct blockade of AT receptors. Recently, a number of selective AT_1 receptor blockers have been released for the treatment of heart failure and hypertension in adults. These agents are particularly useful in adult patients who develop coughing when taking ACE inhibitors. This side effect is much less common in infants and children. The prototype is losartan. Experience with these agents in infants is extremely relatively limited at present. However, based on theoretical considerations and results obtained from clinical trials in adults, these agents may prove to be useful in the pediatric population. Use of these agents in pediatric patients with connective tissue disease such as Marfan and Loeys-Dietz syndromes is a subject of current investigation.

■ ALDOSTERONE RECEPTOR ANTAGONISTS

Enhanced activity of the renin-angiotensin system with increased synthesis of aldosterone is a hallmark of congestive heart failure. Aldosterone may be involved in the pathogenesis of a variety of deleterious responses observed in the heart failure syndrome. Aldosterone plays an important role in promoting the abnormal collagen production and interstitial fibrosis that occurs in chronic congestive heart failure. Therapy with ACE inhibitors has been assumed to block both angiotensin II and aldosterone production. However, recent data in adults suggest that aldosterone production may "escape" despite the appropriate use of an ACE inhibitor. An escape of aldosterone production has several potentially important consequences, including sodium retention, potassium and magnesium loss, excessive myocardial collagen production, ventricular hypertrophy, myocardial norepinephrine release, endothelial dysfunction, and a decrease in serum high-density lipoprotein cholesterol. Administration of the aldosterone antagonist, spironolactone, to patients with heart failure treated with conventional therapy (including an ACE inhibitor) results in increased diuresis and symptomatic improvement. Spironolactone has been used for years as a potassium-sparing diuretic in infants with heart failure. Whether additional benefit is derived from inhibiting the other effects of aldosterone in infants remains to be determined.

■ HORMONES

Nesiritide

Nesiritide is a recombinant B-type natriuretic peptide that has been studied in adults with acutely decompensated heart failure. It is administered intravenously and produces vasodilation, increases glomerular filtration rate, inhibits renal sodium reabsorption, and promotes diuresis. Despite considerable investigation in the adult population, the role and efficacy of nesiritide is controversial. Several studies in children suggest nesiritide may increase urine output and reduce levels of neurohormonal markers of heart failure. Some centers use nesiritide acutely for infants with low cardiac output following cardiac surgery and for infants with severely depressed cardiac function due to cardiomyopathy. Additional studies are needed to determine the safety and efficacy of nesiritide in neonates with heart disease.

Thyroxine and Triiodothyronine

A number of neuroendocrine changes occur in heart failure (Chapter 11), during critical illness and following surgical procedures. Thyroid hormone secretion is reduced in critically ill adults and children following cardiac surgery. These changes in thyroid hormone levels are referred to as "nonthyroidal illness syndrome" and generally have not been thought to represent true hypothyroidism. However, this concept is controversial and some authorities suggest that these patients may have acquired true central hypothyroidism as a consequence of their critical illness or surgical procedure. Some centers routinely administer either thyroxine or triiodothyronine in the postoperative period if thyroid stimulating hormone is elevated, circulating thyroid hormone levels are reduced, and the infant exhibits persistent or refractory low cardiac output. However, little published information exists regarding the safety, efficacy, and long-term effects of thyroid hormone administration to neonates in the early post-cardiac surgery period. Additional studies are required to determine the significance of these changes in thyroid hormone levels and the role, if any, of routine thyroid hormone therapy in this setting.

Vasopressin

Vasopressin is a potent vasoconstrictor that acts directly on the vasculature via V1 receptors and indirectly by potentiating the vasoconstrictor effects of catecholamines. The responses to vasopressin are preserved in the presence of acidosis or hypoxia. Cardiopulmonary bypass is known to evoke a systemic inflammatory response that can result in low cardiac output and vasodilatory shock. The first line of therapy in this setting is infusion of catecholamines such as dopamine or norepinephrine. However, shock persists in some infants despite maximal supportive therapy. This clinical syndrome mimics that seen in patients with septic shock, which has been associated with depressed levels of vasopressin in adults and children. Based on results from studies demonstrating a beneficial effect of vasopressin infusion in patients with vasodilatory septic shock, several investigators have administered vasopressin to infants with vasodilatory shock following cardiopulmonary bypass. In general, the reported results are favorable and it appears that vasopressin can be an effective adjunct to more conventional therapy in this setting. However, additional studies are required to more fully define the indications, safety, and efficacy of vasopressin in infants with heart disease.

■ β-ADRENERGIC RECEPTOR BLOCKERS

β-Blockers can be classified as first generation, nonselective for β_1 and β_2 blockade (eg, propranolol); second generation with relative selectivity for β_1 receptors (eg, metoprolol and atenolol), and third-generation drugs (selective or nonselective) with potentially important ancillary properties (eg, carvedilol and bucindolol). β-Blockers are not interchangeable, therapy must be carefully initiated and monitored, and published experience in pediatric patients is limited. The most commonly used β-blockers in infants are propranolol, atenolol, and esmolol.

Propranolol

Propranolol was the first commercially available β-adrenergic blocker in the United States. Subsequently, many β-blockers have been developed and are available for commercial use. However, propranolol has been most widely used and there is published experience with this drug in pediatric patients. Propranolol is available for oral or intravenous administration, but if intravenous β-blocker therapy is necessary, the short-acting β-adrenergic blocker, esmolol (see following text) should be used because of the risk of severe hypotension and bradycardia associated with the administration of intravenous propranolol.

Propranolol is used in infants for management of supraventricular tachycardia, some forms of ventricular arrhythmias, treatment of congenital long QT syndromes, and hypertrophic cardiomyopathy. In the past, propranolol was sometimes used in an attempt to reduce the frequency and severity of hypercyanotic episodes in infants with tetralogy of Fallot. Now most patients undergo surgical correction or palliation if hypercyanotic episodes occur. Some infants with critical pulmonary stenosis will benefit from a short course of propranolol after relief of pulmonary valve stenosis until the infundibular hypertrophy improves.

Propranolol is well absorbed after an oral dose, although it undergoes extensive first-past hepatic metabolism, reducing the bioavailability to approximately 30% to 40%. Class-dependent effects of β-adrenergic blockers include depression of contractility, atrioventricular block, bronchospasm, and sleep disturbances. Propranolol should be avoided if possible in infants with significant pulmonary disease. Chronic use of propranolol in infants appears to be safe and well tolerated. However, infants are at risk for developing hypoglycemia if their oral intake is restricted because of other illnesses or other conditions. Blood glucose should be monitored in infants receiving propranolol who are unable to feed normally.

Atenolol

Atenolol is relatively selective for β_1-adrenergic receptors. This agent has the advantage of requiring only once or twice a day administration because of a longer half-life (8-10 h). Fewer central nervous system effects occur with atenolol than with propranolol because atenolol does not cross the blood-brain barrier, but the clinical implications in neonates and young infants are unclear. An atenolol suspension can be prepared by many pharmacies and this drug is well tolerated.

Esmolol

Esmolol is a β_1-selective adrenergic blocker with a short plasma half-life (approximately 5-10 min). The indications and precautions for esmolol are similar to those described for propranolol. The major difference is that because of the short half-life, esmolol is administered by continuous intravenous infusion. Thus, the dose is easier to titrate and if adverse effects occur, the duration of toxicity will be quite short. Esmolol is generally used for short periods of time in acute care settings (ie, cardiac catheterization laboratory, postoperative recovery unit, neonatal intensive care nursery).

Carvedilol

Carvedilol is a third-generation β-adrenergic receptor blocker that blocks β_1-, β_2-, and α_1-adrenergic receptors. In addition, it exhibits antioxidant, anti-inflammatory, and antiapoptotic activities. Experience with carvedilol in infants with heart failure is described in Chapter 11. Although promising, additional studies are necessary to

define the potential role of carvedilol in managing neonates with heart disease.

■ PROSTAGLANDIN E$_1$

Prostaglandin E$_1$ (PGE$_1$) is used to dilate the ductus arteriosus in newborns with cardiac defects in which maintaining adequate pulmonary or systemic blood flow is dependent upon a patent ductus arteriosus. The common indications for PGE$_1$ therapy include pulmonary atresia, critical pulmonary stenosis, transposition of the great arteries, coarctation of the aorta, interrupted aortic arch, critical aortic stenosis, and hypoplastic left heart syndrome. Administration of PGE$_1$ should be strongly considered very early in the management of infants in whom a ductus-dependent cardiac defect is suspected. A good example is the infant with signs of congenital heart disease who is born at a center without tertiary-care cardiac services. In this case, it is advisable to begin PGE$_1$ therapy before transport and more definitive delineation of the cardiac status. This can be lifesaving and conversely, withholding therapy can be disastrous if the ductus arteriosus closes in a patient with a ductus-dependent defect. Although not entirely benign, PGE$_1$ can be administered safely and if the infant is subsequently found not to have significant structural heart disease, the infusion can be discontinued.

PGE$_1$ has a short half-life and must be given by continuous intravascular infusion. Although the intravenous route is preferred, it can be given via an umbilical arterial catheter, if necessary. Because these infants are critically dependent upon the infusion for maintaining ductus patency, a reliable intravenous line is essential. Thus, the use of a central venous (umbilical venous) catheter is recommended whenever possible. In addition to effects on the ductus arteriosus, PGE$_1$ dilates the systemic and pulmonary vascular beds. Thus, a potential side effect is hypotension due to arteriolar dilation. In these cases, reduction in the dose is generally sufficient to reverse the fall in blood pressure. If this is not possible, small fluid boluses (5-10 mL/kg) are often effective. Another potentially serious adverse effect is apnea. Administration of a high dose or an inadvertent bolus of PGE$_1$ will most certainly induce apnea. Thus, whenever PGE$_1$ is administered, personnel and equipment necessary to support ventilation must be available. Infusion pumps with a continuous action should be used and the intravenous line containing the drug must not be flushed. Additional side effects include fever, irritability, edema, and cutaneous flushing.

SUGGESTED READINGS

Drug Dosage Reference

Taketomo CK, Hodding JH, Kraus DM. *Pediatric Dosage Handbook.* 16th ed. Hudson, OH: Lexi-Comp, Inc.; 2009.

Pharmacology of Specific Drugs and Drug Classes

Balaguru D, Auslender M. Vasodilators in the treatment of pediatric heart failure. *Prog Pediatr Cardiol.* 2000;12(1):81-90.

Grenier MA, Fioravanti J, Truesdell SC, et al. Angiotensin-converting enzyme inhibitor therapy for ventricular dysfunction in infants, children and adolescents: a review. *Prog Pediatr Cardiol.* 2000;12(1):91-111.

Hougen TJ. Digitalis use in children: an uncertain future. *Prog Pediatr Cardiol.* 2000;12(1):37-43.

Latifi S, Lidsky K, Blumer JL. Pharmacology of inotropic agents in infants and children. *Prog Pediatr Cardiol.* 2000;12(1):57-79.

Lechner E, Hofer A, Mair R, et al. Arginine-vasopressin in neonates with vasodilatory shock after cardiopulmonary bypass. *Eur J Pediatr.* 2007;166:1221-1227.

Lowrie L. Diuretic therapy of heart failure in infants and children. *Prog Pediatr Cardiol.* 2000;12(1):45-55.

Ricci Z, Stazi GV, Di Chiara L, et al. Fenoldopam in newborn patients undergoing cardiopulmonary bypass: controlled clinical trial. *Interact Cardiovasc Thorac Surg.* 2008; 7:1049-1053.

Shekerdemian L. Perioperative manipulation of the circulation in children with congenital heart disease. *Heart.* 2009; 95:1286-1296.

Shih JL, Agus MSD. Thyroid function in the critically ill newborn and child. *Curr Opin Pediatr.* 2009;21:536-540.

Steinhorn RH, Kinsella JP, Pierce C, et al. Intravenous sildenafil in the treatment of neonates with persistent pulmonary hypertension. *J Pediatr.* 2009;155:841-847.

Ward RM, Lugo RA. Cardiovascular drugs for the newborn. *Clin Perinatol.* 2005;32:979-997.

CHAPTER 13

Care of the Postoperative Patient

■ INTRODUCTION

To avoid the cumulative morbidity and mortality associated with initial palliative procedures followed by later repair, primary corrective surgery has become increasingly common for patients with congenital heart disease. One result of this trend is that an increasing number of cardiac surgery procedures are performed on neonates and even on premature infants. Optimal care of these infants requires specialized knowledge of the unique structural and functional characteristics of neonatal organ systems and is best accomplished by a multidisciplinary team including cardiology, cardiac surgery, neonatology, anesthesia, and critical care. The purpose of this chapter is to review general principles of care for these infants. The physiology and surgical procedures pertinent to specific defects are discussed in Chapters 6 through 8.

■ CLASSIFICATION OF CARDIAC SURGERIES

Cardiac surgery procedures are classified as to whether they are open or closed and whether they are corrective or palliative (Table 13-1). "Open" refers to those procedures in which cardiopulmonary bypass is used; bypass is not used in "closed" procedures. Palliative procedures are performed in patients in whom complete correction of the cardiac defects is not possible or not feasible because of comorbidities. Palliated patients have residual intracardiac shunting or other hemodynamic abnormalities. In most institutions, palliative procedures are only performed for infants with a functional single ventricle (eg, hypoplastic left heart syndrome, tricuspid atresia) or for those with poorly developed pulmonary arteries.

■ **TABLE 13-1.** Classification of Cardiac Surgery Procedures

Closed: Cardiopulmonary bypass is not used.
  Palliative—Pulmonary artery band, systemic-to-pulmonary artery shunt
  Corrective—Repair of aortic coarctation, ligation of patent ductus arteriosus
Open: Cardiopulmonary bypass is used.
  Palliative—Stage I Norwood procedure, Damus-Kaye-Stansel procedure
  Corrective—Repair of transposition of the great arteries, tetralogy of Fallot, total anomalous pulmonary venous connection, truncus arteriosus, ventricular septal defect

Examples of palliative and corrective procedures are provided, but these lists are not comprehensive.

Most corrective procedures, for example, for truncus arteriosus or transposition of the great arteries, are performed by use of cardiopulmonary bypass. Venous blood is siphoned to a reservoir of the heart-lung bypass machine, which also collects blood drained from the operative field by suction catheters. Blood is pumped through an oxygenator, a heat exchanger, and a filter and then returned to the patient's ascending aorta through an aortic cannula. The patient is always fully anticoagulated with heparin while on bypass.

Hypothermia extends the safe duration of cardiopulmonary bypass in neonates and infants. Metabolic activity and thus, oxygen consumption, are decreased. "Deep" hypothermia involves cooling to about 18°C. For many years surgeons combined deep hypothermia with either low-flow bypass (25%-50% of normal flow) or more commonly, with no bypass flow, arresting the heart (deep hypothermic circulatory arrest). Deep hypothermic circulatory arrest provided the surgeon with a bloodless and relaxed heart not attached to multiple cannulas that may distort the surgical field. This technique allowed intricate surgical procedures to be performed and markedly improved survival of infants with complex congenital defects. Unfortunately, neurologic and developmental morbidities are increasingly being recognized in survivors (Chapter 14), and longer duration of deep hypothermic circulatory arrest is associated with a greater incidence of adverse neurologic outcomes. Alternate perfusion strategies include moderate hypothermia with normal or increased pump flow or deep hypothermia with intermittent perfusion. A more recently described approach during aortic arch reconstruction is antegrade cerebral perfusion, which involves directing blood flow to the cerebral circulation via a cannula in the innominate artery. Further clinical studies and continued refinements in technique are necessary to optimize neurologic outcomes.

Although cardiopulmonary bypass allows for correction of complex cardiac defects, morbidity associated with its use impacts care of the postoperative patient, particularly neonates. Blood cells are exposed to excessive shear forces and to artificial surfaces. Despite filtration, microembolization of gas bubbles and platelet clumps occurs. Nonpulsatile perfusion and hypothermia per se may also incite injury. Tissue ischemia is present to some extent and subsequent reperfusion injury occurs. These and other factors combine to cause a systemic inflammatory response, with activation of the complement system, leukocytes and the endothelium together with induction of cytokines, chemokines, and endotoxin, that results in increased capillary permeability, tissue edema, and multisystem dysfunction. This response is exaggerated in newborn infants compared to that in older children. Total body water increases, transient myocardial dysfunction occurs, pulmonary vascular resistance may increase, gas exchange is impaired, and stress and hormonal responses often cause fluid and electrolyte abnormalities. In order to limit this systemic inflammatory response, steroids are usually administered in the operating room and various ultrafiltration techniques are used during rewarming or after cardiopulmonary bypass to remove small molecular weight inflammatory mediators. Hemodilution may occur in part because of the priming volume required in the bypass circuit. This decreases oxygen delivery, decreases oncotic pressure resulting in further fluid extravasation, and dilutes clotting factors, contributing to postoperative coagulopathy. Maintenance of a hematocrit of about 25% to 30% during bypass seems to be optimal for hypothermia-induced alterations in blood viscosity and also for maintaining oncotic pressure and oxygen-carrying capacity.

■ TIMING OF SURGERY

In general, cyanotic infants can be stabilized by administration of PGE$_1$ and other supportive measures. Surgery can be scheduled on a semi-elective basis after careful evaluation is complete. Two exceptions are noteworthy: surgery is the only effective therapy for neonates with obstructed total anomalous pulmonary venous return and should be performed as soon as the diagnosis is established;

additionally, patients with d-transposition of the great arteries who have a restrictive patent foramen ovale often need emergency balloon atrial septostomy because of profound hypoxemia. This procedure can be performed at the bedside with echocardiographic guidance. After successful septostomy these infants are usually stable and corrective surgery should be delayed only if end-organic damage has occurred.

Infants who present with shock because of left heart obstructive lesions (eg, coarctation of the aorta, hypoplastic left heart syndrome) also can be stabilized by administration of PGE_1 and other supportive care. These infants may have sustained end-organ damage (most commonly, to the kidneys or liver) because of decreased perfusion. Deferring surgery while organ function recovers allows for complete evaluation of the infant and decreases surgical morbidity and risk. However, surgical intervention should be undertaken if there is evidence of ongoing organ injury despite maximal medical therapy.

■ TRANSPORT AND ARRIVAL FROM THE OPERATING ROOM

All personnel responsible for care of the infant after surgery must understand the anatomic defect(s) and be familiar with the preoperative evaluation and course. Upon return from the operating room information must be provided regarding (1) intraoperative findings; (2) the exact procedure performed; (3) length of time on cardiopulmonary bypass, aortic cross-clamp time, level of hypothermia, and circulatory arrest time; (4) available postoperative hemodynamic and echocardiographic data especially regarding residual lesions; (5) complications including arrhythmias and bleeding, (6) location of catheters, tubes, and temporary pacing wires; (7) vasoactive infusions; (8) other medications; and (9) airway and ventilatory status.

The personnel transporting the infant must work harmoniously with staff in the ICU to ensure a careful and efficient admission of the patient to the ICU. Maintenance of adequate oxygenation and ventilation, and uninterrupted delivery of vasoactive drugs are critically important. About 15 minutes after the patient is placed on the ventilator (or earlier if clinically indicated), initial laboratory studies should be obtained. This often includes arterial blood gas, complete blood count, serum electrolytes and glucose, ionized calcium, and coagulation profile. A chest radiograph and often an electrocardiogram are obtained as soon as possible.

A comprehensive assessment should be performed as soon as possible, including a physical examination focusing on cardiovascular and respiratory function, and review of data from bedside monitors, postoperative orders, and laboratory data as available. The family should be updated and allowed to visit as soon as is feasible.

■ MONITORING

Although variation exists among institutions, most infants have continuous monitoring of their heart rate, rhythm, blood pressure, oxygen saturation, and respiratory rate after cardiac surgery. Most infants have an arterial line. End-tidal CO_2 monitoring is valuable in patients who are mechanically ventilated. Near-infrared spectroscopy (NIRS) monitoring estimates the concentration of oxygen in tissues by comparing the tissue's absorption of two wavelengths of light corresponding to hemoglobin carrying oxygen and hemoglobin without oxygen. NIRS leads placed on the forehead and in the paravertebral region over a kidney allow assessment of blood flow to the brain and kidneys, respectively.

Infants who have been on cardiopulmonary bypass usually have one or more intracardiac catheters for monitoring and infusions. Temporary pacing wires are often placed on the epicardial surface of the atrium and/or ventricle. The data obtained allow more precise measurement of hemodynamic variables thereby providing a rational basis for therapy. Nevertheless, the information obtained should be viewed as an adjunct to rather than a substitute for careful serial physical examinations to assess cardiac output.

A right atrial (RA) catheter may be advanced via a central vein or placed through the RA appendage. RA catheters are used to measure central venous pressure which may reflect intravascular volume status. In addition to volume overload, other causes of increased RA pressure include decreased right (or single) ventricular compliance, tricuspid valve regurgitation or a residual left ventricular to RA shunt, and cardiac tamponade. RA saturation can also be measured but may not represent a true mixed venous sample because of streaming of venous inflow within the atrium and because it is mixed with left atrial blood in the single ventricle patient. When blood can be obtained from a site that is a reasonable estimate of mixed venous saturation (the superior vena cava is usually the best source), an arteriovenous oxygen saturation difference of less than 30% indicates adequate cardiac output.

A left atrial (LA) catheter may be placed via the LA appendage or through the right superior pulmonary vein. The LA pressure provides indirect data regarding functioning of the systemic ventricle as long as the systemic atrioventricular valve is neither regurgitant nor stenotic. LA pressure also rises and falls with intravascular volume status. The oxygen saturation in the LA should be about 100%. Decreased LA saturation can be caused by right-to-left atrial shunting or by pulmonary venous desaturation secondary to abnormal gas exchange (eg, atelectasis).

A pulmonary artery (PA) catheter, inserted through a purse string structure in the right ventricular outflow tract, is used by some institutions to monitor selected infants at high risk for pulmonary arterial hypertension. High pressure and a higher saturation than that obtained in the right atrium is suggestive of a residual left-to-right shunt in a patient with two ventricle physiology. Residual shunting can usually be assessed easily by echocardiography.

■ GENERAL PRINCIPLES OF POSTOPERATIVE CARE BY SYSTEM

Cardiovascular

Decreased Cardiac Output

Myocardial dysfunction is common after surgery in young infants, especially neonates. One or more of the following factors may be involved:

- *Preoperative myocardial dysfunction*—This is most common in patients with left heart obstructive lesions such as aortic coarctation.

- *Effects of cardiopulmonary bypass*—As discussed in the preceding text, a prominent systemic inflammatory response frequently occurs and may adversely affect myocardial function. At times inadequate myocardial perfusion occurs during surgery. Lastly, a ventriculotomy, if performed, may lead to regional myocardial dysfunction. If these intraoperative events lead to a low-output state, their effects usually peak 6 to 12 hours after surgery. Physical examination will disclose tachycardia, hypotension, and cool extremities with decreased perfusion. Decreased urine output, lactic acidosis, and pleural effusions may be present. It is critically important to anticipate this reproducible and potentially lethal phenomenon and to intervene immediately. Infusion of volume and administration of inotropic and afterload reducing agents are often necessary. Serial physical examinations and frequent evaluation of hemodynamic and metabolic data are necessary to assess the response to therapeutic interventions.

- *Residual anatomic lesions*—The operative assessment of cardiac anatomy and function is done by direct inspection, blood gas and pressure measurements, and imaging. The use of transesophageal echocardiography in the operating room after surgery has reduced the incidence of unsuspected residual anatomic lesions. Nevertheless, if the postoperative course does not conform to that expected, investigation should be undertaken to assess for residual or previously undiagnosed anatomic defects. This certainly includes echocardiography but may also involve magnetic resonance imaging and/or cardiac catheterization.

- *Arrhythmias*—Abnormal heart rhythms such as atrioventricular block and tachycardias are relatively common in the postoperative period and may contribute to inadequate cardiac output. Diagnosis and treatment of rhythm disorders is discussed in Chapter 10. The neonate is relatively dependent on heart rate to maintain cardiac output. Therefore bradycardia associated with atrioventricular block will markedly decrease cardiac output and pacing should be instituted promptly via the transthoracic pacing wires. Junctional ectopic tachycardia is the most common tachyarrhythmia and results in loss of atrioventricular synchrony. Infants who are symptomatic from rapid heart rates should be treated immediately.

- *Electrolyte and hormonal disturbances*—Hypocalcemia and hypomagnesemia depress myocardial contractility and should be treated appropriately. Some have postulated that administration of glucocorticosteroids improves refractory hemodynamic instability in stressed neonates who may have an inappropriate or abnormal adrenal response to stress after cardiac surgery. Similarly, decreased concentrations of triiodothyronine, the biologically active hormone in cardiac myocytes, may contribute to low cardiac output syndrome after bypass; some have advocated administration of triiodothyronine. Neither of these therapies has been shown to be efficacious in a clinical trial, but both are used empirically at times.

Support of the Circulation

The primary goals in the initial postoperative period are to optimize cardiac output and blood flow distribution by maintaining optimal heart rate, preload, afterload, and contractility. As discussed earlier, bradycardia adversely affects cardiac output in neonates and should be treated. Preload must be optimized by assessing intravascular volume. Vasodilator agents can be used to decrease afterload as indicated. Contractility is increased by administration of inotropic agents as needed. Care must be taken to avoid adverse effects of these medications. Increased inotropy is associated with increased myocardial energy requirements. Tachycardia may occur and results in decreased diastolic filling time which can decrease myocardial blood flow. Additionally, excessive doses of sympathomimetic amines may predispose to junctional ectopic tachycardia. Despite these concerns, inotropic agents are quite useful for treating myocardial dysfunction and are discussed in detail in Chapter 12. Treatment with these agents should be titrated to maintain adequate end-organ perfusion and not to just a certain level of blood pressure. The physical examination, urine output, plasma acid load, and systemic arteriovenous difference should be assessed repeatedly to evaluate the adequacy of the cardiac output. The choice of inotropic agent is often empiric. The combination of milrinone and dopamine is frequently used to increase cardiac output, maintain appropriate perfusion pressure without an excessive increase in afterload, and improve myocardial relaxation. If increased doses of these agents fail to adequately improve cardiac output, epinephrine in low doses (0.01-0.05 µg/kg/min) is often effective, especially for infants with relative bradycardia or who are chronically stressed. The dose is increased as indicated.

Mechanical support of the circulation. Extracorporeal membrane oxygenation (ECMO) is the most commonly used mode of mechanical circulatory support for neonates and infants with heart disease both before and after surgery. ECMO should be considered for patients thought to have reversible causes of low cardiac output who are not responding to maximal medical therapy. In addition to maintaining adequate systemic blood flow, ECMO facilitates myocardial recovery as ventricular wall tension is decreased and coronary perfusion is improved. This modality can also serve as a bridge to cardiac transplantation. The reported survival rates after ECMO cannulation are 35% to 60% in pediatric patients with heart disease. Patients who fail to wean from bypass are at increased risk of life-threatening bleeding when placed on ECMO. Typical indications for ECMO are shown in Table 13-2. Contraindications include significant neurologic deficit, end-stage or irreversible systemic disease, major bleeding, and inaccessible vessels for cannulation. Some consider important renal or hepatic dysfunction to be a relative contraindication. Aggressive evaluation for residual anatomic lesions including possible cardiac catheterization is critical

---

■ TABLE 13-2. Indications for ECMO

Severe ventricular dysfunction (pre- or postoperative)
Failure to wean from cardiopulmonary bypass
Pulmonary arterial hypertension refractory to medical therapy
Acute systemic-pulmonary shunt malfunction
Arrhythmias refractory to medical management and associated with hemodynamic compromise
Cardiac arrest

ECMO, extracorporeal membrane oxygenation.

---

for patients who are placed on ECMO because of failure to wean from bypass.

A few longer term support devices are available in some centers for those patients who fail to wean from ECMO and who are awaiting cardiac transplantation. The Berlin heart is the most common device used in neonates and infants. This is a pneumatically driven pulsatile device which can provide univentricular (right or left) or biventricular support. The inlet is a cannula placed through the apex of the ventricle and the outlet is to the aorta or pulmonary artery. Advantages of a ventricular assist device compared to ECMO include decreased trauma to blood cells which decreases the need for anticoagulation, decreased risk of infection, and greater patient mobility. The major disadvantage is that these devices do not provide respiratory support.

Pulmonary Arterial Hypertension

Pulmonary arterial (PA) hypertension is an important cause of morbidity and mortality in infants after cardiac surgery. The pulmonary vascular bed is very reactive in young infants, especially neonates during the first few days after cardiac surgery. Acute increases in PA pressure may precipitate life-threatening right heart failure. Patients at highest risk include those with documented increased pulmonary vascular resistance, systemic ventricular dysfunction associated with increased ventricular end-diastolic pressure, and pulmonary venous hypertension of other causes. Conditions known to increase PA pressure, such as acidosis, hypoxia, hypercarbia, cold stress, and agitation from pain should be prevented if possible, and be treated aggressively if they occur. Concomitant pulmonary disease including infection, atelectasis, and reactive airways disease further predisposes the infant to acute increases in PA pressure and also prolongs the period of time that the infant is vulnerable. Sedation, mild hyperventilation, ventilation to maintain normal functional residual capacity, inspired oxygen as needed to avoid alveolar hypoxia, adequate hematocrit, and infusion of agents such as milrinone are often efficacious.

Infants who fail to respond to this treatment may benefit from inhaled nitric oxide (NO). When administered via inhalation, NO acts as a selective pulmonary vasodilator and does not cause systemic hypotension that often results from intravenously administered vasodilators. Patients with a history of pulmonary venous hypertension (eg, obstructive total anomalous pulmonary venous connection, congenital mitral stenosis) are particularly responsive to NO but this agent is also beneficial in patients after repair of defects associated with pulmonary arterial hypertension (eg, truncus arteriosus, atrioventricular septal defect). Weaning of NO can be facilitated by pretreatment with sildenafil, which can be continued for weeks to months as indicated clinically.

Respiratory

Ventilation and respiratory mechanics have important effects on the hemodynamic status of neonates, especially after cardiac surgery. Infants with preexisting myocardial dysfunction as a result of lesions such as severe aortic coarctation and those who have undergone open-heart procedures benefit from a period of maximal ventilatory support while myocardial function recovers. Sedation and occasionally neuromuscular blockade are continued for a period of time after arrival in the ICU. Knowledge of whether the surgery performed was corrective or palliative is essential to setting goals for systemic oxygenation. The oxygen saturation should be about 75% to 85% in patients after a palliative procedure such as a systemic-to-pulmonary artery shunt or a stage I Norwood procedure. For infants at risk for PA hypertension, ventilation is often adjusted to maintain a mild respiratory alkalosis, and the amount of inspired oxygen is weaned slowly. Caution must be used when manually ventilating or suctioning these infants as these maneuvers may precipitate an acute increase in PA pressures and may lead to hemodynamic instability. Some advocate for the administration of additional sedation before suctioning and for increasing the level of inspired oxygen during suctioning. Relatively high levels of positive end-expiratory pressure and large tidal volumes are sometimes necessary to recruit end-expiratory lung volumes after bypass in neonates. Overinflation should be avoided

because this compresses the pulmonary microcirculation and increases pulmonary vascular resistance.

Mechanical ventilation is continued until postoperative bleeding has ceased, the sternum is closed, the hemodynamics are stable, postoperative diuresis has occurred if the patient became fluid overloaded, atelectasis and secretions are minimal, and the patient is capable of protecting the airway. Failure to wean from the ventilator can result from several different problems. First, residual hemodynamic abnormalities such as residual shunts may play a role and should be evaluated by echocardiography and possibly by magnetic resonance imaging or cardiac catheterization. Severe fluid overload decreases chest wall compliance which compromises ventilation. Airway abnormalities (eg, bronchomalacia), pleural effusions, and alveolar disease are relatively common. Rarely, paralysis or paresis of a hemidiaphragm may be present (see following text). Finally, prolonged mechanical ventilation and poor nutrition can weaken respiratory muscles.

Fluids and Electrolytes

Preoperative renal dysfunction and the inflammatory response to bypass cause many infants to develop excess total body water during and immediately after surgery. Total fluid intake should be restricted often to 50% to 65% of maintenance requirements. Urine output is usually at least 1 mL/kg/h immediately after surgery but often decreases markedly 6 to 12 hours later. Total fluid intake and output must be monitored carefully to maintain adequate intravascular volume. Losses which occur as a result of capillary leak and bleeding must be replaced using infusions of crystalloid, colloid, or blood products.

Fluids containing 10% dextrose are generally administered and serum glucose should be measured frequently. Sodium chloride needs are minimal (1-2 mEq/kg/d). Hyponatremia usually reflects excess total body water rather than a sodium deficit. Potassium chloride should not be administered until urine output is adequate. Calcium is an important determinant of myocardial contractility and hypocalcemia impairs myocardial function. Ionized calcium should be monitored frequently. Transfusion of citrate-anticoagulated blood and DiGeorge syndrome (with parathyroid deficiency) are other important causes of hypocalcemia.

Diuretics are usually begun 12 to 24 hours after surgery. Maintenance of an adequate cardiac output by judicious volume replacement and administration of inotropic agents and vasodilators is important to achieve a good response to diuretic agents. At times a continuous infusion of furosemide (0.1-0.4 mg/kg/h) promotes a slow but steady diuresis that is often better tolerated than the sudden large diuresis that may result from a bolus dose of diuretic. Diuretic-induced electrolyte losses always occur and the resulting electrolyte abnormalities, for example, hypokalemia, hypocalcemia, and metabolic alkalosis must be treated aggressively. At times fulminant renal failure related to persistent low output occurs. Peritoneal dialysis, hemofiltration, or hemodialysis may be necessary and will assist in removing excess body water.

Nutrition

Adequate caloric intake is very important because debilitated and critically ill infants with limited fat reserves frequently have increased energy demands after cardiac surgery. Parenteral nutrition may be necessary to provide adequate nutrition for patients too unstable to tolerate enteral feeding. Continuous nasogastric feeding is often begun at very low rates of 2 to 5 mL/h ("trophic feeds") and then advanced as tolerated. Infants at risk for aspiration may be fed with a continuous infusion of formula via a naso-duodenal tube. Feedings should be advanced to 110 to 130 kcal/kg/d as tolerated. Care must be taken in infants who are at risk for bowel ischemia because necrotizing enterocolitis can occur especially in neonates who have (1) left-sided obstructive lesions; (2) systemic-to-pulmonary artery shunts with wide pulse pressures associated with retrograde flow in the mesenteric arteries during diastole; or (3) a history of hypotension or severe hypoxemia. Malrotation occurs frequently in patients with heterotaxy syndrome; feeding intolerance should be investigated early in these patients.

Analgesia and Sedation

Stress responses to pain and noxious stimuli adversely affect hemodynamics and may precipitate an acute increase in PA pressure. The choice of agent is empiric but relatively large doses of narcotic and sedative drugs, often fentanyl and midazolam, are usually administered during the first 48 hours after surgery and then weaned to allow effective spontaneous ventilation. Precise control of pCO_2 and pH, and therefore, pulmonary vascular resistance, is much easier in a well-sedated patient. All infants who are receiving neuromuscular blocking agents must also be given narcotic and sedative medications. Unexplained tachycardia is often a sign of inadequate sedation or

analgesia in these patients. Infants who have a long course in the ICU will require increasing dose of medications as they become tolerant. Administration of oral agents such as methadone, valium or other benzodiazepines facilitates weaning of these medications.

Hematologic

Blood should be administered to neonates who are cyanotic after palliative procedures to keep the hematocrit greater than 40% to 45%. An adequate hematocrit should also be maintained for all critically ill infants to maximize systemic oxygen delivery. Irradiated blood products should be used for infants with known or suspected DiGeorge syndrome because of the risk of graft-versus-host disease in this population.

Coagulopathy is often present in neonates after cardiopulmonary bypass and can be caused by incomplete reversal of anticoagulation, dilution of clotting factors, increased consumption of clotting factors, or loss of clotting factors in the presence of significant pleural drainage. This should be monitored closely in the immediate postoperative period by following clotting studies, platelet counts, and by assessing bleeding. Fresh frozen plasma and platelets should be transfused as indicated.

■ SELECTED COMPLICATIONS

Excessive Bleeding

Bleeding, especially from the chest tubes, should be monitored closely. A volume of more than 5 mL/kg/h is cause for concern and may reflect bleeding from a discrete site but more often is caused by diffuse oozing as a result of coagulopathy. Reoperation is sometimes necessary if bleeding does not resolve with transfusion of fresh frozen plasma and platelets. Chest tube output should become serous within 8 to 12 hours after surgery.

Open Sternum

At times, closing the sternum causes marked increases in diastolic pressure because of edema of the heart and lungs after complex open procedures in young infants. In these cases the sternum is left open and the overlying skin is closed or a barrier dressing is placed. Neuromuscular blockade and mechanical ventilation are continued until after the sternum is closed. The sternum is usually closed 2 to 4 days after surgery when the edema resolves and the infant is hemodynamically stable.

Cardiac Tamponade

Fluid accumulation within the pericardial space eventually causes the pericardial pressure to exceed atrial and ventricular diastolic pressures. This impairs cardiac filling and causes decreased stoke volume. Echocardiography may show diastolic collapse of the right or left ventricle.

In the immediate postoperative period, pericardial compliance is low and myocardial edema further limits the potential space. Cardiac tamponade because of undrained intrapericardial bleeding may occur precipitously. Often an abrupt cessation in mediastinal chest tube output signals obstruction by a clot. This is accompanied by tachycardia, hypotension, increased filling pressures, and poor perfusion. Widening of the superior mediastinal shadow may be seen on the chest radiograph. Opening the sternum emergently is the appropriate treatment.

Later in the postoperative period, fluid accumulation is often serous and may be related to postpericardiotomy syndrome (see following text). Slow fluid accumulation gradually distends the pericardial sac and allows the pericardial space to accommodate a great deal of fluid. Cardiomegaly may be seen on the chest radiograph. Sometimes effusions are seen on a routine echocardiographic examination in asymptomatic patients. Other patients develop signs and symptoms of tamponade and pericardiocentesis is necessary.

Fever

Fever occurring during the first 12 to 18 hours after surgery sometimes reflects low cardiac output. Although febrile, patients typically have cool extremities and decreased peripheral perfusion. The fever should be treated aggressively and every effort should be made to increase cardiac output.

After the immediate postoperative period, infection is the most common cause of fever. The following should be considered:

- *Respiratory*—Infection may be caused by nosocomial organisms, aspiration, or preexisting subclinical infection.
- *Intravascular catheter*—Bacteremia and sepsis from intravascular catheters is relatively common, especially in debilitated infants. The catheter usually should be removed but sometimes intravenous antibiotics alone are effective in patients with limited vascular access.
- *Urinary tract infection*—Urinary catheters are routinely placed to facilitate monitoring of urine output after surgery. These catheters should be removed as soon as

possible. Urinalysis and urine culture should be obtained in postoperative patients with fever.
- *Wound infection*—Reoperation increases the risk of postoperative wound infections. *Staphylococcus aureus* is the most common causative organism. Erythema and seropurulent drainage is suggestive of a superficial wound infection. These can usually be treated with antibiotics alone. Mediastinitis is a much more serious infection, and is characterized by persistent fever, purulent drainage from the sternotomy incision, leukocytosis, and possibly instability of the sternum. In unclear cases, imaging the mediastinum with CT or ultrasound may demonstrate an abscess or accumulation of fluid. Surgical debridement and irrigation are required in conjunction with antibiotic therapy directed at the specific organism. If sternal osteomyelitis is present, antibiotics must be administered for 4 to 6 weeks.

Postpericardiotomy Syndrome

Postpericardiotomy syndrome is an inflammatory process likely mediated by an autoimmune response to cardiac antigens exposed during surgery. Fever, anorexia, and malaise occur usually 5 to 10 days after surgery. The erythrocyte sedimentation rate and C-reactive protein are increased. A pericardial effusion is often present. If the effusion is large, pericardial tamponade with associated respiratory distress, tachycardia, narrow pulse pressure, jugular venous distention, and hepatomegaly may occur. Mildly affected patients are placed on nonsteroidal anti-inflammatory agents. Patients with symptomatic effusions require pericardiocentesis.

Diaphragmatic Paralysis

Hemidiaphragmatic paresis or paralysis caused by phrenic nerve injury during cardiac surgery may not be obvious while the patient is receiving positive pressure ventilation. This problem is most common after aortic arch reconstruction, systemic-to-pulmonary artery shunts, and procedures requiring hilar dissection. This condition should be considered in any patient who fails extubation and does not have other problems. Ultrasonography of diaphragmatic motion will establish the diagnosis. Treatment is conservative initially as many patients will gradually recover enough function to tolerate extubation. The patient who requires prolonged ventilator support may need plication of the diaphragm.

Chylothorax

Disruption of the thoracic duct and intrathoracic lymphatic channels at the time of surgery can result in a chylothorax. A chylous effusion will not be apparent until the patient begins eating a reasonable amount of fat. Chyle often appears milky and usually contains 2000 to 200,000 lymphocytes/μL, > 3 g/dL protein, and > 110 mg/dL triglyceride.

Therapy involves evacuation of the pleural space using chest tubes and elimination of long-chain fatty acids in the diet. Patients are usually placed on a low-fat diet. Several formulas contain primarily medium chain triglycerides and can be useful. The low-fat diet is generally continued for 6 weeks.

SUGGESTED READINGS

General Postoperative Care

Hoffman TM, Wernovsky G, Atz AM, et al. Efficacy and safety of milrinone in preventing low cardiac output syndrome in infants and children after corrective surgery for congenital heart disease. *Circulation.* 2003;107(7): 996-1002.

Hovels-Gurich HH, Vazquez-Jimenez JF, Silvestri A, et al. Production of proinflammatory cytokines and myocardial dysfunction after arterial switch operation in neonates with transposition of the great arteries. *J Thorac Cardiovasc Surg.* 2002;124(4):811-820.

Lee JE, Hillier SC, Knoderer CA. Use of sildenafil to facilitate weaning from inhaled nitric oxide in children with pulmonary hypertension following surgery for congenital heart disease. *J Intensive Care Med.* 2008;23(5):329-334.

Levy JH, Tanaka KA. Inflammatory response to cardiopulmonary bypass. *Ann Thorac Surg.* 2003;75(2):S715-S720.

Mackie AS, Booth KL, Newburger JW, et al. A randomized, double-blind, placebo-controlled pilot trial of triiodothyronine in neonatal heart surgery. *J Thorac Cardiovasc Surg.* 2005;130(3):810-816.

Mascio CE, Myers JA, Edmonds HL, Austin EH, III. Near-infrared spectroscopy as a guide for an intermittent cerebral perfusion strategy during neonatal circulatory arrest. *ASAIO J.* 2009;55(3):287-290.

Schwalbe-Terilli CR, Hartman DH, Nagle ML, et al. Enteral feeding and caloric intake in neonates after cardiac surgery. *Am J Crit Care.* 2009;18(1):52-57.

Suominen PK, Dickerson HA, Moffett BS, et al. Hemodynamic effects of rescue protocol hydrocortisone in neonates with low cardiac output syndrome after cardiac surgery. *Pediatr Crit Care Med.* 2005;6(6):655-659.

Mechanical Support of the Circulation During Surgery

Amir G, Ramamoorthy C, Riemer RK, Reddy VM, Hanley FL. Neonatal brain protection and deep hypothermic circulatory arrest: pathophysiology of ischemic neuronal injury and protective strategies. *Ann Thorac Surg.* 2005; 80(5):1955-1964.

Dominguez TE, Wernovsky G, Gaynor JW. Cause and prevention of central nervous system injury in neonates undergoing cardiac surgery. *Semin Thorac Cardiovasc Surg.* 2007;19(3):269-277.

Goldberg CS, Bove EL, Devaney EJ, et al. A randomized clinical trial of regional cerebral perfusion versus deep hypothermic circulatory arrest: outcomes for infants with functional single ventricle. *J Thorac Cardiovasc Surg.* 2007;133(4):880-887.

Malhotra SP, Hanley FL. Routine continuous perfusion for aortic arch reconstruction in the neonate. *Semin Thorac Cardiovasc Surg Pediatr Card Surg Annu.* 2008:57-60.

Newburger JW, Jonas RA, Soul J, et al. Randomized trial of hematocrit 25% versus 35% during hypothermic cardiopulmonary bypass in infant heart surgery. *J Thorac Cardiovasc Surg.* 2008;135(2):347-354.

Ohye RG, Goldberg CS, Donohue J, et al. The quest to optimize neurodevelopmental outcomes in neonatal arch reconstruction: the perfusion techniques we use and why we believe in them. *J Thorac Cardiovasc Surg.* 2009; 137(4): 803-806.

Reddy VM, Hanley FL. Techniques to avoid circulatory arrest in neonates undergoing repair of complex heart defects. *Semin Thorac Cardiovasc Surg Pediatr Card Surg Annu.* 2001;4:277-280.

Mechanical Support of the Circulation After Surgery

Allan CK, Thiagarajan RR, del Nido PJ, Roth SJ, Almodovar MC, Laussen PC. Indication for initiation of mechanical circulatory support impacts survival of infants with shunted single-ventricle circulation supported with extracorporeal membrane oxygenation. *J Thorac Cardiovasc Surg.* 2007; 133(3):660-667.

Bautista-Hernandez V, Thiagarajan RR, Fynn-Thompson F, et al. Preoperative extracorporeal membrane oxygenation as a bridge to cardiac surgery in children with congenital heart disease. *Ann Thorac Surg.* 2009;88(4): 1306-1311.

Blume ED, Laussen PC. Cardiac mechanical support therapies. In: Allen HD, Driscoll DJ, Shaddy RE, Feltes TF, eds. *Moss and Adams' Heart Disease in Infants, Children and Adolescents.* Philadelphia, PA: Lippincott Williams & Wilkins; 2008:481-495.

Fiser RT, Morris MC. Extracorporeal cardiopulmonary resuscitation in refractory pediatric cardiac arrest. *Pediatr Clin North Am*. 2008;55(4):929-941.

Morris MC, Ittenbach RF, Godinez RI, et al. Risk factors for mortality in 137 pediatric cardiac intensive care unit patients managed with extracorporeal membrane oxygenation. *Crit Care Med*. 2004;32(4):1061-1069.

Pauliks LB, Undar A. New devices for pediatric mechanical circulatory support. *Curr Opin Cardiol*. 2008;23(2):91-96.

Stiller B, Lemmer J, Schubert S, et al. Management of pediatric patients after implantation of the Berlin Heart EXCOR ventricular assist device. *ASAIO J*. 2006; 52(5): 497-500.

Thiagarajan RR, Laussen PC, Rycus PT, Bartlett RH, Bratton SL. Extracorporeal membrane oxygenation to aid cardiopulmonary resuscitation in infants and children. *Circulation*. 2007;116(15):1693-1700.

CHAPTER 14

Neurology of Congenital Heart Disease: Brain Development, Acquired Injury, and Neurodevelopmental Outcome

■ INTRODUCTION

Dramatic advances in echocardiography, cardiopulmonary bypass, surgical technique, and intensive care now allow most patients with congenital heart defects to undergo surgery during the neonatal period or infancy. With these advances mortality declined, but caretakers, patients, and families observe a significant burden of neurodevelopmental impairment in survivors. A natural assumption was that adverse neurologic outcome was directly related to brain injury sustained during neonatal surgical intervention, leading to a seminal study in the late 1980s. The Boston Circulatory Arrest Trial compared two methods of vital organ support in infants undergoing open-heart surgery to repair d-transposition of the great arteries. Consequently, much of what is known about the relationship between complex heart disease and neurodevelopmental outcome has been gleaned from this study. Importantly, it is apparent that injury to the brain may occur during fetal life, at birth, preoperatively, intraoperatively, and postoperatively. In fact, the interplay between the brain and the circulation is complex, occurring at many levels. This chapter will review mechanisms influencing neurologic outcome including: (1) shared genetic and developmental pathways; (2) physiologic effects of congenital heart lesions on brain blood flow; and (3) timing, appearance, and mechanism of acquired brain injuries. We will summarize how these pathogenic mechanisms result in a neurodevelopmental "signature" of congenital heart disease. Finally, we will speculate on how these mechanisms suggest strategies of neuroprotection, repair, and recovery that may improve outcome.

■ GENETIC CONTRIBUTION TO ADVERSE OUTCOME

Shared Genetic Pathways in Brain and Heart Development

Certain aspects of heart and brain development occur simultaneously in the human fetus (summarized in Chapter 1 for heart and following text for brain). Many vertebrate organs undergo related developmental events (eg, cell fate determination, cell migration, dorsal/ventral patterning, left/right asymmetry, area specification, etc). Thus, it is not surprising that similar genes share important and similar developmental roles in both organs (Table 14-1). This includes genes such as members of the transforming growth factor-β family including bone morphogenic proteins, fibroblast growth factor family members, notch and notch-ligands, sonic hedgehog, vascular endothelial growth factor, and neuregulins. Disruption of shared fundamental genetic pathways that result in cardiac defects will affect brain development as well.

Common Genetic Syndromes With Congenital Heart Disease

It is apparent that congenital heart disease may occur within the context of a genetic syndrome. Often, but not exclusively, these syndromes also include abnormal neurodevelopment.

Notable examples of genetic syndromes with both congenital heart disease and neurodevelopmental impairment include trisomy 21 (Down syndrome), 22q11 deletion (DiGeorge and velocardiofacial syndrome), monosomy X (Turner), Jacobsen, and Williams syndromes. Despite well-characterized chromosomal microdeletions, identifying a specific gene or limited set of genes that accounts for any one component (eg, cardiac or brain) of the syndrome is challenging. The 22q11 deletion syndrome is a good example. The causative microdeletion encompasses three megabases of DNA, representing 30 to 40 genes and the syndrome is notably highly heterogeneous with regards to all potential components of the syndrome (eg, parathyroid, immune deficiency, conotruncal cardiac defects, and neurodevelopmental outcome). Even when known genetic or malformation syndromes are excluded, a large prospective study of the determinants of 1-year neurodevelopmental outcome identified genetic syndromes, unsuspected at birth, to be among the most potent predictors of adverse outcome. The list of single gene defects contributing to congenital heart disease and/or neurodevelopmental impairment is likely to grow quickly with the advent of large-scale genomics projects.

Patient-Specific Genetic Risk Modifiers

Beyond the direct effects of single genes or shared genetic pathways in genetic syndromes, patient genotype can influence neurodevelopmental outcome as "risk modifiers" of the response to brain injury. This is perhaps best described for alleles of apolipoprotein E in which the Apo ε4 allele is associated with adverse outcome in many conditions in adults (eg, Alzheimer disease, traumatic brain injury, stroke, and subarachnoid hemorrhage). In infants with congenital heart disease, however, the Apo ε2 allele is associated with worse outcome. Interestingly, polymorphisms of inflammatory cytokines, including interleukin-6, have been associated with poor outcome in the form of cerebral palsy in term newborns. This issue has not been examined despite observations that inflammatory cytokines, including interleukin-6, are increased after surgery and associated with postoperative cardiovascular morbidity.

■ BRAIN DEVELOPMENT IS DELAYED IN PATIENTS WITH CONGENITAL HEART DISEASE

Human Brain Developmental Timeline

Human cardiac development begins during the first postconceptual days with rhythmic contractions of a primitive heart tube beginning by embryonic day 23 and a

■ **TABLE 14-1.** Genes With Identified Role(s) in Both Heart and Brain Development

Gene	Function in cardiac development	Function in brain development	Syndrome or isolated CHD
BMP-2	Cardiac looping	Neural cell fate commitment	
Nkx2.5	Cardioblast cell fate commitment, chamber septation	Neural cell fate commitment	Holt-Oram, ASD, VSD, TOF
TBX5	Left ventricular specification	Cortical area specification, axon guidance	Holt-Oram
Sonic hedgehog (SHH)	Left/right asymmetry	Neural cell fate commitment	
FGF8	Left/right asymmetry	Cortical area specification	
Nodal	Left/right asymmetry	Cell migration, axon guidance	
Lefty1	Left/right asymmetry	Neural cell fate commitment, left/right asymmetry	Heterotaxy
ZIC1	Left/right asymmetry	Neural progenitors proliferation, neural crest and roof plate specification, holoprosencephaly, cerebellar development	Heterotaxy
Pitx2	Left/right asymmetry	Left/right asymmetry	
GATA4	Heart tube formation	Astrocyte proliferation	ASD, VSD
Smad2	Endocardial cushion, valve formation	Axon development	
TGF-β	Endocardial cushion, valve formation	Anterior/dorsal patterning	
COUPTFII	Atrial specification	Area specification—caudal ganglionic eminence, migration	
MEF2C	Right ventricular specification	Neural stem cell differentiation, maturation	
Neuregulin/ erb2/erb4	Chamber maturation	Synapse formation	
NF-1	Myocardial growth	Glial differentiation	
Pax3	Neural crest	Cortical area specification	
VEGF/ Neuropilin-1	Neural crest	Angiogenesis, axon guidance	
ET-1	Neural crest	Sensory neuron neurotransmitter, modulation of hypothalamic neurosecretory system, and neurovasculature	
TFAP2B	Neural crest	Regulates monoaminergic gene expression in neural crest cells in midbrain, hindbrain, and spinal cord	Char
Notch/Jagged	Cardiac progenitor cell fate determination	Neural cell fate commitment	Alagille, aortic stenosis/ bicuspid aortic valve
TBX1	Outflow tract, pharyngeal arch development, aortic arch patterning	Learning and memory (prepulse inhibition)	DiGeorge
Retinoic acid/ RXRa	Outflow tract, pharyngeal arch development, aortic arch patterning, chamber maturation	Pleomorphic: Neurogenesis, ventral/lateral neural tube patterning, cortical area specification, synaptic plasticity	

(Continued)

■ **TABLE 14-1.** Genes with Identified Role(s) in Both Heart and Brain Development (*Continued*)

Gene	Function in cardiac development	Function in brain development	Syndrome or isolated CHD
Foxc1	Neural crest, outflow tract/ secondary heart field development	Neurogenesis, cerebellar development	
Ras-MAPK	Pulmonary valve development, cardiomyopathy	Pleomorphic: Learning memory, neuronal survival/death, plasticity	Noonan, Cardio-facio-cutaneous, Costello
Elastin/ Limk1, Cyln2, Fzd9; Gtfll	Elastin: Valve formation	Limk1, Cyln2: Regulation of neuronal cytoskeleton—growth cone motility, dendrite formation, synaptogenesis; Fxd9: hippocampal development; Gtf2i: visuospatial processing	Williams-Beuren
PROSIT240	Ventricular septation	Cerebellar development	d-TGA

BMP, bone morphogenic protein.

morphologically mature heart formed by day 50, or gestational week 7 (reviewed in Chapter 1). In contrast, brain development extends over a much longer time period, with morphologic events (cell proliferation, migration, axon pathfinding, and target selection) occurring in the first two trimesters, followed by a prolonged period of refinement of connections that occurs both in the third trimester and early postnatal period.

A primitive neural tube forms by five gestational weeks with identifiable radial glia, the neural stem cell. Corticogenesis, the process of production and migration of neurons from regions of proliferation to their targets in specific neocortical layers, occurs from week 7 through week 18, although a mature six-layered cortex does not appear until week 26. Axon outgrowth, pathfinding, target selection, and innervation all take place after production and migration of neurons. Formation of connections between thalamus and cortex requires a transient population of early born neurons, referred to as subplate neurons because of their location as a discrete layer below the cortical plate. In humans, thalamocortical pathfinding takes place between the histological emergence of the subplate at the end of the first trimester and the appearance of cholinesterase positive fibers in the subplate at weeks 17 to 20 (earlier for somatosensory versus visual cortex). Thalamocortical fibers accumulate during a "waiting period" from week 17 through weeks 22 to 26 before innervating the cortical plate.

Most morphologic events of brain development are completed by the end of the second trimester. The third trimester involves a period of dramatic brain growth and refinement of connections that is dependent upon endogenous and spontaneous neuronal activity arising at multiple levels. In the visual system, this endogenous activity takes the form of spontaneous waves of neuronal activation that sweep across and tile the retina and are transmitted to thalamus and cortex. This patterned activity sculpts developing neural circuits into mature, precise patterns. Ocular dominance columns in the visual system, representing nonoverlapping eye-specific innervation are a representative example of such a patterned circuit and form the basis of binocular vision. In higher primates, ocular dominance columns have fully formed by birth before onset of visually driven activity. At a gross morphologic level, the third trimester is characterized by development of secondary and tertiary gyri. At a cellular level, brain growth involves elaboration of dendritic arbors and formation of corticocortical connections. Myelination of fiber tracts also begins during fetal life, with a characteristic caudal to cranial pattern beginning with deep structures, such as the tegmentum and cerebellar peduncles. By the end of the third trimester, myelination extends to the posterior limb of the internal capsule and involves the motor fibers of the pyramidal tract. In neocortex, myelination begins in the optic radiations and occipital white matter after birth, before extending to the frontal lobes by 9 months of age.

Brain development continues after birth, with sensory-driven activity now influencing the refinement of connections. For a brief period of time (critical period), soon after the onset of vision, deprivation of visually evoked activity leads to permanent loss of visual acuity in the deprived eye, a process referred to in humans as amblyopia that represents a form of neural plasticity. In humans, amblyopia is usually observed only after 6 months of age. Weeks of deprivation can lead to substantial loss of visual acuity between 6 to 18 months and months of deprivation can have an effect until 8 years of age.

Fetal Circulation in Congenital Heart Disease: Effects on Cerebral Blood Flow

The fetal circulation is unique in a number of respects that impact cerebral blood flow. As reviewed in detail in Chapter 3, vascular and cardiac blood flow patterns in the normal fetus direct the most highly saturated blood from the ductus venosus and left hepatic vein via the foramen ovale to the left heart and, subsequently, to the cerebral circulation. In contrast, in d-transposition of the great arteries, the aorta arises from the right ventricle and thus receives the relatively desaturated blood from the superior vena cava, lower body, and coronary sinus. The left ventricle delivers the more highly saturated blood to the lungs, lower body, and placenta. In hypoplastic left heart syndrome, the fetal circulation is characterized by admixture of all venous streams in the right atrium and ventricle. The ascending aorta is only a very small vessel, delivering blood in a retrograde direction to the coronary arteries. The aortic arch is also hypoplastic, and shows flow reversal to supply the brain and upper body (Chapters 3 and 8). The effects of these abnormal flow patterns on brain development are uncertain but may be very different, despite the fact that both decrease the oxygen content of the blood delivered to the brain. In d-transposition of the great arteries, the pulsatility and perfusion pressure of the cerebral arterial circulation are normal. On the other hand, in hypoplastic left heart syndrome, the hypoplastic isthmus and aortic arch may function as resistors, decreasing the pulsatility and perfusion pressure to the cerebral circulation. This cannot easily be overcome by the cerebral circulation, particularly early in gestation, and may explain the finding of a recent study showing that ascending aortic diameter predicts the degree of microcephaly in newborns with hypoplastic left heart syndrome.

Blood flow to the fetal brain is estimated to be almost one quarter of the combined ventricular output in the third trimester. Autoregulation of fetal cerebral blood flow is thought to redistribute blood flow to the brain in the setting of placental insufficiency, a phenomenon referred to as "brain sparing" resulting in a pattern of overall somatic growth restriction with relative preservation of head growth. In the setting of congenital heart disease with decreased oxygen content in the cerebral arterial blood, similar mechanisms can be invoked to decrease the cerebral to placental resistance ratios and thus preserve cerebral blood flow. However, low cerebral blood flow has been measured in newborns with hypoplastic left heart syndrome and d-transposition of the great arteries using magnetic resonance imaging (MRI). Newborns with certain forms of congenital heart disease have smaller head circumferences, which may be an indicator of impaired brain growth. The issue is complex, however. The different patterns of alterations in cerebral blood flow are associated with different patterns of growth disturbance. Newborns with d-transposition of the great arteries tend to have small head circumference with normal birth weight whereas those with hypoplastic left heart syndrome are smaller in all dimensions, but head volume is disproportionately decreased. Surprisingly, infants with isolated aortic coarctation have a greater head volume relative to birth weight.

Magnetic Resonance Imaging Identifies Delayed Brain Development Before Surgery

Advanced MRI provides the highest resolution conventional images of brain anatomy and acquired brain lesions. These techniques can also be used to measure brain development and to investigate brain metabolism and microstructure. Proton MR spectroscopic imaging measures resonance from N-acetyl groups (predominantly N-acetylaspartate), lactate, creatine, and tetramethylamines (predominantly choline containing compounds). N-acetylaspartate is found predominantly in neurons (cell body and axon), so that changes in N-acetylaspartate reflect neuronal metabolic integrity. Particularly relevant to studies of brain development is the observation that N-acetylaspartate increases consistently with advancing cerebral maturity, providing a developmental brain "growth chart."

Another advanced technique is diffusion tensor imaging which provides a sensitive measure of regional brain microstructural development. It characterizes the three-dimensional spatial distribution of water diffusion in each voxel of the MR image. With increasing brain maturation, brain water content diminishes and developing neuronal and glial cell membranes increasingly restrict

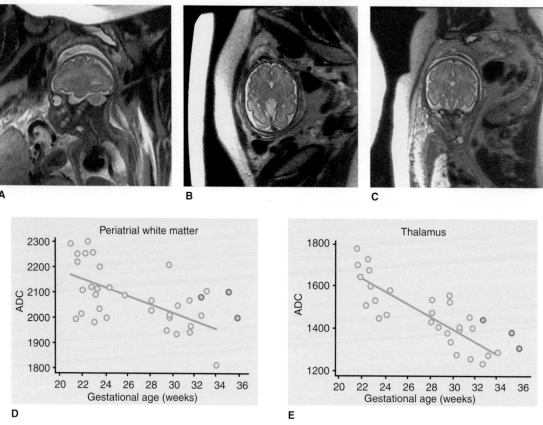

FIGURE 14-1. Fetal MRI and diffusion imaging detects delayed brain development in congenital heart disease. A-C. Sagittal, axial, and coronal T2 images at 31 weeks in a fetus with prenatal diagnosis of hypoplastic left heart syndrome. The brain is morphologically normal. **D-E.** Average diffusivity coefficient (ADC) is plotted against gestational age for periatrial white matter (D) or thalamus (E). Values for three fetuses with hypoplastic left heart syndrome (*orange*) are compared with a control cohort without congenital heart disease (*green*). The regression line was fit to the control population. Average diffusion is higher in fetuses with hypoplastic left heart syndrome, indicating a relative delay in development.

proton diffusion resulting in a consistent decrease in average diffusivity over time in gray and white matter regions (Figure 14-1).

Recently, using both advanced imaging modalities, brain metabolism, and microstructure were characterized as measures of brain maturation in term newborns with d-transposition of the great arteries or single ventricle physiology before heart surgery and compared to control infants. Relative to the normal control newborns, newborns with congenital heart disease had 10% lower N-acetylaspartate/choline ratios and 4.5% higher average diffusivity. Comparing these data to values obtained from normal fetuses suggests that term newborns with congenital heart

disease have a delay in brain development of approximately 1 month, equivalent to an infant born prematurely at 34 to 36 weeks. Thus, data from this study suggest that abnormal brain development precedes surgery in these newborns.

Brain development can also be assessed at a macroscopic, morphologic level. In a similar study examining structural brain development, preoperative MRIs from term newborns with d-transposition of the great arteries or hypoplastic left heart syndrome were reviewed to assign a "total maturation score" describing myelination, cortical folding, involution of glial cell migration bands, and the presence of germinal matrix tissue (Figure 14-2).

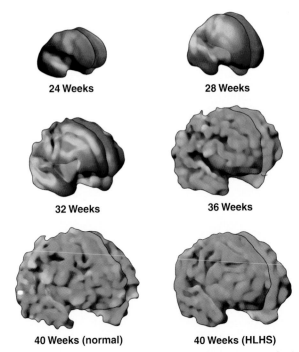

24 Weeks 28 Weeks

32 Weeks 36 Weeks

40 Weeks (normal) 40 Weeks (HLHS)

FIGURE 14-2. Macroscopic brain development—cortical folding. Three-dimensional reconstructions of cortical white matter volumes from MRI scans taken at 24 weeks to term gestation showing the development of cortical folding and surface curvature. The white matter surface from a term newborn with hypoplastic left heart syndrome displays noticeably less cortical folding and smoother surface curvature than a term newborn without heart disease.

Consistent with the data described in the preceding paragraphs, the maturation score was delayed, corresponding to a delay of 1 month in structural brain development compared to normative data in infants without congenital heart defects. These in vivo observations using quantitative MR methods are consistent with neuropathology data showing that newborns with congenital heart disease are more likely to be microcephalic and to have an immature cortical mantle.

Fetal Brain MRI

The concept that delayed postnatal brain development occurs as a result of disordered fetal cerebral blood flow suggests two predictions: (1) delayed brain development begins during fetal life and (2) different forms of congenital heart disease will manifest different degrees of delayed development. Fetal brain ultrasound studies suggest that the decline in head growth begins after

mid-gestation in fetuses with hypoplastic left heart syndrome. A study comparing brain volumes and proton MR spectroscopic images from fetuses with congenital heart disease and normal fetuses between 25 and 37 gestational weeks showed definitive evidence for delayed fetal brain development. No differences were found between controls and fetuses with heart defects during the second trimester. During the third trimester, a progressive impairment of brain volumes was observed, particularly in those fetuses with left-sided obstruction. Additionally, larger delays in the expected increase in N-acetylaspartate/choline ratio and greater impairment of growth in brain volume were noted in fetuses with aortic atresia and no antegrade blood flow in the aortic arch. These observations support the concept that brain development is impaired during fetal life because of impaired fetal cerebral blood flow, oxygen and substrate delivery, and that compensatory mechanisms (brain sparing effect) are inadequate.

■ ACQUIRED BRAIN INJURY: WHITE MATTER INJURY AND STROKE

Neonates with congenital heart disease are also at risk of discrete acquired brain injury in the perioperative period that may be exacerbated by delayed brain development.

Imaging Characteristics of Acquired Brain Injury

Focal brain abnormalities (or "injuries") in the term newborn can be clearly and reliably detected with conventional MRI, and with greater resolution than with either ultrasound or computed tomography. Further, the extent of MRI abnormalities corresponds closely to histopathological changes found on postmortem examination. The most common brain injuries observed in newborns with congenital heart disease are white matter injury (defined in more detail in the following text) and small focal strokes (less than one-third to two-thirds of the arterial distribution, Figure 14-3). It is important to recognize that the strokes and white matter injuries identified by MRI in these research studies are largely clinically silent and overlooked with routine clinical screening cranial ultrasounds. These patterns of brain injury are uncommon for term newborns experiencing hypoxic ischemic injury. Instead, newborns with birth asphyxia present with two different patterns of brain injury: parasagittal watershed injury or the "basal ganglia pattern" with injury to deep grey nuclei, indicative of partial or total ischemia, respectively. These patterns are

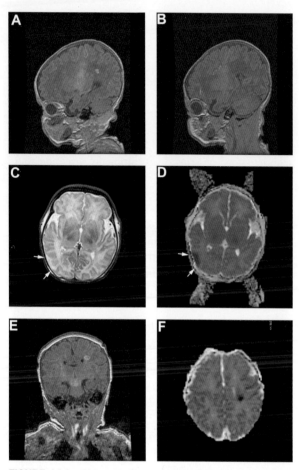

FIGURE 14-3. MRI patterns of injury. A, B. Moderate white matter injury in a newborn with hypoplastic left heart syndrome is seen on sagittal T1 images in the postoperative scan. White matter injuries appear as small, focal areas of T1 hyperintensity (brightness). **C, D.** Term newborn with hypoplastic left heart syndrome imaged postoperatively at day of life 17, after a modified Norwood procedure. A small middle cerebral artery distribution infarct is seen as cortical T2 hyperintensity (white arrows in C) and corresponding reduced diffusion (white arrows in D) in the right parietal-occipital lobe. **E, F.** Term newborn with transposition of the great arteries imaged preoperatively after a balloon atrial septostomy. A single focus of T1 hyperintensity is seen in the periatrial white matter on the coronal SPGR sequence (E). This same focus has reduced water diffusivity on the average diffusivity (Dav) map (F, dark spot). This spot is larger than the typical solitary white matter lesion and may represent a small embolic stroke.

seen rarely in newborns with congenital heart disease, and usually occur after cardiac arrest or severe shock.

Stroke is defined as "a focal area of diffusion restriction in an arterial territory," a definition that incorporates both imaging characteristics and presumed embolic mechanism. Stroke is distinguished from white matter injury based upon imaging characteristics, the latter characterized by "punctate periventricular lesions associated with T1 hyperintensity (brightness) with or without restriction of water diffusion." Larger injuries (> 5 mm) in the white matter may represent either focal embolic strokes or large, atypical confluent white matter injuries.

Identification of white matter injury in term newborns with cardiac defects was unexpected because this pattern was thought to be restricted to premature newborns with brain injury (periventricular leukomalacia). The early descriptions of periventricular leukomalacia referred to extensive cystic necrotic lesions that were frequently accompanied by white matter atrophy reflected in enlargement of the lateral ventricles. The cystic lesions were characteristically symmetric and located adjacent to the anterior and posterior horns of the lateral ventricles. However, with the increasing use of magnetic resonance imaging tools, focal or diffuse noncystic white matter injuries are emerging as the predominant lesions whereas cystic lesions account for less than 5% of injuries in some series.

Advanced MRI techniques such as diffusion tensor imaging and spectroscopy are useful for evaluating acute injury as well as measuring brain development. Quantitative and qualitative morphometric techniques (eg, deformation morphometry and analysis of curvature) have been useful for predicting outcomes following premature birth. Studies evaluating these techniques in newborns with congenital heart disease are in progress.

Risk Factors for Preoperative Brain Injury

Several relatively large prospective studies have been performed using pre- and postoperative brain MRI to determine the frequency of acquired brain injury and associated risk factors in newborns with congenital heart disease. Preoperative brain injury in the form of white matter injury or stroke is present in 28% to 39% of such newborns. Risk factors for preoperative brain injury are summarized in Table 14-2 and include hypoxemia and time to surgery, preoperative base deficit, preoperative cardiac arrest, and balloon atrial septostomy. The risk of balloon atrial septostomy has not been observed in all studies, perhaps because of confounding association with hypoxia, a common indication for the procedure. These risk factors not surprisingly represent brain injury occurring as the consequence of hypoxia and ischemia related to intracardiac shunting and ductal-dependent circulation. The delayed

■ **TABLE 14-2.** Risk Factors for Brain Injury

Preoperative	Intraoperative	Postoperative
Low arterial hemoglobin saturation	Prolonged total circulatory arrest (> 40 min)	Low blood pressure
Length of time to surgery	Decreased cerebral oxygen saturation (NIRS)	Low arterial PaO_2
Catheter-based procedure (eg, balloon atrial septostomy)	Cardiopulmonary bypass strategy (regional cerebral perfusion)	Prolonged cerebral regional oxygen saturation (NIRS < 45% for > 3 h)
Preoperative base deficit	Air or particulate emboli	Morphologically immature brain (total maturation score)
Preoperative cardiac arrest	Inflammation	Single ventricle physiology
Morphologically immature brain (total maturation score)		

brain development as measured by the "total maturation score" detailed in the preceding text may explain the observed predisposition of term newborns with congenital heart disease to white matter injury following hypoxic ischemic stress.

Risk Factors for Intraoperative Brain Injury

Proposed risk factors for intraoperative brain injury relate predominantly to the method of cardiopulmonary bypass and/or hypothermic total circulatory arrest (Table 14-2). Most neuroprotective trials have involved manipulating some component of cardiopulmonary bypass. The Boston Circulatory Arrest Trial compared two methods of vital organ support in infants undergoing open-heart surgery to repair d-transposition of the great arteries. d-transposition of the great arteries is an optimal lesion to study the effects of acquired perioperative brain injury as the cardiac anatomy is anatomically homogenous with few associated genetic or malformation syndromes that might contribute independently to neurodevelopmental outcome. Neonates with this condition undergo complete repair in the neonatal period; normal cardiovascular physiology is reestablished with low mortality and excellent long-term cardiac functional outcome. Although deep hypothermic circulatory arrest, which provides the surgeon with an empty and relaxed heart, clearly allowed intricate surgeries to be performed, there was concern at the time regarding late adverse neurologic outcome and the "safe" duration of circulatory arrest was unknown. An alternative method (low-flow bypass) was felt to maintain some amount of brain oxygen delivery, while still allowing the surgeon a relatively bloodless field. Equipoise emerged from concerns that low-flow bypass prolonged the exposure to

pump-related sources of injury including embolism and inflammation.

This study enrolled 171 infants into a single-center, randomized clinical trial comparing deep hypothermic total circulatory arrest with low-flow cardiopulmonary bypass. All of the early outcome variables pointed to a benefit of low-flow bypass compared to circulatory arrest. The variables suggesting greater neurologic injury in the circulatory arrest group included more frequent postoperative seizures, higher serum levels of brain-specific enzymes (creatine kinase), worse 1 year motor outcome (Bayley scales of infant development—psychomotor development index), and abnormalities on neurologic examination. No differences were found in cognitive development (Bayley—mental development index) or magnetic resonance imaging at 1 year of age. Importantly, these differences between the groups disappeared when the patients were assessed at older ages, but both groups remained below population norms for performance on standardized tests. Children treated with circulatory arrest consistently scored worse on tests of motor function, especially fine motor dexterity and speech apraxia. Children in the low-flow bypass group showed more impulsivity and difficulty with attention, especially at 8 years of age. An important observation that has implications for all studies of neurodevelopment in patients with congenital heart disease was that testing at 1 year of age was only modestly predictive of outcome at 8 years with poor sensitivity and positive predictive value.

A number of other differences among the groups emerged as predictors of adverse outcome, including seizures. Presence of a ventricular septal defect was associated with worse outcome at all ages, and apart from socioeconomic status, explained the largest percentage of variance in the scores (3.2% compared with 0.3% for treatment group assignment). Interestingly, surgery was performed at older ages in infants with d-transposition of the great arteries and ventricular septal defect (2-3 weeks of age) compared with d-transposition of the great arteries and intact ventricular septum (1 week of age).

Other variables examined include circulatory arrest versus low-flow bypass, hypothermic blood pH management (alpha stat versus pH stat), hemodilution/hematocrit (25% vs 35%), and maintaining regional cerebral perfusion during aortic arch reconstruction. None of these studies has identified definitively improved neurologic outcomes. Patients who underwent regional cerebral perfusion tended to have the worse outcome, and this technique was associated with new postoperative injury on brain MRI. These results suggest that although risks remain during the intraoperative period, a major burden of risk for acquired injury occurs outside of the operative period but the possibility that unidentified intraoperative risk factors contribute cannot be excluded.

Risk Factors for Postoperative Brain Injury

Risk factors for postoperative brain injury (Table 14-2) include hypotension and hypoxemia related to low cardiac output syndrome, defined as a combination of clinical signs (tachycardia, oliguria, cold extremities, or cardiac arrest) and a $\geq 30\%$ difference in arterial-mixed venous oxygen saturation or lactic acidosis (> 4 mg/dL). Multiple studies have identified hypotension as a risk for new postoperative white matter injury including low systolic blood pressure on admission, low mean blood pressure during postoperative day 1, and low diastolic blood pressure during postoperative days 1 to 2. One study showed that low regional cerebral oxygen saturation ($< 45\%$) measured by cerebral near-infrared spectroscopy for longer than 3 hours in the postoperative period was a risk for new ischemic injury. However, this has not been confirmed in subsequent studies. In many series, single ventricle physiology carries a higher risk of postoperative brain injury, which correlates with the higher postoperative hemodynamic instability, morbidity, and mortality seen in these patients. Decreased postoperative systemic venous oxygen saturation, indicative of low cardiac output, is a risk factor for poor neurodevelopmental outcome at 1 year.

■ NEURODEVELOPMENTAL OUTCOME

Transposition of the Great Arteries

Formal intelligence testing of children with d-transposition of the great arteries repaired in the neonatal period shows IQ scores that are in the normal range and only slightly below population norms (8-year WISC-III Full-Scale mean IQ 97.1 + / − 15.3). Despite relatively modest differences in IQ from the population average and overall good general health status, a high percentage of children (1 in 5) in the Boston Circulatory Arrest study were judged to have behavioral problems by parents and teachers; 37% required remedial education services and 10% had repeated a grade.

Hypoplastic Left Heart Syndrome

Patients with single ventricle physiology usually require a three-staged surgical approach with exposure to cyanosis and embolic risk over the first few years of life. As one might expect, reported outcomes are worse than for d-transposition patients, but still fall within the normal range. In the largest series reported to date (N = 83), the mental development index is 90 (range 50-129) at 1 year of age. The median psychomotor development index is lower 73 (range 50-117). This pattern is seen in virtually every study of neurodevelopmental outcome at 1 year of age and likely represents a performance assessment heavily weighted toward the ability to walk. Other smaller studies report similar values with a trend toward slight improvement with more contemporary series. Risk factors for poor neurodevelopmental outcome are similar to those discussed earlier and include the presence of genetic syndrome, younger gestational age at birth, preoperative instability (increased base deficit, need for preoperative intubation), and postoperative instability (lower superior vena cava saturation). As the children are assessed at older ages, the prevalence of subtle abnormalities increases, with many children (~30%) needing special education services.

Neurodevelopmental Signature of Complex Congenital Heart Disease

Mortality rates for most congenital cardiac defects have fallen below 10%, with hospital mortality for many lesions < 3%. These children grow up with overall physical and psychosocial health status similar to the general population. However, despite intelligence testing in the normal population range, many have such a prevalence of pervasive but subtle cognitive problems that some have termed as "neurodevelopmental signature of complex congenital heart disease." These children show behavioral and attention problems that are often not detected on standardized testing but result in poor school performance. This developmental signature in many ways resembles problems observed in survivors of premature birth. Among a large cohort of infants who were followed prospectively after undergoing surgery as infants, abnormalities on neurologic examination at school entry were present in 28%, although less than 5% were severe. Most of the abnormalities involved fine motor coordination and tone. Cognitive difficulty and behavioral problems were identified in 30%.

■ CONCLUSION

In this chapter, we have reviewed the major risk factors for adverse neurologic outcome, noting that they vary in both timing and mechanism. Some patient-specific factors, such as genetic defects that result in both abnormal heart and brain development, and parental education and socioeconomic status, may not be amenable to intervention. However, other factors have been identified that may provide opportunities for intervention at different stages, including during fetal life, and before, during, and after surgery. Trials are under way to assess fetal interventions to improve left ventricular growth in prenatally diagnosed aortic stenosis, to prevent progression to hypoplastic left heart syndrome and the resulting cerebral perfusion abnormalities during fetal life. Another potential opportunity for investigation involves determining the optimal time for surgery. The identification of delayed brain development as a risk for perioperatively acquired injury suggests the possibility of delaying nonemergency surgery. The issue is complicated, however, because the longer the surgery is delayed in newborns with d-transposition of the great arteries, the greater the likelihood of white matter injury. Other studies have shown that both younger and older ages at surgery are risk factors for injury. The combination of brain immaturity and vulnerability to white matter injury suggests that neuroprotection must be tailored toward the immature brain. In animal models, the preoligodendrocytes, precursors to the cells responsible for forming white matter and myelinating the brain, are uniquely vulnerable to hypoxia ischemia through specific mechanisms of glutamate excitotoxicity and oxidative stress. Despite

well-performed trials with long-term follow-up, no cardiopulmonary bypass strategy has emerged as being clearly superior.

Although a wealth of information is emerging from sensitive advanced MRI studies, the relationship of perioperative acquired brain injury to long-term neurodevelopmental outcome has yet to be determined. In the premature infant and term infant with birth asphyxia, advanced MR imaging is the most sensitive study for detection of acquired injuries and is predictive of neurodevelopmental outcome. Studies examining whether perioperative MRI findings predict outcome in large cohorts of newborns with congenital heart disease are urgently needed. At the same time, for MRI to become sufficiently sensitive for establishing early outcome variables for use in interventional trials, investigators must determine which MRI method and findings are most sensitive to late outcome, when to perform MRIs in the course of the infant's treatment, and how to describe the findings in a coherent, reproducible, and uniform manner.

Finally, although many patients show subtle or even pronounced neurodevelopmental deficits, it is clear that many are not receiving appropriate rehabilitation services (speech, occupational, or physical therapy). Caretakers should ensure that at risk patients are evaluated and advocated for provision of appropriate services as early recognition and intervention will improve late functional outcome.

SUGGESTED READINGS

Andropoulos DB, Hunter JV, Nelson DP, et al. Brain immaturity is associated with brain injury before and after neonatal cardiac surgery with high-flow bypass and cerebral oxygenation monitoring. *J Thorac Cardiovasc Surg*. 2009 Nov 10.

Bellinger DC, Jonas RA, Rappaport LA, et al. Developmental and neurologic status of children after heart surgery with hypothermic circulatory arrest or low-flow cardiopulmonary bypass. *N Engl J Med*. 1995 Mar 2;332(9):549-555.

Bellinger DC, Wypij D, Duplessis AJ, et al. Neurodevelopmental status at eight years in children with dextro-transposition of the great arteries: the Boston Circulatory Arrest Trial. *J Thorac Cardiovasc Surg*. 2003 Nov;126(5):1385-1396.

Bellinger DC, Wypij D, Kuban KC, et al. Developmental and neurological status of children at 4 years of age after heart surgery with hypothermic circulatory arrest or low-flow cardiopulmonary bypass. *Circulation*. 1999;100(5):526-532.

Counsell SJ, Allsop JM, Harrison MC, et al. Diffusion-weighted imaging of the brain in preterm infants with focal and diffuse white matter abnormality. *Pediatrics*. 2003 Jul;112(1 Pt 1):1-7.

Dent CL, Spaeth JP, Jones BV, et al. Brain magnetic resonance imaging abnormalities after the Norwood procedure using regional cerebral perfusion. *J Thorac Cardiovasc Surg*. 2006 Jan;131(1):190-197.

Donofrio MT, Bremer YA, Schieken RM, et al. Autoregulation of cerebral blood flow in fetuses with congenital heart disease: the brain sparing effect. *Pediatr Cardiol*. 2003 Sep-Oct;24(5):436-443.

du Plessis AJ. Mechanisms of brain injury during infant cardiac surgery. *Semin Pediatr Neurol*. 1999;6(1):32-47.

Ferriero DM: Neonatal brain injury. *N Engl J Med*. 2004 Nov 4;351(19):1985-1995.

Galli KK, Zimmerman RA, Jarvik GP, et al. Periventricular leukomalacia is common after neonatal cardiac surgery. *J Thorac Cardiovasc Surg*. 2004 Mar;127(3):692-704.

Gelb BD. Genetic basis of syndromes associated with congenital heart disease. *Curr Opin Cardiol*. 2001 May; 16(3): 188-194.

Glenn OA. Normal development of the fetal brain by MRI. *Semin Perinatol*. 2009 Aug;33(4):208-219.

Goldmuntz E: DiGeorge syndrome: new insights. *Clin Perinatol*. 2005 Dec;32(4):963-978, ix-x.

Hoffman GM, Mussatto KA, Brosig CL, et al. Systemic venous oxygen saturation after the Norwood procedure and childhood neurodevelopmental outcome. *J Thorac Cardiovasc Surg*. 2005 Oct;130(4):1094-1100.

Jonas RA, Newburger JW, Volpe JJ. *Brain Injury and Pediatric Cardiac Surgery*. Boston, MA: Butterworth-Heinemann; 1996.

Karl TR, Hall S, Ford G, et al. Arterial switch with full-flow cardiopulmonary bypass and limited circulatory arrest: neurodevelopmental outcome. *J Thorac Cardiovasc Surg*. 2004 Jan;127(1):213-222.

Kostovic I, Vasung L. Insights from in vitro fetal magnetic resonance imaging of cerebral development. *Semin Perinatol*. 2009 Aug;33(4):220-233.

Licht DJ, Shera DM, Clancy RR, et al. Brain maturation is delayed in infants with complex congenital heart defects. *J Thorac Cardiovasc Surg*. 2009 Mar;137(3):529-536; discussion 36-7.

Licht DJ, Wang J, Silvestre DW, et al. Preoperative cerebral blood flow is diminished in neonates with severe congenital heart defects. *J Thorac Cardiovasc Surg*. 2004 Dec; 128(6): 841-849.

Limperopoulos C. Disorders of the fetal circulation and the fetal brain. *Clin Perinatol*. 2009 Sep;36(3):561-577.

Mahle WT, Tavani F, Zimmerman RA, et al. An MRI study of neurological injury before and after congenital heart surgery. *Circulation*. 2002 Sep 24;106(12 suppl 1):I109-I114.

Majnemer A, Limperopoulos C, Shevell MI, et al. A new look at outcomes of infants with congenital heart disease. *Pediatr Neurol*. 2009 Mar;40(3):197-204.

Majnemer A, Limperopoulos C, Shevell M, et al. Developmental and functional outcomes at school entry in children with congenital heart defects. *J Pediatr*. 2008 Jul;153(1):55-60.

McGrath E, Wypij D, Rappaport LA, et al. Prediction of IQ and achievement at age 8 years from neurodevelopmental status at age 1 year in children with d-transposition of the great arteries. *Pediatrics*. 2004 Nov;114(5):e572-e576.

McQuillen PS, Barkovich AJ, Hamrick SE, et al. Temporal and anatomic risk profile of brain injury with neonatal repair of congenital heart defects. *Stroke*. 2007 Feb;38(2 suppl):736-741.

McQuillen PS, Ferriero DM. Perinatal subplate neuron injury: implications for cortical development and plasticity. *Brain Pathol*. 2005 Jul;15(3):250-260.

McQuillen PS, Ferriero DM. Selective vulnerability in the developing central nervous system. *Pediatr Neurol*. 2004 Apr;30(4):227-235.

Ment LR, Hirtz D, Huppi PS. Imaging biomarkers of outcome in the developing preterm brain. *Lancet Neurol*. 2009 Nov;8(11):1042-1055.

Meyer-Lindenberg A, Mervis CB, Berman KF. Neural mechanisms in Williams syndrome: a unique window to genetic influences on cognition and behaviour. *Nat Rev Neurosci*. 2006 May;7(5):380-393.

Miller SP, Ferriero DM. From selective vulnerability to connectivity: insights from newborn brain imaging. *Trends Neurosci*. 2009 Sep;32(9):496-505.

Miller SP, McQuillen PS, Hamrick S, et al. Abnormal brain development in newborns with congenital heart disease. *N Engl J Med*. 2007 Nov 8;357(19):1928-1938.

Newburger JW, Jonas RA, Wernovsky G, et al. A comparison of the perioperative neurologic effects of hypothermic circulatory arrest versus low-flow cardiopulmonary bypass in infant heart surgery. *N Engl J Med*. 1993; 329(15): 1057-1064.

Rosenthal GL. Patterns of prenatal growth among infants with cardiovascular malformations: possible fetal hemodynamic effects. *Am J Epidemiol*. 1996 Mar 1;143(5):505-513.

Rudolph AM. *Congenital Diseases of the Heart: Clinical-Physiological Considerations*. 3rd ed. Chichester, United Kingdom; Hoboken, NJ: Wiley-Blackwell; 2009.

Sherlock RL, McQuillen PS, Miller SP, et al. Preventing brain injury in newborns with congenital heart disease. Brain imaging and innovative trial designs. *Stroke*. 2008 Nov 6.

Tabbutt S, Nord AS, Jarvik GP, et al. Neurodevelopmental outcomes after staged palliation for hypoplastic left heart syndrome. *Pediatrics*. 2008 Mar;121(3):476-483.

Wernovsky G. Current insights regarding neurological and developmental abnormalities in children and young adults with complex congenital cardiac disease. *Cardiol Young*. 2006 Feb;(16 suppl 1):92-104.

Woodward LJ, Anderson PJ, Austin NC, et al. Neonatal MRI to predict neurodevelopmental outcomes in preterm infants. *N Engl J Med*. 2006 Aug 17;355(7):685-694.

Epidemiology, Etiology, and Genetics of Congenital Heart Disease

■ INTRODUCTION

Knowledge of the occurrence and etiology of congenital defects is essential to improvements in diagnosis, management, and genetic counseling. Congenital heart disease refers to structural abnormalities of the heart or intrathoracic great vessels that impact the function of the cardiovascular system. This chapter summarizes current knowledge regarding epidemiology and etiology of congenital heart disease. Information regarding the etiology of inherited cardiomyopathies and arrhythmias is presented in Chapters 9 and 10, respectively.

■ EPIDEMIOLOGY

Epidemiologic studies seek to measure disease frequency and to establish associations between disease states and a multitude of other variables such as heart defects and maternal diabetes. These observational studies establish statistical associations (*but not cause and effect*) that are useful for (1) developing diagnostic screening studies; (2) defining

heritability and recurrence risk; (3) evaluating the contribution of candidate genes identified in high-risk families or experimental models to disease in the general population; (4) characterizing environmental risk factors; (5) developing testable hypotheses regarding etiology and pathogenesis; and (6) planning for effective delivery of health care services.

All epidemiologic studies begin with measures of disease frequency. The two most common measures are prevalence and incidence.

- Prevalence is the proportion of the population at risk affected by disease at a given point in time. Prevalence excludes those who have already died from the disease, those in whom the disease has been cured or has spontaneously resolved, and those with undetected disease. Prevalence answers the question, "how many people have this disease in this place, at this time?"

- Incidence is expressed as a rate and is defined as the number of new cases among those at risk within a population over a certain period of time. Incidence answers the question, "how often does this disease occur?" For congenital heart disease, the total population at risk includes all embryos. However, even with advances in fetal echocardiography, the true incidence of congenital heart disease is difficult to measure. Many cardiovascular defects are associated with spontaneous abortion and stillbirth so that many of those embryos are never known to have heart disease. The prevalence of congenital heart disease is estimated to be about 15% in fetuses that have been spontaneously aborted and about 8% in stillborn infants. Based on these data, it is apparent that the true incidence of congenital heart disease is much greater than that reported in studies of the frequency of congenital heart disease at birth. Although incidence at birth is most frequently reported and is probably the most useful concept for the clinician, this figure must be interpreted with caution because the entire population with congenital heart disease is not considered. Consequently, the importance of chromosomal and genetic factors which are associated with spontaneous abortion or stillbirth will be underestimated.

Counting congenital heart disease cases after birth depends on the accurate detection of persons with various cardiac defects, and the accuracy of detection depends on the method used. No one method is completely accurate. Some studies have relied on data from medical records and birth/death certificates, which are known to be inaccurate. Others have relied on physical examination alone, in which case the training and skill of the examiner will certainly affect the results. More recently, some investigators have included results of echocardiograms, cardiac catheterizations, cardiac surgeries, and autopsies to increase diagnostic accuracy.

Once a case of congenital heart disease has been identified, the method of naming and classifying the defects will affect the results of epidemiologic studies. Classifying defects based on developmental mechanisms may reveal important pathophysiologic relationships among heterogeneous lesions. Unfortunately no universally agreed-upon nomenclature and classification scheme exists. It is difficult, if not impossible, to compare results from studies that have used different systems. For example, the same infant with pulmonary stenosis, a ventricular septal defect, and a malaligned ventricular septum may be classified as having tetralogy of Fallot, or as having double-outlet right ventricle with pulmonary stenosis. This will affect the relative proportion of patients having each of these defects. Currently, international collaborations of

clinicians are working to develop consensus-based nomenclature and classification systems, and to map defects across different existing systems.

Difficulties in calculating prevalence also result from determining the denominator or reference population. Characterizing an entire population at risk for developing congenital heart disease is quite difficult so a representative sample or subgroup is often selected. The process of selection must ensure that bias is not introduced. For example, studying only patients seen at a tertiary care center will be biased toward patients with more serious conditions.

■ INCIDENCE OF CONGENITAL HEART DISEASE

Multiple studies have been published reporting the birth incidence of congenital heart disease. The overall incidence ranges from about 2 to 20 cases per 1000 live births and depends largely on the number of trivial lesions included. In general, the incidence is 3 per 1000 for clinically severe conditions which require surgical or catheter intervention, excluding atrial septal defects and noncritical coarctation. The incidence of more moderate defects (atrial septal defect, mild to moderate aortic stenosis/insufficiency, moderate pulmonic stenosis or insufficiency, complicated but not large ventricular septal defects) is another 3 per 1000. The reported incidence increases to a total of 9 to 20 per 1000 when milder conditions such as small septal defects and mild pulmonic stenosis are included. Of note, this does not include isolated bicuspid aortic valves which have an estimated incidence of 9 to 14 per 1000.

Attempts have also been made to define the birth incidence of individual heart defects. These efforts have also been hampered by the lack of a uniform naming and classification scheme. The results also are affected by whether patients with chromosomal abnormalities such as trisomy 21 and other important noncardiac defects were included. The Baltimore-Washington Infant Study (BWIS) was a case-control study designed to provide comparative genetic and environmental data on the families of infants with congenital heart disease and the families of control infants. Data from the BWIS are shown in Table 15-1. The prevalence of ventricular septal defect increased during the time this study was performed (1981-1989) as a result of detection of tiny defects by color Doppler imaging. Indeed, differences in the relative frequency and prevalence of various defects in more recent studies are driven primarily by inclusion of milder conditions such as small septal defects and

■ **TABLE 15-1.** Live Birth Incidence (per 10,000) of Selected Defects: Baltimore-Washington Infant Study[a]

	Prevalence	Relative frequency (%)
Ventricular septal defects		
Membranous	9.87	25.2
Muscular	4.73	12.1
Pulmonary valve stenosis	3.76	9.6
Atrioventricular septal (canal) defects		
Down syndrome	2.32	5.9
Normal chromosomes	0.97	2.5
Atrial septal defect	3.21	8.2
Transposition of the great arteries	2.64	6.7
Tetralogy of Fallot	2.60	6.6
Hypoplastic left heart syndrome	1.79	4.6
Heterotaxia/l-loop	1.44	3.7
Coarctation of the aorta	1.39	3.5
Patent ductus arteriosus	0.88	2.2
Aortic stenosis	0.82	2.1
Bicuspid aortic valve	0.74	1.9
Total anomalous pulmonary venous connection	0.66	1.7
Pulmonary atresia	0.58	1.5
Ebstein anomaly	0.47	1.2
Tricuspid atresia	0.36	0.9

[a]Calculated from Ferencz C, Loffredo CA, Correa-Villaseñor A, Wilson PD. Perspectives in Pediatric Cardiology. vol 5. Genetic and Environmental Risk Factors of Major Cardiovascular Malformations: The Baltimore-Washington Infant Study 1981-1989. Armonk, NY: Futura; 1997.

mild valve stenosis that are detected by echocardiographic examination. A decline noted in the incidence of hypoplastic left heart syndrome may be the result of therapeutic pregnancy terminations or direct referral of prenatally detected cases to a surgical center outside of the study area.

■ RISK FACTORS FOR CONGENITAL HEART DISEASE

Genetic Factors

Among the 2659 infants identified with congenital heart disease in the BWIS, 26.5% had a noncardiac malformation. Noncardiac abnormalities were identified in only 0.7% of infants in the control group. Noncardiac defects

were more common in infants with atrioventricular septal defect and conotruncal abnormalities and less common in those with simple transposition of the great arteries and right and left heart obstructive lesions. Chromosomal abnormalities (not including deletion 22q11 syndrome) were present in 12% of patients and trisomy 21 was present in about 10% of all patients with congenital heart disease. A recognizable syndrome was present in 6% of infants with congenital heart disease. Data such as these and the fact that clustering of heart defects in some families has been recognized since the 1950s are suggestive that genetic factors play a role in the etiology of some defects.

Techniques for Detection of Genetic Alterations

The search for genetic alterations contributing to congenital heart disease either as part of a syndrome or in isolation has progressed rapidly over the past decade. These efforts have been aided dramatically by advances in molecular genetic techniques (Table 15-2). If a chromosomal location of a possible disease gene can be identified by linkage analysis techniques, then positional cloning is used to identify the gene. Identification of a disease gene once a disease locus is defined has been greatly facilitated by The Human Genome Project. Rapidly improving sequencing techniques will also benefit these efforts. Studies of large families with inherited congenital heart disease have provided important insight into the genetic basis of some defects. However, small family size is more typical, which markedly diminishes the power and utility of linkage analysis since the number of affected patients is small (autosomal recessive traits are especially difficult to detect in small pedigrees). Additional factors that hinder the identification of a genetic basis for specific congenital heart defects include incomplete penetrance (a person with the disease gene may not have the disease), variable expressivity (different phenotypes seen in persons with the same disease gene), genetic heterogeneity (different genetic etiologies for similar phenotypes), and decreased reproductive capability in persons with some malformations. Despite these issues, studies of first-degree relatives have detected previously undiagnosed defects and have strengthened the notion that a genetic component plays an important role even in sporadic congenital heart disease.

Candidate gene screening techniques take advantage of the increased understanding of normal cardiogenesis by assessing for mutations in relevant genes in patients with congenital heart disease. This technique can be combined with linkage analysis; candidate genes relevant to

■ **TABLE 15-2.** Molecular Genetic Techniques Available to Assist in Identification of Congenital Heart Disease Genes

Technique	Comments
Standard metaphase karyotype analysis	Widely available. Useful for evaluation of chromosome number, eg, trisomy or monosomy (Turner syndrome, 45,X). Small chromosomal abnormalities may be missed.
High-resolution banding (Giemsa staining)	Will detect relatively large duplications, translocations between chromosomes, and interstitial or terminal deletions.
Fluorescence in situ hybridization (FISH)	Biotinylated test and control DNA probes are hybridized with metaphase chromosomes. Useful for smaller structural abnormalities such as microdeletions. Newly developed fluorescent DNA probes for interstitial chromosomal regions allow detection of abnormalities in the subtelemore-telomere regions. Not practical for application on a genome-wide level.
Linkage analysis	Linkage analysis used to identify chromosomal location of a disease gene by mapping of a gene by analysis of its proximity to another locus on the same chromosome. Need large family pedigree (usually at least 10 affected family members). All family members must be carefully phenotyped.
Genome-wide association studies	Compares the frequency of a specific allele (single nucleotide polymorphisms or haplotype) in affected individuals and in unaffected controls. Greatly facilitated by completion of the Human Genome Project, the International HapMap Project, and rapid automated array techniques.
Comparative genomic hybridization (chromosomal microarray analysis)	Used to identify submicroscopic chromosome copy number variations (potential genetic risk factor) across the entire genome.
High-throughput sequencing, "next generation" deep sequencing	Sequencing techniques are being developed that sequence the entire genome and that are faster and less costly.

cardiogenesis residing on a particular region of a chromosome identified by linkage analysis can be evaluated for mutations. Candidate gene techniques are unfortunately limited by the fact that not all relevant cardiogenesis genes are known. Genome-wide association studies may provide information regarding whether certain haplotypes occur more often in patients with certain defects. The utility of these studies may be limited by the relatively small number of available congenital heart disease patients. Whether copy number variations (arising from microdeletions or microduplications) that have been identified in some patients with dysmorphic features and mental retardation contribute to congenital heart disease remains to be determined.

Role of Genetics in Congenital Heart Disease

Even though human cardiovascular genetics is in the early phase of gene discovery, insights provided by studies thus far show an important genetic contribution to congenital

heart disease. DNA testing for many of the relevant genes is gradually transitioning from the research laboratory to clinical availability. The list of genetic abnormalities contributing to congenital heart disease will continue to grow quickly. Clinicians are advised to consult the gene tests website (http://www.genetests.org) for updates on currently available testing. Specific chromosomal abnormalities (Table 15-3) and single gene disorders (Table 15-4) associated with syndromic congenital heart disease have been described. The specific genetic abnormality has not been identified for other examples of syndromic congenital heart disease (Table 15-5). Additionally, the genetic etiology of some nonsyndromic defects has also been described (Chapter 1) but this accounts for a small minority of cases.

In general, chromosomal abnormalities and single gene defects likely account for less than 15% of congenital heart disease. However, even for these so-called "sporadic" defects, epidemiologic studies show an increased precurrence

■ TABLE 15-3. Selected Chromosomal Abnormalities Causing Genetic Syndromes Associated With Congenital Heart Disease[a]

Syndrome	Incidence	Prevalence of CHD (%)	Types of CHD	Noncardiac features	Comment
Aneuploidy syndromes					
Trisomy 21	1/800	40-50	AVSD (60%), VSD, AS, TOF, PDA	Hypotonia, joint laxity, flat facial profile, slanted palpebral fissures, dysplasia of midphalanx of fifth finger, GI malformations	No association known between genes in critical region on chromosome 21 and CHD.
Trisomy 18	1/6000	> 95	VSD, polyvalve disease, DORV, TOF	Intrauterine growth retardation, polyhydramnios, hypertonicity, prominent occiput, short sternum, rocker-bottom feet, clenched hand with overlapping fingers	Median survival 18 days. Both proximal and distal regions of 18Q are required for full expression of the phenotype.
Trisomy 13	1/10,000-1/15,000	80	DORV, TOF, ASD, VSD, PDA, polyvalve disease	Holoprosencephaly, apnea, microcephaly with sloping forehead, microphthalmia, colobomata of iris, cleft lip and palate, polydactyly	
Turner (monosomy X)	1/2500-1/5000	25-30	BAV (30%), coarctation (10%-20%), mitral valve anomaly, HLHS	Short stature, short and webbed neck, broad chest, lymphedema, cubitus valgus, horseshoe kidney	CHD critical region not defined.
Deletion syndromes					
Deletion 22q11[b]	1/6000	75-80	TOF, IAA-B, truncus arteriosus, VSD, aortic arch abnormalities	Cleft palate, velopharyngeal incompetence, long and slender limbs, hypocalcemia, T-cell dysfunction	90% of patients test positive for a microdeletion of whom 6%-28% inherit the deletion. Marked variability in expression within families.
Deletion 7q11 (Williams-Beuren)	1/10,000	55-80	Supravalvar AS and PS, coronary artery stenosis, peripheral PS	Depressed nasal bridge, epicanthal folds, long philtrum, large mouth, stellate pattern in the iris, characteristic loquacious personality	90% have de novo submicroscopic deletion that encompasses elastin and other genes. Abnormalities in elastin account for vascular manifestations.

(Continued)

279

■ **TABLE 15-3.** Selected Chromosomal Abnormalities Causing Genetic Syndromes Associated With Congenital Heart Disease[a] (*Continued*)

Syndrome	Incidence	Prevalence of CHD (%)	Types of CHD	Noncardiac features	Comment
Deletion 4p (Wolf-Hirschhorn)	1/50,000	50	ASD, VSD,	Intrauterine growth retardation, microcephaly, hypertelorism, hypotonia, hypospadias	
Deletion 11q (Jacobsen)	1/100,000	55	VSD, left ventricular outflow tract obstruction including hypoplastic left heart syndrome	Intrauterine growth retardation, hypotonia in infancy, prominent forehead, epicanthal folds, hypertelorism, urologic abnormalities, abnormal platelets	
Deletion 5p (cri-du-chat)	< 1/200,000	20-60	VSD, ASD	Low birth weight, catlike cry, hypotonia, hypertelorism, downward slanting of palpebral fissures	The reader is urged to consult online resources such as Online Mendelian Inheritance in Man (http://www.ncbi.nlm.nih.gov/omim) for new data.

[a]Selected examples of more common conditions are shown in the table.

[b]Previously known as DiGeorge, velocardiofacial, and CATCH-22 syndromes.

AS, aortic stenosis; ASD, atrial septal defect; AVSD, atrioventricular septal defect; BAV, bicuspid aortic valve; CHD, congenital heart disease; DORV, double-outlet right ventricle; GI, gastrointestinal; HLHS, hypoplastic left heart syndrome; IAA-B, type B interrupted aortic arch; PDA, patent ductus arteriosus; PS, pulmonary stenosis; TOF, tetralogy of Fallot; VSD, ventricular septal defect.

■ **TABLE 15-4.** Selected Single Gene Disorders Associated With Syndromal Congenital Heart Disease[a]

Disorder	Incidence	Inheritance	Prevalence of CHD (%)	Types of CHD	Noncardiac features	Comment
Alagille	1/70,000	AD	> 90	Peripheral and valvar PS, TOF	Decreased intrahepatic interlobular bile ducts, chronic cholestasis, typical facial features, vertebral arch defects	90% have mutations in the Notch ligand *JAGGED-1*
Cardio-facio-cutaneous		AD	75	Valvar PS, hypertrophic cardiomyopathy	Macrocephaly with prominent forehead, bitemporal narrowing, shallow orbits, sparse, curly hair, skin abnormalities	Gain of function mutations in RAS-MAPK pathway
CHAR		AD	20–70	PDA	Supernumerary nipple, fifth finger anomalies	50% have mutations in *TFAP2B* gene which encodes a transcription factor expressed in neural crest cells
CHARGE association	1/12,000	AD	60–90	TOF, DORV, AVSD, aortic arch abnormalities	Colobomata of iris, choanal atresia, retardation of mental and somatic development, genital and ear anomalies	70% have mutations in a chromodomain helicase DNA-binding gene which is highly expressed in neural crest
Costello		AD	60–75	Valvar PS, hypertrophic cardiomyopathy, atrial tachycardia (30%)	Curly hair, coarse facies, hyperextensibility	Gain of function mutations in *HRAS* gene which encodes a protein involved in regulation of cell division
Ellis-van Creveld		AR	60	ASD, AVSD, common atrium	Short stature, hypoplastic nails, dental anomalies, polydactyly	66% have mutations in novels genes (EVC and EV2) with unknown function
Holt-Oram	1/100,000	AD	75	ASD, VSD, atrioventricular conduction delay	Upper limb defect	75% have mutations in *TBX5* gene which encodes a transcription factor
LEOPARD		AD	85	Hypertrophic cardiomyopathy, PS, arrhythmias	Multiple lentigines	Allelic to Noonan syndrome

■ TABLE 15-4. Selected Single Gene Disorders Associated With Syndromal Congenital Heart Disease[a] (*Continued*)

Disorder	Incidence	Inheritance	Prevalence of CHD (%)	Types of CHD	Noncardiac features	Comment
Loeys Dietz		AD	>95	Arterial tortuosity and aneurysm, PDA, mitral valve prolapse	Craniosynostosis, hypertelorism, bifid uvula, micrognathia	Caused by mutations in genes encoding type I and II receptors for transforming growth factor beta
Marfan	1/5000	AD	80	Aortic dilation and dissection, mitral valve prolapse	Arachnodactyly, pectus deformities, lens dislocation often not present in infancy	Caused by mutations in fibrillin-1 gene. Poor genotype-phenotype correlation
Noonan	1/1000-1/2500	AD	80-90	Valvar PS, hypertrophic cardiomyopathy	Short stature, downslanting palpebral fissures, short and webbed neck, pectus deformities, bleeding diathesis	Mutations in several genes encoding proteins in the Ras-mitogen activated protein kinase pathway
Smith Lemli Opitz	1/30,000	AR	45	ASD, VSD, AVSD, TAPVC	Intrauterine growth retardation, microcephaly, ptosis of eyelids, genital abnormalities, syndactyly of second and third toes	Mutations in *DHCR7* which encodes a protein involved in cholesterol synthesis. Role in cardiogenesis unknown

[a]Selected examples of more common conditions are shown in the table. Newer data are available through resources such as Online Mendelian Inheritance in Man (http://www.ncbi.nlm.nih.gov/omim).

AD, autosomal dominant; AR, autosomal recessive; AS, aortic stenosis; ASD, atrial septal defect; AVSD, atrioventricular septal defect; BAV, bicuspid aortic valve; CHD, congenital heart disease; DORV, double-outlet right ventricle; HLHS, hypoplastic left heart syndrome; IAA-B, type B interrupted aortic arch; MAPK, mitogen activated protein kinase; PDA, patent ductus arteriosus; PS, pulmonary stenosis; TAPVC, total anomalous pulmonary venous connection; TBX, T-box transcription factor; TGFBR, transforming growth factor beta receptor; TOF, tetralogy of Fallot; VSD, ventricular septal defect.

■ TABLE 15-5. Disorders Associated With Syndromal Congenital Heart Disease[a]

Disorder	Prevalence of CHD (%)	Types of CHD	Noncardiac features	Comment
Kabuki syndrome	45-55	ASD, VSD, left ventricular outflow tract obstruction	Long palpebral fissures, arching eyebrows, large protruding ears, joint hyperextensibility, prominent fingertip pads	Autosomal dominant
PHACES association	90	Coarctation, aortic arch anomalies including interruption	Hemangiomas, posterior fossa malformations	
Goldenhar syndrome (hemifacial microsomia)	30	TOF, VSD	Asymmetric facies, malformed ears including microtia, vertebral and renal anomalies	Part of a spectrum of craniofacial anomalies
Heterotaxy	95	Ambiguous situs, transposition, AVSD, pulmonary and systemic venous anomalies	Malrotation, spleen abnormalities	Abnormalities in right-left axis. Various chromosome abnormalities observed in isolated cases
VATER association	50	Multiple	Vertebral defects, tracheo-esophageal fistula with esophageal atresia, radial dysplasia, renal anomalies	Likely several pathogenetic mechanisms

[a]Selected examples of more common conditions are shown in the table. The reader is urged to consult online resources such as Online Mendelian Inheritance in Man (http://www.ncbi.nlm.nih.gov/omim) for new data.

Abbreviations as in Table 15-4.

(number of affected relatives at the time of birth) and recurrence risk for congenital heart disease within families (see following text) which supports the concept of genetic predisposition. Nevertheless, only 2% to 4% of patients with isolated defects have a family history of congenital heart disease. Malformations in the vast majority of these patients are therefore likely multifactorial in origin and result from the interaction of complex environmental and genetic factors (Figure 15-1). These complex conditions are likely caused by one or more "susceptibility genes" which may be influenced by various "modifier genes," epigenetic factors, hemodynamic phenomena, and environmental factors. The presence of different polymorphisms of these genes may directly affect normal development or may induce biological alterations that predispose to the adverse effects of other factors.

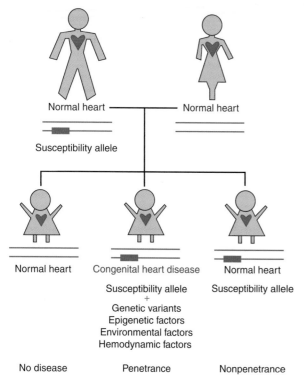

FIGURE 15-1. Model of multifactorial origin of congenital heart disease. A parent may harbor a genetic predisposition to disease (susceptibility allele) and transmit this genetic risk to offspring. However, this would result in heart defects only in conjunction with variants in other genetic loci or with epigenetic factors, resulting in disease penetrance. The susceptibility allele alone may not be sufficient to cause disease in offspring (nonpenetrance), but the individual would still transmit increased risk to offspring. *Adapted from Shieh J, Srivastava D. Circulation. 2009;120(4):269-271.*

Attributes of the Infants

In the BWIS, infants with isolated defects such as atrial and ventricular septal defects, right- and left-sided obstructive lesions, and simple transposition were similar in birth weight to the control infants. In contrast those infants with complex defects such as atrioventricular septal defects, functional single ventricle, and complex transposition were much smaller than the control infants. Additionally, decreased fetal growth was commonly found in infants with any cardiac defect who also had noncardiac malformations.

Gender differences in the prevalence of specific defects have been noted consistently. Left heart obstructive lesions, transposition of the great arteries, pulmonary atresia, and tricuspid atresia occur more frequently in boys. Patent ductus arteriosus, atrial septal defect, atrioventricular septal defect, and Ebstein anomaly of the tricuspid valve occur more often in girls. The reasons for these gender differences are not known.

Racial and ethnic group differences in the prevalence of congenital heart disease have been reported in some studies. Most of these are likely the result of incomplete case ascertainment and differences in the distribution of risk factors in the populations; true racial or ethnic differences have not been identified.

Environmental Factors

Considerable attention has been focused on environmental factors that might increase risk of congenital heart disease in offspring. The most common risk factors identified in the BWIS were a positive family history and maternal pregestational diabetes. Notably, toxic and infective embryopathies accounted for less than 1% of cases.

A variety of environmental factors have been variably associated with congenital heart disease. Caution is necessary when interpreting these studies because associations identified from observational studies may be spurious because of chance, bias, or confounding factors. Recall bias is a problem because exposure to most factors is assessed after the birth of the child. Confounding occurs, for example, when an apparent association between a maternal condition and congenital heart disease in an infant is the result of the medication taken by the mother for that condition.

Many exposures have been investigated and the more common ones thought to be associated with increased risk for congenital heart disease are shown in Table 15-6. Maternal pregestational insulin-dependent diabetes increases the risk of fetal malformation. In the BWIS study the overall risk of heart defects was 3.2 times higher if

■ **TABLE 15-6.** Environmental Risk factors Associated With Congenital Heart Disease

Maternal Illness
    Diabetes (pregestational)
    Febrile illness, influenza
    Phenylketonuria (poorly controlled)
    Rubella
Maternal therapeutic and recreational drug exposures
    Anticonvulsants
    Thalidomide
    Vitamin A congeners (retinoic acid)
Alcohol[a]
Smoking[a]
Obesity[a]
Other maternal exposures
    Solvents and varnishes

[a]Inconsistent findings regarding causation.

■ **TABLE 15-7.** Indications for Genetic Evaluation

Patient
    Multiple congenital anomalies
    Dysmorphic facial features or skeletal abnormalities
    Abnormal prenatal diagnostic test
    Abnormal newborn screening test
    Perinatal death
Family history
    Congenital heart disease
    Genetic disorder
    Congenital anomalies
    Miscarriages, still births, neonatal deaths

maternal pregestational diabetes was present. The most common defects were double-outlet right ventricle, truncus arteriosus, tetralogy of Fallot, and ventricular septal defect. In addition, offspring of mothers with overt diabetes were 18 times more likely to have cardiomyopathy (Chapter 9) than offspring of mothers without diabetes. Lack of adequate glycemic control is correlated with the risk of congenital heart disease. No definite increased risk of congenital heart disease is associated with gestational diabetes.

■ GENETIC COUNSELING

Indications for Genetics/Dysmorphology Evaluation

Clinicians caring for patients with congenital heart disease should be aware of the need to assess a newly diagnosed patient for relevant associated anomalies. Identification of a recognizable syndrome will assist in determining the need for genetic testing and in evaluating the patient for other anomalies. Additionally, identification of a syndrome may indicate the need for genetics testing in other family members and will allow more accurate risk assessment of recurrence of congenital heart disease in future children.

A complete physical examination should include an assessment for dysmorphic features. Genetics evaluation including examination by a geneticist and cytogenetic testing is often indicated (Table 15-7). Chest and abdominal

radiographs may identify abnormalities in situs. Upper gastrointestinal series, abdominal ultrasound, liver-spleen scan, and head imaging studies are obtained as indicated. A complete family history should be taken and should include pregnancy loss, ethnic origin, and consanguinity. Recent studies have shown that first-degree family members may have subclinical cardiovascular defects. For example, the parents of a male child with hypoplastic left heart syndrome have a greater than 25% likelihood of having a bicuspid aortic valve. Thus, echocardiographic study of first-degree relatives may be indicated.

Certain congenital heart defects are frequently associated with genetic abnormalities. For example, 60% of infants with atrioventricular septal defects have trisomy 21. Tetralogy of Fallot is associated with more than 50 syndromes, the most common being deletion 22q11 syndrome. This syndrome is present even more frequently in patients with defects such as interrupted aortic arch type B (Table 15-8). Patients with heart defects highly associated with syndromes may need evaluation for the presence of a genetic abnormality even in the absence of dysmorphic features.

Recurrence Risks

Questions regarding causation are directly relevant to the risk of recurrence and the parents of any child with congenital heart disease will have questions about the risk of recurrence in subsequent pregnancies or in their grandchildren. Additionally, as more patients with heart defects survive to reproductive age, questions about recurrence come directly from patients. Unfortunately, accurate genetic counseling requires knowledge regarding causation

■ **TABLE 15-8.** Estimated Frequency of 22q11 Deletions in Congenital Heart Disease

Defect	Estimated Deletion Frequency (%)
Interrupted aortic arch type B	50-89
Ventricular septal defect	10
With normal aortic arch	3
With aortic arch anomaly[a]	45
Truncus arteriosus	34-41
Tetralogy of Fallot	8-35
Isolated aortic arch anomalies	24
Double-outlet right ventricle	< 5
Transposition of the great arteries	< 1

[a]Includes right aortic arch, abnormal branching pattern, cervical location, and/or discontinuous pulmonary arteries.

Reprinted with permission: *Circulation.* 2007;115:3015-3038. ©2007 American Heart Association, Inc.

■ **TABLE 15-9.** Relative Risk of Recurrence by Congenital Heart Defect (CHD) by Family History of CHD[a]

Heart defect	Relative risk[b]
Heterotaxy	79.1
Conotruncal defect	11.7
Atrioventricular septal (canal) defect	24.3
Anomalous pulmonary venous return	0
Left ventricular outflow tract obstruction	12.9
Right ventricular outflow tract obstruction	48.6
Atrial septal defect	7.07
Ventricular septal defect	3.41
Patent ductus arteriosus (term)	4.80
Overall same heart defect	8.15

[a]Data adapted from Øyen et al. *Circulation.* 2009;120:295-301.

[b]Reference was index persons with a heart defect who had a first-degree relative without a heart defect.

and the direct cause of most congenital heart disease is not known. The availability of prenatal diagnosis, including amniocentesis and chorionic villus sampling for chromosomal diagnosis, and fetal echocardiography (beginning at about 16 wk gestation) for evaluation of cardiac structure, should be communicated. The long-term goal of genetic counseling is educational; information regarding risk and prenatal diagnosis must be presented in a balanced manner and decisions regarding reproduction should be left to the patient and family.

Many studies have attempted to assess the recurrence risk to siblings and offspring of patients with congenital heart disease. Study results often conflict and interpretation is confounded by methodologic differences in patient ascertainment, diagnostic techniques, morphologic classification of defects, and identification of chromosomal abnormalities and syndromic features. Clearly, the recurrence risk will vary among specific types of defects and within different kindred. Risk will be determined in part by the specific genetic and environmental contributions to each defect such as the presence of additional affected family members and the presence of known genetic or syndromic risk factors.

The recurrence risk for a sibling is at least 2% to 3% and increases substantially if more than one sibling is affected. The recurrence risk to offspring of parents with congenital heart disease averages 2% to 4%. However, multiple studies have shown that recurrence risks vary depending on the exact defect. Most recently, Øyen et al reported recurrence risk ratios from zero among 228 patients with anomalous pulmonary veins to 79 in 359 patients with heterotaxy (Table 15-9). For persons with isolated heart defects, the overall relative risk of recurrence for the same defect was 8.15. Interestingly, same-sex twins (some of which are monozygotic) showed about a threefold higher relative risk of recurrence than unlike-sex twins. These data strongly suggest a genetic component even to sporadic congenital heart disease. Future research, which characterizes genes and gene defects in family pedigrees, will provide more definitive information.

SUGGESTED READINGS

Botto LD, Correa A, Erickson JD. Racial and temporal variations in the prevalence of heart defects. *Pediatrics.* 2001; 107(3):E32.

Botto LD, Goldmuntz E, Lin AE. Epidemiology and prevention of congenital heart defects. In: Allen HD, Driscoll DJ, Shaddy RE, Feltes TF, eds. *Moss and Adams' Heart Disease in Infants, Children, and Adolescents.* Vol 1. Philadelphia, PA: Lippincott Williams & Wilkins; 2008:524-545.

Clayton DG, Walker NM, Smyth DJ, et al. Population structure, differential bias and genomic control in a large-scale, case-control association study. *Nat Genet.* 2005;37(11): 1243-1246.

Cordell HJ, Clayton DG. Genetic association studies. *Lancet.* 2005;366(9491):1121-1131.

Ferencz C, Loffredo CA, Correa-Villasenor A, Wilson PD. Perspectives in Pediatric Cardiology. Vol 5. Genetic and Environmental Risk factors of Major Cardiovascular Malformations: The Baltimore-washing Infant Study 1981-1989. Armonk, NY: Futura; 1997.

Ferencz C, Loffredo CA, Rubin JD, Magee CA. Perspectives in Pediatric Cardiology. Vol 4. Epidemiology of Congenital Heart Disease: The Baltimore-Washington Infant Study 1981-1989. Mount Kisco, NY: Futura;1993.

Ferencz C, Boughman JA, Neill CA, Brenner JI, Perry LW. Congenital cardiovascular malformations: questions on inheritance. Baltimore-Washington Infant Study Group. *J Am Coll Cardiol.* 1989;14(3):756-763.

Goldmuntz E, Lin AE. Genetics of congenital heart disease. In: Allen HD, Driscoll DJ, Shaddy RE, Feltes TF, eds. *Moss and Adams' Heart Disease in Infants, Children, and Adolescents.* Vol 1. Philadelphia, PA: Lippincott Williams & Wilkins; 2008:545-572.

Hoffman JI, Kaplan S. The incidence of congenital heart disease. *J Am Coll Cardiol.* 2002;39(12):1890-1900.

Jenkins KJ, Correa A, Feinstein JA, et al. Noninherited risk factors and congenital cardiovascular defects: current knowledge: a scientific statement from the American Heart Association Council on Cardiovascular Disease in the Young: endorsed by the American Academy of Pediatrics. *Circulation.* 2007;115(23):2995-3014.

Jones K. *Smith's Recognizable Patterns of Human Malformation.* 6th ed. Philadelphia, PA: Elsevier Sanders; 2005.

Øyen N, Poulsen G, Boyd HA, Wohlfahrt J, Jensen PK, Melbye M. Recurrence of congenital heart defects in families. *Circulation.* 2009;120(4):295-301.

Pierpont ME, Basson CT, Benson DW, Jr., et al. Genetic basis for congenital heart defects: current knowledge: a scientific statement from the American Heart Association Congenital Cardiac Defects Committee, Council on Cardiovascular Disease in the Young: endorsed by the American Academy of Pediatrics. *Circulation.* 2007;115(23):3015-3038.

Pollex RL, Hegele RA. Copy number variation in the human genome and its implications for cardiovascular disease. *Circulation.* 2007;115(24):3130-3138.

Shephard TH, Lemire RJ. *Catalog of Teratogenic Agents.* 12th ed. Baltimore, MD: John Hopkins University Press; 2007.

Tegnander E, Williams W, Johansen OJ, Blaas HG, Eik-Nes SH. Prenatal detection of heart defects in a non-selected population of 30,149 fetuses—detection rates and outcome. *Ultrasound Obstet Gynecol.* 2006;27(3):252-265.

Reference Web Sites

Clinical Teratology Web. (http://depts.washington.edu/terisweb/). University of Washington, Seattle; 2010.

Gene Reviews. (http://www.ncbi.nlm.nih.gov/sites/ GeneTests/review?db=genetests). University of Washington, Seattle; 2010.

GeneTests. Medical Genetics Information Resource (http://www.genetest.org). University of Washington, Seattle; 2010.

National Newborn Screening and Genetics Resource Center (http://genes-r-us.uthscsa.edu/index.htm). University of Texas San Antonio, San Antonio; 2010.

Online Mendelian Inheritance in Man (OMIM, http://www.ncbi.nlm.nih.gov/omim). Johns Hopkins University, Baltimore; 2010.

Index

Page references followed by *f* indicate figures; those followed by *t* indicate tables.